Xenobiosis

'It's all a matter of the dose'
(*quintessence of the Paracelsian doctrine*)

Xenobiosis
Foods, drugs and poisons in the human body

Adrien Albert

DSc (Lond), PhD Medicine (Lond)
Fellow of the Australian Academy of Science
Professor Emeritus, Department of Chemistry
Australian National University, Canberra
Research Professor, Department of Pharmacological Sciences
School of Medicine, State University of New York, Stony Brook

London   New York
Chapman and Hall

First published in 1987 by Chapman and Hall Ltd
11 New Fetter Lane, London EC4P 4EE
Published in the USA by Chapman and Hall
29 West 35th Street, New York, NY 10001

Printed in Great Britain at the
University Press, Cambridge

ISBN 0 412 28800 1 (hb)
ISBN 0 412 28810 9 (pb)

British Library Cataloguing in Publication Data

Albert, Adrien
    Xenobiosis: foods, drugs and poisons
    in the human body.
    1. Xenobiotics
    I. Title
615.7   QP529

    ISBN 0–412–28800–1
    ISBN 0–412–28810–9 Pbk

Library of Congress Cataloging in Publication Data

Albert, Adrien.
    Xenobiosis: foods, drugs, and poisons in the human body.

    Bibliography: p.
    Includes indexes.
    1. Xenobiotics—Metabolism.   2. Biotransformation
(Metabolism)   I. Title. [DNLM: 1. Biotransformation.
2. Drugs—metabolism.   3. Food.   4. Poisons.   QU 120
A333x]
QP801.X45A43   1987   615.9   87–11646
ISBN 0–412–28800–1
ISBN 0–412–28810–9 (pbk.)

Contents

Preface

This book deals with the chemical and pharmacological behaviour of foreign substances in the human body. That statement at once raises two questions: What are 'foreign substances' and Where is 'in'? Each question requires an immediate if provisional answer which can be refined as we proceed.

The word *xenobiotic* was coined by H. S. Mason and his colleagues at the University of Oregon Medical School who wrote:

> 'We would like to call the components of this chemical environment, which are foreign to the metabolic network of an organism, *xenobiotic* compounds, from the Greek *xenos* and *bios* (stranger to life).' (Mason, North and Vanneste, 1965).

The present treatment is divided into three parts: foods, drugs, and poisons. The essentially foreign nature of food may not be immediately apparent but will be explained in Part One. A drug is defined here as a medication, a term which will be enlarged on in Part Two, but drugs of dependence and poisons generally will appear in Part Three.

A substance inserted into an aperture of the human body cannot, according to the anatomists, be said to be *inside* the body until it has crossed a semipermeable membrane. Thus a dose of liquid paraffin (mineral oil), introduced into the mouth, then excreted quantitatively from the rectum, is strictly considered not to have been *in* the body.

This book began as a course of lectures which I regularly give in the Department of Chemistry of the Australian National University. They are attended by students in the year in which they graduate with Honours. These are students who are developing a strong interest in the interface between chemistry and biology. On graduation they move on to interesting work in health and the environment, some with their feet implanted on the teaching and research ladder, and others bound for administrative positions. These are areas where there is an increasing demand for graduates with interdisciplinary background. Many opportunities for attractive employment are afforded by the steadily increasing allocations being made by governments to ensure the purity of foods, drugs, air, water and indeed the whole environment. This book is offered as a rational, broadly based introduction to toxicology in its widest aspects, to provide a firm base for later specialization. Aspiring xenobiologists may enjoy attempting the exercises marked 'Follow-up', which are placed near the end of some chapters.

I thank Professor R. N. Warrener for encouraging these studies, also the following colleagues in the Australian National University who have kindly read the manuscript: Professor D. J. Mulvaney (Prehistory and Anthropology), Dr Tessa Raath (Botany), Professor D. P. Craig, Drs J. H. Bradbury, W. D. Holloway, M. Rasmussen and B. K. Selinger (Chemistry). It is a pleasure to acknowledge help from Professor Pierre Magot, Institut de Police Scientifique, Université de Lausanne, Switzerland, and from Dr Ruth English and her co-nutritionists in the Australian Commonwealth Department of Health.

A. A.
Canberra

1
Introduction to the concept: Xenobiosis

Xenobiosis is defined here as *The behaviour of foreign substances in the human body*. The treatment of these foreign substances is divided into foods, drugs and poisons. To some readers this listing of food as a foreign substance may make it seem the odd man out! Yet intimations that foods, drugs and poisons were fundamentally related began to be realized as early as the sixteenth century. This idea was clearly expressed by the noted Swiss sage and physician Paracelsus (1493–1541) in the third of his *Sieben Defensiones* (1538), as follows:

'Wenn ihr jedes Gift recht ausslegen wolt, was ist, das nit Gift ist? Alle Dinge sind Gift, und nichts ist ohne Gift; allein die Dosis machts, dass ein Ding kein Gift sei. Zu exempel, ein jegliche Speise und ein jeglich Getränk, wenn es über seine Dosis eingenommen wird, so ist es Gift; das beweist sein Ausgang. Ich gebe auch zu, dass Gift Gift sei; dass es aber darum verworfen werden solle, das darf nicht sein.'

Which is in translation:

'What is not a poison? All things are poisons, and nothing is without toxicity. Only the *dose* permits anything not to be poisonous. For example, every food and every drink is a poison if consumed in more than the usual amount: which proves the point. I admit that a poison *is* a poison; but that is no reason for condemning it outright.'

The advance of knowledge in the present century has helped to separate the three classes, yet many areas of overlap remain, and these are of increasing concern to Health Authorities.

Let us consider the familiar substance, ethanol which is popularly known, if vaguely, as *alcohol*. This can act as a food, a powerful medicine, or as a poison, depending on the dose; thereby necessitating entries in all three Parts of this book. A similar split treatment must be accorded oxygen which, at the 1 in 5 dilution that exists in the air we breathe, is a healthy and necessary item for combustion of the food we eat; at a higher concentration it finds cautious employment in medicine; but pure oxygen is poisonous and its multiple toxic effects will be described in Chapter 11. Those indispensable safeguards to our health, the oil-soluble vitamins, are quite poisonous in small excess, and many people suffer chronic illnesses through their heavy consumption of fats and of salt – items normally found on the dinner table. Quite apart from such preventable details, we shall see how *too much* of even the purest and most praiseworthy foods can endanger health and shorten the expectation of life.

Lack of variety in the diet is another common source of illness. Because foods are such very complex mixtures of various chemical substances, some of which are poisons but commonly consumed below the threshold level, any specialization in diet can raise a noxious constituent (e.g. the goitrogens in cabbage or the methanol in pineapple) above that threshold. This fact does not indicate that we should drop these foods from our diet, but that we should take pains to diversify it – *It's all a matter of the dose.*

Finally even the foods that are innocuous to the majority of eaters can be health-endangering to a significant minority. For example many people are made chronically ill by cereals such as wheat (whether eaten as bread or as goods made from its flour) because of sensitivity to a protein (p. 78). The risks that the cholesterol in dairy products poses seem to be confined to one sector (although a significant one) of the population. Apart from these dangers there are the *allergies* (e.g. to bananas, tomatoes, seafood, or poultry) to one or more of which many people are subject.

The loosely-defined borderline that separates foods from medicaments (drugs) is displayed not only by ethanol. Consider for instance the caffeine beverages (tea, coffee, cola) which are in reality drugs with no nutritive value, but are commonly consumed at the meal table; consider also the excess doses of purified vitamins taken by enthusiasts. Another example is the eating of bran, at the breakfast table, for its medicinal effects.

Yet a fundamental difference between a food and a drug does exist. We eat our foods with the knowledge that they will all be combusted within us in less than four hours and that, apart from the pleasures of eating (not lightly to be discounted) our meals will provide us with energy, storable for later spending, as well as the potential for growth and repair. A drug on the other hand is designed not to be wasted metabolically: its molecule should remain intact long enough to repair an abnormal state of the body or even, as is expected of an anaesthetic, to temporarily create one.

The difference between a drug and a poison also deserves careful thought. Until the present century, there was not much margin between the effective dose of a drug and its maximum tolerated dose. Therapy was often a battle whose outcome depended on which cells could hold out longest or renew themselves first. Ehrlich's introduction of the *therapeutic index* in 1911 provided for the first time a measure of the degree of selectivity of each drug. This desirable quality – *selectivity* – consists of being able to affect selected cells without harm to others, a subject which will be developed in Chapter 9. More recently the principles that can confer selectivity on the drug molecule, which differ from those on which the *activity* of the drug rests, have been defined. As a result we have some highly selective drugs (and are well on the way to discovering more of them) that are far removed from the class of poisons. Even so, the dose needs careful observance.

Because foods, drugs, and poisons often display a marginal overlap between their apparently distinct classes, an overlap that has often proved as dangerous as it is surprising, it is clearly in the public interest to group all three categories as *xenobiotics*. The study of xenobiosis impinges strongly on many economic, legal, and other social issues of our times, with possible extensions to philosophy or even politics. None of these are subjects in which I have expertise so I shall not introduce them. On the other hand those readers who are heading their careers towards any of these wider territories may be glad of the foundation of verifiable facts that this book can provide.

So different are the circumstances of the different nations, and of different sectors of the population in any one nation, that some readers may find an initial difficulty in setting to one side their own xenobiotic preferences, particularly for food. However to enjoy these studies and to get the most out of them objectivity is essential.

Further reading

Xenobiotic Metabolism: Nutritional Effects (Finley and Schwass, 1985). This is a scientific assessment of how our choice of foods can prevent or encourage the onset of chronic disease.

Xenobiotica, (Taylor and Francis, London). This periodical was started in 1971 by Professor D. V. Parke (University of Surrey, England) to investigate the fate of foreign substances in biological systems.

PART ONE
Foods

'Metron ariston'
Moderation is best

(inscribed in the Temple of Apollo at Delphi)

2

Introduction to Part One: Foods as foreign substances

How we enjoy eating! Yet we seldom remind ourselves that almost everything we swallow is foreign to the human body. This means that we have to perform work on food before we can begin to use it for energy, growth or repair. In other words we have to spend energy before we can start to get energy. The assimilable portion of food consists mainly of carbohydrate, lipids (fats) and proteins – exactly the three classes of matter that the human body requires. Unfortunately the carbohydrates, lipids and proteins contained in foods differ from those which constitute our tissues, so that they have to be broken down to very small chemical fragments before we can begin to use them. Thus the starches in our food, with their molecular weights varying from 50 000 to 400 000, have to be split to glucose (MW 180) before they can be converted to the body's storage carbohydrate – glycogen – with molecular weight ranging from 1 to 10 million.

This state of affairs prompts an unconventional but necessary question: Would our nutrition proceed more economically if we were to consume human food? The answer is not far to seek. As infants all of us imbibed mother's milk which is composed of human protein, human carbohydrate and human lipids. Yet, convenient though it may appear for us to have stored and used these nutrients directly in our little bodies, the interposition of membranes and of biochemical barriers made such a short-cut quite impossible. Nor does the adult body provide a pathway for the direct assimilation of human flesh, nutritious though it is known to be*.

---

* Sixteen survivors from an unprovisioned plane that crashed in the Andes on October 12, 1972 (most of them young footballers) were rescued in excellent physical condition after 10 weeks, thanks to the availability of 29 other passengers who died in the crash (Read, 1974).

8   Foods as foreign substances

An acceptable meaning for the word 'food' should be established at this stage of our introduction. *The Concise Oxford Dictionary* (7th edn, 1982) defines it as 'Substance(s) taken into the body to maintain life and growth', and *Webster's Ninth New Collegiate Dictionary* (1984) states that food is 'Material consisting essentially of protein, carbohydrate and fat, used in the body of an organism to sustain growth, repair and vital processes and to furnish energy; *also* such foods together with supplementary substances (as minerals, vitamins, and condiments)'.

Apart from these constituents all foods contain many minor components, some of which supply the characteristic flavours whereas others are frankly toxic (poisonous), at least if consumed in excess of the usual domestic serving (see for example cabbage, p. 66). Other common constituents, usually present only in small proportion, include the nucleic acids and dietary fibres (see p. 31, 27).

Oxygen of course is an essential food adjunct, for without a steady supply of this element combustion of what we eat could not take place. So insatiable is our appetite for this nutrient that we renew its intake some 20 times a minute, even during sleep! Although oxygen cannot be thought of as foreign to the human body even a small excess is toxic. Hence the concentration of *free* oxygen is kept low as follows. At rest an adult absorbs about 250 ml of oxygen per minute from the room's air. Of this the blood carries only 0.3 ml per 100 ml as *free* oxygen whereas the fraction bound to haemoglobin is 19 ml per 100 ml (Green, 1976). Water is another essential nutritional factor but no xenobiotic!

We shall now need to memorize the calorific values of food components: That of carbohydrates is conveniently remembered as 16, of lipids 37 and of proteins 17 – all in kilojoules per gram (kJ/g)* (Royal Society, 1972). In kilocalories (popularly called *calories*) the rough equivalents are 3.75, 9 and 4 kcal/g respectively. It is important to note that the calorific value of lipids exceeds twice that of the other two main food constituents. Children resynthesize dietary protein into body protein whereas adults combust most of it and void the nitrogen content, with loss of energy, in the urine. High protein foods are the most expensive foods, and hence a high protein diet is uneconomic for adults.

Never before in human history has so large a proportion of citizens, at least in the more prosperous countries, become aware that overconsumption of food even when it is of supreme quality lowers resistance to chronic disease and tends to shorten an active and enjoyable life. One curious byproduct of this awareness is the trend to advertise food as 'naturally pure', 'low calorie', 'salt reduced', 'vitamins and minerals enriched', or 'free from all additives'. Small, but elegant shops boldly announce that they sell only 'Health Foods' implying that the abundance of attractive, lower-priced food in the markets is not equally healthy! Fortunately in many countries the wholesomeness of food and the purity of

---

* Ethanol, in small doses, produces 29 kJ/g, but as the dose is increased the body can usually do little to increase its capacity for combusting it (p. 25).

ambient air and drinking water are stringently inspected and controlled by statutory Government agencies.

2.1 Our debt to Early man: the hazardous evolution of man's diet

'I eat as much meat as possible', said the young fellow at the dinner party, 'our ancestors were hunters, and so we need mainly meat'.

'Not so', replied the medical student sitting opposite, 'the human gut is so long compared to that of carnivores that it seems designed for a mainly vegetarian diet'. Who was right?

In order to trace foundations for contemporary food choices and customs let us step back into prehistory, a study which scientific dating methods have rescued from former vagueness. Indeed since the radiocarbon method was launched in 1949, this and other physical and chemical methods have been effectively applied to anthropological and archeological problems to yield what pre-historians judge to be reasonably precise dates over the entire range of evolution (Young, Jope and Oakley, 1981).

The most basic fact to emerge is this: Life is no newcomer to planet earth. The casts of innumerable bacteria, alive 3.5×10^9 years ago, have been discovered in deposits in Australia, Canada, China and South Africa. Their complexity of structure and diversity of type indicate that life began on Earth still earlier (Schopf, 1983; Awramik, Schopf and Walter, 1983).

More relevant to our enquiry is that hominids – man-like creatures who walked on two legs and eventually learnt how to make fine tools – have roamed the earth for at least 3.5 million years. Our own race *Homo sapiens* seems to have emerged comparatively recently, about 40 000 years ago during the last of the ice ages (Washburn and McCown, 1978; Daniel, 1978).

Prehistorians consider that *all* humans lived by hunting, fishing and the gathering of plants and shellfish until about 10 000 years ago when the agricultural revolution began. Excavated remains indicate that these early 'hunter-gatherers' practised much more gathering than hunting, apparently because gathering was quicker and safer, and a pleasant activity in which the whole family could share.

'It seems reasonable to conclude that before agriculture began, most people were gatherers rather than hunters, and that the bulk of their food was either plants or (where available) shellfish' (Harlan, 1975).

Early man must have chosen his food primarily by availability and taste, but equally important would be freedom from ill effects after the meal. Sadly, but inevitably, countless numbers of our ancestors sacrificed themselves in finding out what is safe to eat. Beyond doubt, the use of plants and shellfish by Early man was greatly restricted by the widespread occurrence of toxic substances in them. We can hardly be surprised that so high a proportion of wild vegetable material is poisonous, because plants cannot flee from their predators. This disadvantage has put them under continual evolutionary pressure to secure their survival by chemical means. To this end, they have accumulated many kinds of substances that repel or discourage attack by microorganisms, insects, or grazing animals (including man). This is where the detoxifying effect of cooking, when discovered, brought a major evolutionary advance (Leopold and Audrey, 1972).

Just who was the world's first cook we may never know; but the improvement of food by cooking seems to have become well established about 40 000 years ago. For a long time it consisted of roasting in ashes. Cooking aided digestion by disintegrating animal tissues and the tight granules of starch of which cereals are largely composed. However in addition (and this is possibly more important) cooking detoxified a great many species of plants that were too poisonous to eat in the raw condition. In particular it inactivated the toxic proteins that are almost universally present in legumes (beans, peas and lentils) and in grains. Thus the many species of two widely-occurring and prolific families, the Leguminosae and the Gramineae (cereal grasses), suddenly became available for enriching man's diet.

These toxic proteins, mainly lectins and inhibitors of proteases, are discussed on pp. 61–62. Further benefits of cooking included the vaporization of irritating volatile oils, and the destruction of cyanogenic toxins (p. 64). It has been suggested that the great increase in population that followed the introduction of cooking owed much to this new detoxifying approach (Leopold and Audrey, 1972). A similar advance was the discovery of grinding, for which the earliest known devices are dated at about 15 000 years ago in the Middle East. Grinding facilitated detoxication by extraction with hot or cold water. For a more detailed account of hunter-gatherers, see Lee and DeVore (1968).

Let us try, briefly, to visualize the eating choices of our ancestors from observations made on some hunter-gatherers who still practise their traditional lifestyle.

The Australian Aborigines

When British people began to colonize Australia in 1788 they found an estimated 300 000 people scattered over an island almost as big as Europe (Harlan, 1975). These dark-skinned Aborigines, to whom agriculture was unknown, have been living in Australia for at least 40 000 years of which the earlier millenia were lived in an ice age. They appear to have had only minimal contact with the outside world before the end of the 18th century (Mulvaney, 1970; Daniel, 1978). They have long been acquainted with the practice of cooking because a 31 000 year old hearthstone has been found in the Willandra Lakes region of NSW (Australian Heritage Commission, 1980).

From the records of explorers in the early 19th century we learn that Aborigines required only 2–4 hours a day to acquire and cook their food (Grey, 1837; Eyre, 1845). Aboriginal people gather and use more than 400 species of

Australian plants belonging to about 250 genera (Irvine, 1957). Tribes who circulate in the dry areas of the continent depend heavily on the pods of *Acacia* (Leguminosae) and the seeds of two cereal grasses (wild rice and millet), all of which are roasted (Harlan, 1975). In riverine Western Australia, Grey (1837) found a mainly vegetarian diet was followed, based on edible roots, usually the yam *Dioscorea*. In a meticulous survey of eating habits among the least disturbed of contemporary Aborigines, namely those inhabiting the Arnhem Land peninsula in the far north of Australia, Meehan (1982) reported a 57:43 proportion of vegetable to animal food was eaten (calculated as kilojoules). This still fully functioning hunting and gathering society actually performed very little hunting, preferring to take their animal component mainly as shellfish and a large lizard called 'goanna'. However, it was noted that a wallaby (small marsupial) would be hunted and speared about every five days in a good season (Meehan, 1982, p. 160). Fish, birds and sugar-grubs were also consumed. Roast yams played the most important part in the diet, supplemented by fruits, nuts and wild honey. Meehan found no lack of food among these coastal people who set a high value on freshness, meticulous preparation and tasteful garnishing.

The Australian Aborigines possessed skill in detoxication. Grey (1837) recounts that some of the crew of Captain Cook's expedition of the 1770s observed the Aborigines eating the large seeds of *Macrozamia*, a primitive gymnosperm of the cycad class. The crew consumed some seeds not knowing that they had first to be treated, and became very ill. Aborigines detoxified these seeds in different ways – by leaching in running water, by fermentation or by roasting. Ground into flour, the seeds formed an important part of the diet in the south (Carr and Carr, 1981). The seeds of other cycads, containing the same poisonous principle (methylazoxymethanol, *2.1*) are eaten in other warm countries where they are similarly detoxified (Liener, 1980).

$$\overset{\displaystyle O}{\overset{\displaystyle \uparrow}{MeN=N\cdot CH_2OH}}$$

Methylazoxymethanol
(2.1)

When living traditionally Aborigines look thin but without malnutrition. Those who have contact with trading posts usually put on weight but lose health (Hetzel and Frith, 1978). To overcome this problem some Aborigines have established their own medical services. In 1980, 21 such clinics were operating employing Aboriginal physicians and nurses. Medical services in the tribal areas provide help for those who in recent years decided to return to their traditional lifestyle (Kirk, 1981). Biochemical tests carried out in Arnhem Land indicated normal levels of (serum) iron, calcium, folate and vitamin B_{12}. No anaemia or vitamin C deficiency was found and cholesterol was low (Casley-Smith, 1958).

The !Kung People of Botswana

Protected by the Kalahari desert from contact with outside influences, these bushmen who dwell in the NW corner of what was formerly called Bechuanaland in a southern part of Africa, live by hunting and gathering; their lifestyle apparently unchanged by the passage of time. There they were studied by Lee and DeVore over a ten year period (1963–1973) (Lee, 1979). In this society hunting confers prestige, but is not much practised because the reward is small for so much effort. Hence plant foods are used for most of the diet (average 70% by weight).

'Meat has come to be regarded as a special treat; when available, it is welcomed as a break from the routine of vegetable foods, but it is never depended upon as a staple. No one ever goes hungry when hunting fails' (Lee, in Lee and DeVore, 1968).

In season they use 105 edible species of plants, consisting of fruits, nuts, berries, roots, bulbs, gums, beans, melons and leafy greens. However 75% of the total kilojoules of their vegetable diet comes from only 14 species; the other kinds are used as garnishes. The most eaten item is the fruit of the mongongo tree (*Ricinodendron*, Euphorbiaceae) whose flesh is rich in carbohydrates whereas the centrally-sited nut (eaten only after roasting) contains 58% of fat and 28% of protein (Lee, 1979).

These bushmen appear thin but not malnourished. There is little dental caries, no hypertension and the serum cholesterol is low (Truswell, 1977).

The Eskimo People

There are today about 60 000 Eskimos living mostly in Alaska and Greenland, but spread in small enclaves across the whole of arctic North America and completely dominating 11 000 km of coastline. From the fossil record they seem to have colonized Alaska about 6000 years ago and then, as the ice barrier retreated, they spread out. Eskimos have efficiently adapted to a particularly inhospitable environment (Laughlin, 1963; Lee and DeVore, 1968; Dumond, 1977). They live mainly on raw walrus meat and fish. At the end of summer a few of them hunt caribou (a large deer). Because of the high latitide very little plant food is available.

The Eskimos are healthy people in spite of their lipid-rich diet and the high ratio of protein to carbohydrate; however they show a tendency to respiratory diseases (Way, 1970; Reinhold and Rice, 1970). Their expectation of life is in general excellent, except where they have formed close contact with other races (Stefansson, 1960; Laughlin, 1968).

The North American Indians

These people are thought to have crossed the then-existing land bridge from Asia about 20 000 years ago; some of them went on to occupy South America. When

European settlers arrived in North America they found the eastern portion under cultivation, whereas the Indians who lived in the plains, and westward to the Pacific coast, were still hunter-gatherers. Baumhoff (1963) has estimated that at that time about a quarter of a million people were living in California on a diet of acorn and fish (or, if inland, of acorn and game) – both of excellent nutritional quality.

The health of the hunter-gatherer

Dunn (1968) remarked:

> 'Many workers have commented on the relatively good nutritional status of hunter-gatherers in comparison with neighbouring agriculturists or urban dwellers'.

Although many of them are reported as being so thin that the rib outlines are visible, this condition is also favoured by healthy athletes in affluent societies. A formerly held opinion that the life of 'Primitive Man' was 'nasty, brutish and short' has been greatly changed by scholarly investigations (Harlan, 1975, p. 31). Some guidance may be extracted from such studies when considering contemporary health problems.

For further reading on health and disease in hunter-gatherers see Elliott and Whelan (1977); and for more information on their diet and nutrition see Truswell (1977).

2.2 Food from the beginning of civilization to the present time

The agricultural revolution

The *agricultural revolution* began about 10 000 years ago, at the end of the last ice age (Washburn and McCown, 1978). Wheat farming at Jericho in the Jordan Rift has left substantial evidence of its practice about this time and cattle were similarly shown to have been domesticated about 8000 years ago at Ali Kosh in Mesopotamia (Daniel, 1978). The first cultivated plants appear to have been cereals and legumes. Because these two kinds of food have incomplete (defined on p. 56) but complementary proteins (p. 64), it is essential that some of each should be eaten in the same meal. The first domesticated animals appear to have been the herbivores that had competed with man for such plants. Thus by becoming a farmer man the gatherer outwitted the herbivores. The crops too gained from the application of the herd's dung.

Orme (1977) has suggested further gains: by becoming stationary for the first time in his existence man could get to know his (now equally stationary) neighbours and this sociability could lead to sharing of supervision and exchange of surplus production – the very beginnings of civilization!

Once man ceased to be mobile he started to accumulate possessions: He built substantial wooden houses and fitted them out with objects too heavy or too fragile for a hunter-gatherer to move about. Clay cooking vessels began to appear and women must have been relieved not to have to carry infants on the endless trek.

Harlan (1975) points out, humorously but with a grain of truth, that crops have not so much been domesticated by man as they have domesticated him! No longer free to roam, he must live near his valuable fields, sheltering them from gales and predatory animals, and attending to their watering, fertilization and reproduction. It was at this time that man began to consume eggs, dairy products, alcoholic beverages and salt.

As the practice of agriculture grew, larger populations came to live closer together; settlements became villages, towns and eventually cities. Usually an elite class arose – a priesthood or aristocracy, that enjoyed feasting – a likely cause of the gross atherosclerosis found in the aorta of Egyptian mummies, and of the angina pectoris and sudden death to which the Roman governing classes were subject (Leibkowitz, 1970). The general population seemed to be healthier on their meagre diets which consisted principally of cereals and legumes, supplemented by beer or wine and (but in Europe only since 1570) potatoes; little animal protein seems to have been regularly consumed.

At the present time, the developing countries of Africa, Asia and the Americas experience much undernutrition which shows as impaired bodily development and apathy. Yet these people are remarkably free from diseases of the cardiovascular and alimentary systems that are so common in the industrialized nations (Ucko and Dimbleby, 1969).

The industrial revolution

The industrial revolution began about 200 years ago and is still only patchily distributed throughout a world in which about three-quarters of the people still live by farming. In what follows we shall sometimes contrast the nutrition of *developing* countries with that of *industrialized* countries but intermediate stages of industrialization also exist. Even in the European Economic Community, which is an association of industrialized countries, the degree of industrialization differs markedly from one country to another and also within one country.

Follow-up

Take a sheet of paper and note, briefly, those items in Section 2.2 which you think relevant to a discussion on contemporary patterns of eating. Do this once again when you have read all of Part One. Meanwhile jot down those food and health questions that you would most like to ask the next prehistorian, anthropologist or archaelogist that you happen to meet.

2.3 The gastrointestinal tract and what it does to food

Before we consider what happens to food *in* the human body let us look at what takes place after a meal has been swallowed but is still, as anatomists insist, on the *outside.* The gastrointestinal tract forms the major part of the alimentary canal which stretches, in one single length, from mouth to anus (Fig. 2.1). It can conveniently be thought of as an elastic tube that is divided into specialized areas, each with its characteristic shape and special functions. These functions are well coordinated by particular divisions of the nervous system and also by the enteric hormones which include secretin, gastrin, somatostatin, cholecystokinin, substance P, vasoactive intestinal polypeptide (VIP) and several prostaglandins.

The sequence of these specialized areas, and the average length of each, are: oesophagus 22 cm; stomach 28 cm (it is 11 cm wide at its widest); duodenum 22 cm; jejunum 240 cm; ileum 330 cm and colon (from ileocaecal valve to anus) 150 cm. The duodenum, jejunum and ileum together constitute the small intestine; the large intestine is also called the colon.

Large amounts of water are required for the digestive process. The salivary glands, stomach, pancreas, and liver pour out five litres each day, of which 4500 ml is resorbed before the ileocaecal valve is reached. Healthy eaters remain as unaware of this deluge as they are of the beating and sweeping movements of the stomach and intestines.

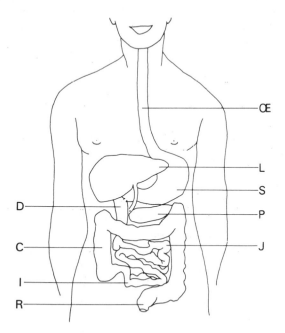

Fig. 2.1 The gastrointestinal tract. OE, oesophagus; S, stomach; L, liver; P, pancreas; D, duodenum; J, jejunum; I, ileum; C, colon; R, rectum.

Digestion

This consists of the hydrolysis of large molecules of food to obtain smaller molecules which can be transported across the membrane that lines the small intestine. In digestion the starch is broken down to glucose, proteins to peptides (and eventually to amino acids), and lipids, which are mainly triglycerides, become hydrolysed to monoglycerides, fatty acids and glycerol.

During eating, food is chewed into a bolus that is passed down the oesophagus into the stomach which, although normally free from acid, now secretes hydrochloric acid and a protease (pepsin) which, at the ruling pH of about 2, cleaves proteins into a mixture of smaller peptides. The arrival of food also initiates peristalsis in the stomach which gently, but thoroughly, mixes the gastric contents and progressively empties them into the duodenum at such a rate that about half of an average meal has been passed through the controlling sphincter (pylorus) in the first half hour. The rate of emptying of the stomach is controlled by enteric hormones. Apart from ethanol, little nutritive matter is absorbable through the stomach wall.

The arrival of acid and lipid in the duodenum induces the wall to secrete enteric hormones into the bloodstream that stimulate the pancreas to release a solution of sodium bicarbonate and several enzymes into the duodenum. The latter include (a) trypsin, chymotrypsin, carboxypeptidase, and elastin, (b) α-amylase and (c) lipase, which respectively digest peptides, starch, and lipids. This pancreatic α-amylase digests starch to a mixture of glucose, maltose and dextrin; related enzymes then digest the maltose and dextrin. Another α-amylase (formerly called ptyalin) also occurs in the saliva, but is rather weak in action. The hormones also stimulate the gall bladder to release the liver-derived bile acids, which assist digestion by emulsifying the water-insoluble lipids. Hormone-activated contractions of the whole of the small intestine unceasingly mix this neutralized 'chyme' (as the meal has now become – a thin, yellow paste), and move it steadily along at a rate that does not exceed that at which *absorptive cells* can extract nutrients.

During the third hour after a meal the jejunum, the centrally located region of the small intestine, secretes its *succus entericus*, a juice that contains enzymes. It furnishes carboxypeptidase, aminopeptidase and dipeptidase (collectively known as 'erepsin') to hydrolyse any recalcitrant peptides; and also disaccharidases to hydrolyse any lingering sucrose, maltose or lactose.

The duodenum is adapted to the absorption of glucose, most of the vitamins, calcium, iron and the products of the digestion of lipids. The jejunum is the principal region for absorbing amino acids, and the ileum for bile salts and vitamin B_{12}. The apparent area of the small intestine's wall is made enormously greater by its subdivision into projections, known as villi, each of which carries numerous absorptive cells. The glucose, glycerol, and amino acids, after absorption, are passed into the portal vein which transports them to the liver (from where we will take up their metabolism in Chapter 3). The medium-chain monoglycerides and aliphatic acids (C_4-C_{12}) are bound to albumin in the absorptive cells and then transferred to the portal vein and liver. However, the long-chain monoglycerides and fatty acids $(C_{16}-C_{18})$ are resynthesized into triglycerides by the absorptive cells, and then coated with protein and phospholipid (lecithin) to form spheres called chylomicrons. These are extruded into the lymphatic system from where they enter the bloodstream and eventually become stored in the fat depots that exist under the skin and in the abdominal cavity. Vitamins A, D, E, and K, as well as cholesterol, follow the triglyceride pattern of absorption.

The epithelial absorptive cells of the small intestine are replaced about every second day. They are digested in the chyme and the products of digestion resorbed, an example of the localized *anthropophagy* that is continually restoring and even reshaping most of the body's tissues. This turnover of the absorptive cells is thought to be in response to bacterial attack.

Everything that the small intestine has failed to absorb now passes through the ileocaecal valve into the colon which maintains two kinds of movement: (a) segmentation without propulsion, a process designed to absorb water and salts, and (b) peristalsis, which occurs principally after meals and propels the faecal mass. This mass weighs about 370 g for those on a vegetarian diet, but approximates to 60 g for the meat eater. It usually contains about 25% of solids, made up of about 8% bacteria, 10% food residues (cellulose and lignin from plants, fibres from meat, undigested fat), and the rest comprises mucus, desquammated epithelium, and the yellow bile pigment known as stercobilin.

The gastrointestinal tract presents a major interface between the germ-laden outside of the body and its sterile inside. The contents of the gut present a hostile environment from which the delicate lining membrane tries to protect itself by a surface coat of mucus, and antibacterial molecules big and small.

Further reading

An Introduction to Human Physiology (Green, 1976).
The Concise Gray's Anatomy (Leonard, 1983).
Human Nutrition and Dietetics (Davidson and Passmore, 1986).
McCance and Widdowson's: The Composition of Foods (Paul and Southgate, 1978).
Davidson's Principles and Practice of Medicine (Macleod, 1984).
Man the Hunter (Lee and DeVore, 1968).
Crops and Man (Harlan, 1975).

Follow-up

Can you work out what *really* troubles those good citizens who, in evident agony, complain of 'indigestion'? Alumina, charcoal, kaolin, liquid paraffin, and bran are indigestible, yet are valued for treating gastrointestinal ailments.

3

The metabolism of foods

In the previous Chapter we reviewed the breakdown of the large food molecules into others that are small enough to be absorbed *from* the gut *into* the human body. Digestion wins no energy from a meal. On the contrary every digestive step is a hydrolysis, a process that consumes energy. The generation of energy requires oxidative phosphorylation, a process that is made available by *catabolism*. *Anabolism* uses a different set of reactions to build up stores of human carbohydrate, lipid and protein. Human catabolism and anabolism, collectively known as *metabolism**, form the substance of this chapter.

Most readers probably have some knowledge of general biochemical metabolism. The present chapter aims to review this subject as it applies to human nutrition, partly for the subject's own interest, but more particularly to provide background for the following chapter which is intended as a major contribution to this study of foods as foreign substances.

3.1 The conversion of digested foods into energy: the storage and release of energy

Carbohydrate

(a) *Glucose*. The catabolism of carbohydrates will be discussed before that of lipids and proteins, because glucose is the body's major fuel. Glucose ends by being completely oxidized to carbon dioxide and water.

In Section 2.3 we saw how glucose (whose main source is dietary starch) was absorbed from the bowel and then transported to the liver. The level of glucose in the bloodstream is maintained at 120 mg/100 ml after meals as follows: Any

---

* Greek *kata* down, *ana* up, *meta* change and *ballein* to throw.

excess glucose triggers secretion (by the pancreas) of insulin, which quickly converts the excess glucose to its polymer, glycogen, which is then stored in muscles and liver. However when through exertion the level of glucose falls below 80 mg/100 ml (4.4 mM) the secretion of glucagon (by the pancreas) and epinephrine (from the suprarenal glands) restores the limiting level by effecting the breakdown of glycogen from liver and muscle respectively.

We shall now review that long sequence of catabolic reactions required for *glycolysis*, i.e. the enzymatic conversion of glucose into pyruvate* with simultaneous synthesis of adenosine triphosphate (ATP). Glycolysis takes place in the cytosol of most cells but particularly in those of the liver and muscles. In the first stage glucose is converted to glucose 6-phosphate (*3.1*) which is isomerized, then changed into fructose 1,6-diphosphate (*3.2*) by fructokinase. This becomes split into glyceraldehyde 3-phosphate (*3.3*).

Up to this point there have been energy losses but no energy gain from the eating of starch. Energy is extracted from the meal, for the first time, by the oxidation of the aldehyde group in *3.3*. This is accomplished by the enzyme known as glyceraldehyde 3-phosphate dehydrogenase, which produces a mixed acid anhydride, namely 3-phosphoglyceroyl phosphate (formerly 1,3-diphosphoglycerate) (*3.4*). This enzyme has as its coenzyme the substance known as NAD which is simultaneously reduced to NADH.

'NAD' is shorthand for nicotinamide adenine dinucleotide (*3.5a*) which is the commonest electron acceptor in the oxidation of fuel molecules. Both of the

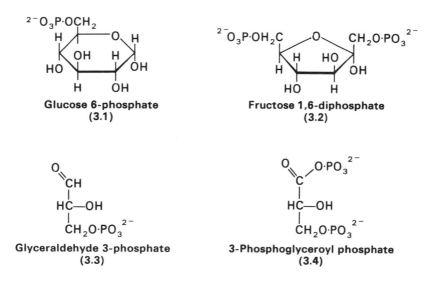

Glucose 6-phosphate
(3.1)

Fructose 1,6-diphosphate
(3.2)

Glyceraldehyde 3-phosphate
(3.3)

3-Phosphoglyceroyl phosphate
(3.4)

---

* The literature of biochemistry is rich in mention of such anions (lactate, citrate etc.) which it assumes to be paired with potassium cations when *inside* cells and with sodium cations otherwise.

electrons lost by the substrate (but only one of its hydrogen atoms, the other being lost as H^+) are transferred to NAD, which thereby becomes nicotinamide adenine dinucleotide hydride (NADH). The nicotinamide portion of NAD is, effectively, a carrier of the hydride anion (H^-). The energy that has been stored by the conversion of NAD to NADH will later be transferred to ATP in the mitochondria, for ATP (*3.6*) is the ultimate storer (and dispenser) of metabolism-won energy.

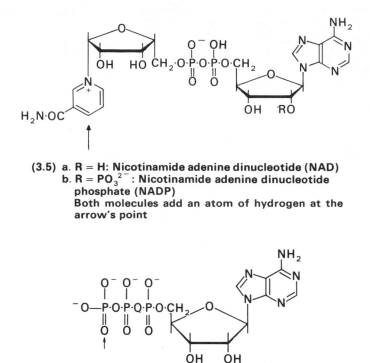

(3.5) a. R = H: Nicotinamide adenine dinucleotide (NAD)
   b. R = PO$_3{}^{2-}$: Nicotinamide adenine dinucleotide phosphate (NADP)
   Both molecules add an atom of hydrogen at the arrow's point

Adenosine triphosphate (ATP)
The phosphate group opposite the arrow's head is lost when ADP is formed
   (3.6)

In the next stage of glycolysis, phosphoglycerate kinase transfers the mixed-anhydride phosphate group of 3-phosphoglyceroyl phosphate *directly* to ADP, thus producing 3-phosphoglycerate (*3.7*) and ATP. In the last stage of glycolysis, 3-phosphoglycerate is converted (in three reactions) into pyruvate (*3.8*). The energy gain, up to this point, i.e. in the conversion of glucose to pyruvate, may be usefully summarized as follows:

$$\text{Glucose} + 2P_i + 2NAD + 2ADP \rightarrow 2\text{Pyruvate} + 2NADH + 2ATP$$

(where P_i stands for inorganic phosphate).

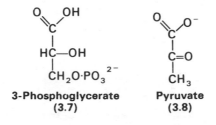

3-Phosphoglycerate   **Pyruvate**
(3.7)   **(3.8)**

Directly or indirectly, the oxidation of one molecule of glucose converts 36 molecules of ADP to ATP. Most of these changes are effected after the entry of pyruvate into the citric acid cycle, which we shall now review. Of the several kinds of organelles which the electron microscope has revealed inside every cell (see Fig. 3.1), the mitochondrion plays an unique and important part by taking up the small molecules into which carbohydrates, lipids and proteins become fragmented, and converting them to energy. This energy is stored as ATP in the mitochondria and released from them on demand.

A mitochondrion (Fig. 3.2) is usually 2–3 μm in length and 1 μm in diameter. It consists of a rather permeable outer membrane, and a far less permeable inner membrane which is indented to form shelves (called *cristae*). These structures enclose two spaces, the intermembrane space and the central matrix or lumen.

The outer membrane contains the enzyme system that oxidatively decarboxylates pyruvic acid (*3.8*) to the acetyl residue (*3.9*). The coenzymes in this complex reaction are dihydrolipoic acid (*3.10*), thiamine pyrophosphate, and NAD. The acetyl residue combines at once with coenzyme A (CoA) (*3.11*) which is a derivative of the vitamin, pantothenic acid. In this operation, one molecule of NADH is formed. Thus:

$$\text{Pyruvate} + \text{CoA} + \text{NAD} \rightarrow \text{Acetyl CoA} + CO_2 + \text{NADH}$$

The acetylcoenzyme A is transferred to the mitochondrial matrix where the reactions of the citric acid cycle (also called the tricarboxylic acid cycle) (*3.12*) take place. An enzyme known as citrate synthetase brings about combination of the acetyl fragment (*3.9*) of CoA (*3.11*) with the oxaloacetate (*3.13*) present in the cycle, thus forming citrate (*3.14*) and liberating CoA. Specific enzymes convert citrate to isocitrate (*3.15*), then oxidize the latter to α-ketoglutarate (*3.16*), with concomitant reduction of NAD to NADH and loss of CO_2.

This α-ketoglutarate is then condensed with coenzyme A to give succinylcoenzyme A, with simultaneous reduction of NAD to NADH and loss of CO_2. Thus, all the carbon atoms of pyruvic acid (and hence of the glucose from which it was formed) have now been burnt away to CO_2, a substance for which the human body has only a limited use; most of it is quickly lost in exhalation. Let us note, though, that a good part of the *energy* supplied by these fuels is stored in the succinylcoenzyme A, to be released through operation of the rest of the cycle, as follows.

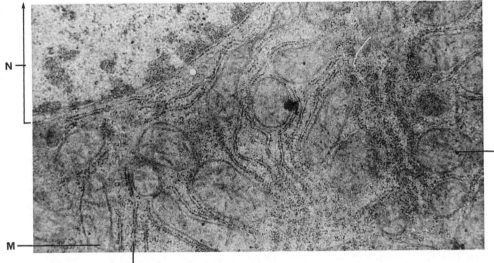

Fig. 3.1 Electron micrograph of rat liver cell. ER, endoplasmic reticulum; M, mitochondria; N, portion of nucleus.

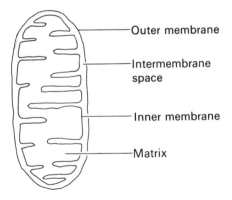

Fig. 3.2 A mitochondrion.

$CH_3CO^\bullet$

Acetyl residue
(3.9)

$$\begin{array}{cc} SH & SH \\ | & | \end{array}$$
$$CH_2CH_2CH(CH_2)_4CO_2H$$

Dihydrolipoic acid
(Thioctic acid)
(3.10)

$$HS \cdot CH_2 \cdot CH_2 \cdot NH \overset{O}{\underset{\uparrow}{\overset{\|}{-}}} C \cdot CH_2 \cdot CH_2 \cdot \underset{H}{N} \overset{O}{\overset{\|}{-}} C \cdot \overset{H}{\underset{H}{\overset{O}{\overset{|}{C}}}} \cdot \overset{OMe}{\underset{Me}{\overset{|}{C}}} \cdot CH_2 \cdot O \cdot (\text{iso-ATP})$$

Coenzyme A (CoA)
Acetylation occurs at the arrow's point
(3.11)

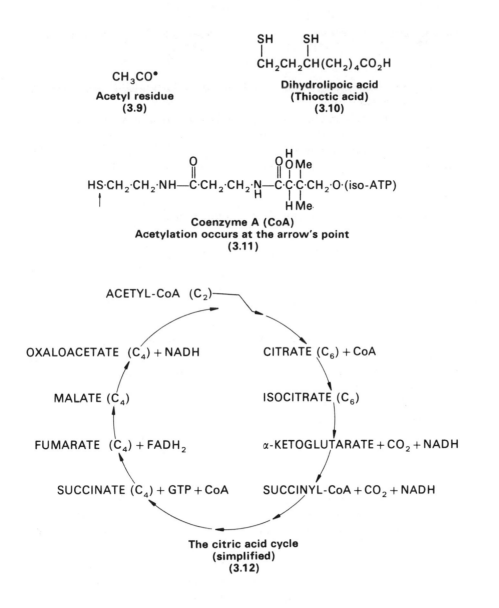

ACETYL-CoA (C_2)

OXALOACETATE (C_4) + NADH   CITRATE (C_6) + CoA

MALATE (C_4) ISOCITRATE (C_6)

FUMARATE (C_4) + FADH$_2$ α-KETOGLUTARATE + CO$_2$ + NADH

SUCCINATE (C_4) + GTP + CoA   SUCCINYL-CoA + CO$_2$ + NADH

The citric acid cycle
(simplified)
(3.12)

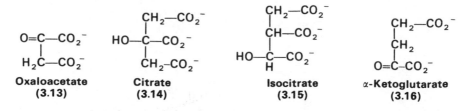

Oxaloacetate (3.13)   Citrate (3.14)   Isocitrate (3.15)   α-Ketoglutarate (3.16)

Succinyl CoA converts guanosine diphosphate (GDP) (available at this point in the cycle) to GTP, thus liberating free succinate (*3.17*) and CoA. (The GTP later gives its newly-won phosphoryl group to ADP, to form ATP). Succinate is oxidized to fumarate (*3.18*) by the enzyme succinate dehydrogenase which uses (ribo)flavine adenine dinucleotide as the hydrogen acceptor (the $FADH_2$ produced in this way is later used to convert ADP to ATP). Fumarate is enzymatically hydrated to malate which is dehydrogenated to oxaloacetate (*3.13*), thus completing one round of the cycle. Thus, a very small amount of oxaloacetate can oxidize an unlimited amount of pyruvate.

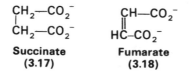

Succinate (3.17)   Fumarate (3.18)

This *oxidative phosphorylation* of ADP takes place in the inner mitochondrial membrane thanks to the *respiratory assembly*, a spaced sequence of enzymes, many of which have cytochrome coenzymes. Because one molecule of NADH can convert three molecules of ADP to ATP and one molecule of $FADH_2$ forms two of ATP, the oxidation of one molecule of pyruvate produces 15 molecules of ATP (one came from GTP). Thus, one molecule of glucose (which gave two of pyruvic acid) produces 36 molecules of ATP, provided we count the 6 molecules of ATP formed during glycolysis. The ATP is stored in the inner mitochondrial membrane.

(*b*) *Sucrose, fructose, lactose and galactose.* Sucrose (cane or beet sugar), a substance entirely foreign to the human body, forms a significant proportion of the diet of people in industrialized countries. The small intestine very rapidly splits it to glucose and fructose, of which the former is quickly and the latter tardily absorbed. Honey contains equal proportions of glucose and fructose and the latter is also contained in many fruits. Fructose is converted in the liver (in several stages) to glyceraldehyde 3-phosphate (*3.3*) at which point it enters the glycolytic pathway, just as glucose does.

Galactose, available only from intestinal hydrolysis of lactose (glucose is simultaneously formed) which is found only in milk, is rapidly absorbed and then converted (in 4 stages) to glucose 1-phosphate which directly enters the glycolytic pathway.

(*c*) *Alcohols*. Glycerol, formed in the small intestine by lipolysis, is absorbed into the blood and slowly converted to dihydroxyacetone phosphate, which supplies its isomer, glyceraldehyde 3-phosphate (*3.3*), to the glycolytic pathway.

Ethanol does not occur naturally in the human body. When consumed, it is rapidly absorbed from both stomach and duodenum, and it becomes distributed throughout the total body water. Over 90% of an ingested amount is slowly metabolized by the liver at a rate that averages 100 mg/kg body-weight per hour, but which varies between individuals from 60–200 mg/kg. The other 10% is lost in breath and urine. After a 30 g dose of ethanol a typical 65 kg man clears it from his blood in 4.6 h (Davidson and Passmore, 1986, p. 497).

Ethanol is mainly metabolized in the cytosol of the liver where it is oxidized first to acetaldehyde by a non-specific dehydrogenase that uses NAD as hydrogen acceptor. This slow stage is followed by a quicker conversion of acetaldehyde to acetyl CoA, which can be used as a source of energy in the citric acid cycle. Thus a small amount of ethanol can replace its caloric equivalent of carbohydrate or lipid as an energy source for steady, undemanding work. However, because ethanol is oxidized only at a slow, invariable rate (and not *on demand* as is the case with glucose), its clearance from the blood cannot be increased by muscular exertion.

Ethanol provides one of the clearest examples of the Paracelsian doctrine that 'It's all a matter of the dose', and we shall find ourselves discussing it again as an enhancer of mood (Section 5.3), as a medicine (Section 8.1) and as a lethal poison (Section 13.2). Here we are concerned only with its use as a food. Formerly, ethanol was used as a dietary supplement for patients being fed exclusively by intravenous drip; many of these had 25 ml of ethanol added to each bottle of carbohydrate solution. Provided the mix is administered slowly, no intoxication occurs (Davidson and Passmore, 1986).

The proportion of ethanol considered suitable for a repast in Biblical times is glimpsed in the First Book of Samuel (25–16):

> 'Then Abigail made haste, and took two hundred loaves, and two bottles of wine, and five sheep ready dressed, and five measures of parched corn, and an hundred clusters of raisins, and two hundred cakes of figs'.

Today, ethanol contributes on average 12% of the food intake of adults in the USA (Lehninger, 1982), and, although this figure varies from country to country (Davidson and Passmore, 1986, p. 72), the intake of ethanol at the expense of other foods is characteristic of many industrialized lands.

Considered as a food, ethanol has four disadvantages: (a) it is not oxidizable on demand (see above) and hence cannot supply energy for heavy work or emergency action, (b) it readily becomes converted to body fat, but cannot form any glucose or glycogen, (c), like sucrose, it is not marketed in forms which supply the vitamins needed (as coenzymes) for its metabolism, and (d) thanks to excise regulations it costs up to 20 times as much as its caloric equivalent of carbohydrate.

The strength of ethanolic drinks varies with geography. Many Arab countries make no use of these beverages. In Britain, beers, wines, fortified wines (e.g. sherry, port) and spirits contain about 3, 9, 15, and 32 g/100 ml respectively (Paul and Southgate, 1978), whereas in the USA, the figures for beer, wine, and 'hard liquor' are 5, 12, and 50 g/100 ml, respectively (Lehninger, 1982). In France, where wine is the principal alcoholic beverage, the content averages 12%. In Australia the Law requires that beer, wine and spirit should contain no less than 1.15, 8 and 37 v/v % respectively of ethanol; in each case the percentage must be declared on the front label in large numerals. Thus each type of beverage is available in a range of strengths and the purchaser can make an informed choice. At present 4 and 12% are popular strengths for beer and wine respectively, but public health education is creating a demand for lower strengths.

(d)   *The pentose phosphate pathway.*   In muscle, practically all of the glucose derived from food enters into glycolysis, whereas in some other tissues, particularly those that synthesize lipids, some of the glucose is diverted into the pentose phosphate pathway. In this alternative route all reactions take place in the cytosol; neither mitochondria nor the citric acid cycle is used. It is thought that the principal use of this pathway is (a) to manufacture NADP, which is as necessary for anabolism as NAD is for catabolism, and (b) to generate D-ribose, which is essential for the biosynthesis of nucleic acids.

This route may be summarized as:

$$\text{Glucose 6-phosphate} + 2\text{NADP} \rightarrow \text{Ribose 5-phosphate} + 2\text{NADPH} + CO_2$$

In detail: glucose 6-phosphate is oxidized (by glucose 6-phosphate dehydrogenase) to 6-phosphogluconate (*3.19*) simultaneously converting one molecule of NADP (*3.5b*) to NADPH. Enzymatic dehydrogenation then gives ribulose 5-phosphate which becomes isomerized to D-ribose 5-phosphate (*3.20*). Besides

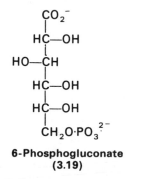

6-Phosphogluconate
(3.19)

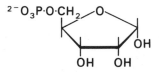

D-Ribose 5-phosphate
(3.20)

forming a significant part of the molecules of NAD, NADP, ATP, and RNA ribose plays an important role in purine biosynthesis.

(e) *Unavailable carbohydrate and dietary fibre.* These were also known, originally, as 'residue' and 'roughage'. Cellulose, the principal supporting material of plants, is a polymerized glucose as are starch and glycogen. Cellulose is not digested by amylase yet bacteria that are often present in the human colon can transform it into a mixture of acetic, propionic and butyric acids, which after absorption can contribute to the caloric intake (Holloway, Tasman-Jones and Lee, 1978; McNeil, 1984). Hemicelluloses, which are mainly polymerized pentoses, are consumed along with cellulose in fruits, vegetables and bran. Although hemicelluloses are not digested in the small intestine they break down to a small extent in the colon. The water-retaining capacity of undigested hemicelluloses is thought to be the factor that prevents constipation (Davidson and Passmore, 1986, pp. 34–38).

Different types of unavailable dietary material seem to benefit *different* parts of the body. The earliest work was on wheat bran, thought to decrease incidence of diverticulitis, haemorrhoids, cancer of the colon and even heart disease (Burkitt and Trowell, 1975). Pectin and guar gum appear to lower blood cholesterol (Kay and Truswell, 1977; Jenkins, *et al.*, 1977). Pectins, which are gelatinous rather than fibrous, occur in fruits and vegetables and are polymers of galacturonic acid. Like lignins and saponins, pectins are thought to bind bile acids in the intestine, thereby preventing their resorption. Because bile acids are formed from cholesterol, the blood level of the latter falls so that functional levels of bile acids can be maintained in the intestine.

The addition of pectin and guar gum to carbohydrate meals decreases the subsequent rise in blood glucose, a phenomenon utilized in some diabetic diets. It is thought that the viscosity of these polysaccharides hinders the absorption of glucose (Jenkins, *et al.*, 1976).

It may take some time for these various indications to become firmly established.

Plant material used in thickening prepared foods include agar (polymerized galactose), alginic acid (polymerized guluronic and mannuronic acids), both of which come from seaweeds; also carob and guar gums (both of which are galactose-mannose polymers obtained from trees). Meat contributes unavailable fibrous protein to the faeces.

(f) *How essential is carbohydrate in the diet?* Although man can convert the glycerol of lipids and the amino acids of proteins into glucose, most nutritionists think that it is healthier for human beings to consume about 50–100 g of their daily energy requirement as starch (Calloway, 1971). A diet devoid of carbohydrate favours ketosis (p. 29), loss of sodium, breakdown of tissue protein and dehydration. These are unpleasant phenomena but not life-threatening. Meat is virtually free from carbohydrate yet some Arctic explorers have lived for a year entirely on meat and managed to keep fit (McClellan and Du Bois, 1930). Again Eskimos get little carbohydrate in their diet, and this was the case with the Andean survivors (p. 7). Other hunter-gatherers in parallel with farming and industrial communities have diets containing about 50% carbohydrate.

Lipids

Most of the lipids made available by a meal are despatched, inside chylomicrons (p. 17), into the bloodstream from where they soon disappear into the *adipose tissue*. The latter is a substantial protein network that extends all over the body, from ankles to cheeks. When loaded with triglycerides it weighs 8–20 kg in normal healthy adults. In response to signals from muscles or liver, lipases in the adipose tissue liberate fatty acids from the triglycerides. These acids, coated with albumin, travel in the bloodstream to the requesting organ. Another important fraction of the blood plasma is low density lipoprotein (LDL) which contains most of the circulating cholesterol in the form of its ester with linoleic acid. This lipoprotein transports the cholesterol to peripheral tissues which need it for viability and growth.

If investigated during, or straight after, a meal it is found that most of the body's energy requirement is being provided by carbohydrate. At other times however the oxidation of fatty acids supplies half of this requirement. In the first step of their utilization, these acids acylate the –SH group in coenzyme A (*3.11*). The products are then acted on by the β-oxidation enzyme complex in the central matrix of the mitochondria (Fig. 3.2). The long chain of the acid becomes shortened in four consecutive reactions to give a carboxylic acid that has two carbon atoms fewer than the original (this shortening takes place at the –COOH end).

Let us follow this process in palmitic acid $[CH_3(CH_2)_{14}CO_2H]$. One turn of the β-oxidation cycle produces one molecule of acetyl CoA, and the energy liberated by the oxidation converts one molecule of FAD (p. 24) to $FADH_2$, and one molecule of NAD to NADH. The complete breakdown of this C_{16} acid requires seven turns of the cycle, and produces 8 molecules of acetyl CoA, and 7 molecules each of $FADH_2$ and NADH. When these two reduced coenzymes give up their stored energy to ADP the equation runs:

$$\text{Palmitoyl CoA} + 7\text{CoA} + 7O_2 + 35P_i + 35\text{ADP} \rightarrow 8\text{acetyl CoA} + 35\text{ATP} + 16CO_2$$

Most of this acetyl CoA enters the citric acid cycle (*3.12*) thus generating a further 12 molecules of ATP. In sum by the complete oxidation of one molecule of palmitoyl CoA to CO_2 and water, 130 molecules of ATP were generated. Yet we have not completed investigating the high calorific value of lipids until we include the energy obtained from the oxidation of the glycerol (p. 25) liberated from triglycerides.

Oleic acid, abundantly present in body fat, presents a special case because of its *cis* 9–10 double bond. When β-oxidation has pared the molecule down to this area a special epimerase comes into play, after which oxidation continues as with palmitic acid. A second epimerase is available to deal with polyunsaturated fatty acids such as linoleic acid.

A small proportion of the acetyl CoA produced from oxidation of the body's palmitic and oleic acids is converted by the liver to a mixture of 'ketone bodies' in which acetoacetate predominates. This is transported by the blood to tissues, such as heart and kidney cortex, where it is the preferred fuel. Liver and brain do not normally use acetoacetate. The tissues which prefer acetoacetate, oxidize it after prior conversion to acetyl CoA. The capacity of using acetoacetate as fuel is lost in starvation and diabetes, so that this ketonic acid accumulates in the blood and is excreted in the urine, a condition known as ketosis.

Many otherwise well-informed people do not realize what a rich contribution of lipid is made by a serving of meat. Thus, a small helping of roast beef will provide 24 g of protein, 21 g of fat, but no carbohydrate. Also extra fat will be taken in with the gravy.

What constitutes a healthy intake of lipids (fat)? In most of the industrialized countries lipids usually contribute about 40% to the total energy production (expressed in kJ). However this may be an unhealthily high ratio for sedentary people (see Section 4.2). Yet, when rationing reduced this figure to 33% in wartime Britain, housewives complained that it was no longer possible to prepare a palatable meal (Davidson and Passmore, 1986, p. 67). This may be a matter of custom because the Hos aboriginals in India, although consuming only 2% of their energy requirements as lipids (to which they have abundant access), show no symptoms of lipid deficiency (Mitra, 1942).

Proteins

Normally proteins provide only about 10% of the body's energy demands because in contrast to what happens to an excess of glucose or fatty acids, most of the amino acids formed by the digestion of protein cannot be stored in the body which carries only a small protein reserve. Expressed briefly, their fate is to lose all nitrogen as ammonia which is converted into urea in the liver and this end-product is voided in the urine. This loss of nitrogen presents the liver cells with a set of α-keto acids which, if not otherwise required, undergo oxidation to carbon dioxide and water via the citric acid cycle (*3.12*).

In detail: most of the twenty common L-amino acids produced in the digestion of proteins, are transaminated, a process in which the amino group is transferred to α-ketoglutarate (*3.16*) (available from the citric acid cycle) which is thereby changed to glutamate (*3.21*) as follows:

$$\alpha\text{-Amino acid} + \alpha\text{-ketoglutarate} \rightarrow \alpha\text{-keto acid} + \text{glutamate}$$

The result is that the nitrogen that was present in *many* kinds of amino acids is now accumulated in only *one* of them, a step that simplifies the next stage.

Glutamate serves as the cell's ammonia-carrier, a necessary function because ammonia is highly toxic to the brain.

All of the ammonia that is not required for anabolism is excreted as urea, through operation of the *urea cycle*. This is a multienzyme process that operates partly in the cytosol and partly in mitochondria. One of the two nitrogen atoms of urea comes from free ammonia, the other from aspartate (*3.22*); the carbon atom comes from carbon dioxide. The cycle starts with conversion of ornithine (*3.23*) to citrulline (*3.24*) by carbamoyl phosphate. The latter is synthesized by the following equation:

$$NH_4^+ + CO_2 + 2ATP \rightarrow H_2N.C(:O).O.PO_3^{2-} + 2ADP + P_i$$

Thus the detoxication of ammonia loses the body much valuable energy from the store of ATP.

The citrulline combines with aspartate to give argininosuccinate, a C_9 structure that loses fumarate (*3.18*) to give arginine (*3.25*). Finally the arginine loses *urea* to give the ornithine with which the cycle began. In the equation the ammonia came largely from glutamate (*3.21*) which, by transamination with oxaloacetate (*3.13*) (available from the citric acid cycle) provides the aspartate component of the urea cycle. Another portion of glutamate is oxidatively deaminated by glutamate dehydrogenase to yield the ammonium ion shown in the equation.

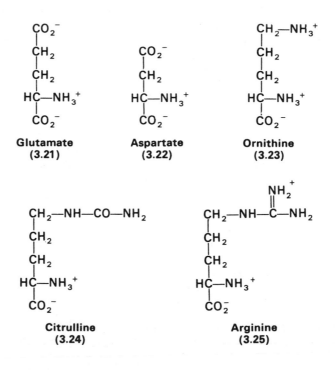

Glutamate
(3.21)

Aspartate
(3.22)

Ornithine
(3.23)

Citrulline
(3.24)

Arginine
(3.25)

Let us return to the α-keto acids. Those derived from alanine, cysteine, glycine, serine and threonine are enzymatically changed to pyruvate (*3.8*) which enters the citric acid cycle (*3.12*) via acetyl CoA. Those derived from isoleucine, leucine and tryptophan are degraded directly to acetyl CoA. Those derived from lysine, phenylalanine and tyrosine are transformed to acetoacetyl CoA which is then degraded to acetyl CoA. The citric acid cycle is entered at the fumarate level by the keto acid derived from aspartate, and this site is also used as an alternative entry for keto acids derived from phenylalanine and tyrosine. The cycle is entered at the succinyl CoA level by the keto acids given by methionine and valine, and this is a second point of entry for those derived from isoleucine and threonine. Finally, the keto acids given by arginine, glutamate, glutamine, histidine and proline enter the citric acid cycle at the α-ketoglutarate level. Amino acids undergoing biosynthesis into protein escape degradation.

Nucleic acids

Nucleic acids are another nitrogen-containing fraction of food and become a significant item of diet when the following are eaten regularly: liver, kidneys, pancreas, anchovies, sardines, fish roe and meat extracts. Nucleic acids are hydrolysed in the duodenum by ribonucleases and deoxyribonucleases secreted by the pancreas. The liberated purine bases (adenine, guanine) and pyrimidine bases (uracil, thymine, and cytosine) then enter the bloodstream. There they mix with identical bases formed by the breakdown of the body's nucleic acids, a process which is taking place constantly in cells. Depending on requirements, new nucleic acids can be synthesized by salvaging this pool of bases. However, if bodily needs are exceeded, the bases are oxidized to uric acid (purines) and urea (pyrimidines) and voided in the urine. When the level of purines and pyrimidines in the bloodstream becomes low, new supplies are synthesized *de novo* in the liver (p. 36).

3.2 The conversion of metabolic fragments into human carbohydrate, lipid and protein

Carbohydrate

Small as the body's store of carbohydrate is (about 160 g of glycogen), this is absolutely essential because every day the brain consumes about 120 g of glucose as its exclusive fuel (Stryer, 1981). In Section 3.1 we noted that any excess of glucose in the blood, during or after meals, triggers a secretion of insulin which converts this sugar to glycogen. An alternative source of the latter is provided for use during periods of starvation or of unusually strenuous work. This gluco*neo*genesis (as it is called) is simply the synthesis of glucose from non-carbohydrate precursors. The principal precursors are lactate, glycerol or amino acids.

Lactate (*3.26*) is formed anaerobically in muscles when the rate of glycolysis exceeds the metabolic rate of the citric acid cycle and respiratory chain. This happens under conditions of great muscular exertion. This lactate cannot be converted to pyruvate (*3.8*) in the muscle but must travel to the liver to find the appropriate enzyme, lactate dehydrogenase. Glucose is formed from this pyruvate by the consecutive action of several enzymes, of which an early product is phospho*enol*pyruvate (*3.27*). This is converted in turn to fructose 1,6-diphosphate and glucose 6-phosphate. According to the body's needs at the time, the latter is converted to glycogen *or* glucose. It is important to note that very few of the enzymes used in glycolysis are capable of taking part in gluconeogenesis, and vice versa; moreover the former group of enzymes use NAD, whereas the latter group use NADP.

Glycerol can be used for gluconeogenesis when it is coursing in the bloodstream following hydrolysis of triglycerides in the liver. It is converted to dihydroxyacetone phosphate which exists in equilibrium with its isomer, glyceraldehyde 3-phosphate (*3.3*). The latter is converted to fructose 1,6-diphosphate and hence to glucose.

Those α-keto acids (derived from amino acids, as described in Section 3.1) that enter the citric acid cycle through acetyl CoA cannot contribute to gluconeogenesis because the pyruvate → acetyl CoA reaction is irreversible. The remaining keto acids, however, enter the citric acid cycle at the points listed on p. 31, and they leave it in the form of phosphoenolpyruvate (*3.27*), between oxaloacetate and citrate.

Neither fatty acids nor ethanol play any part in gluconeogenesis. In fact heavy consumption of ethanol actually inhibits this process.

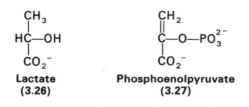

Lactate
(3.26)

Phosphoenolpyruvate
(3.27)

Lipids

A healthy (70 kg) man has reserves of lipids capable of producing about 400 000 kJ, which is enough to sustain life during at least three weeks' abstention from eating. For comparison, the protein store (mainly in muscle) can yield about 100 000 kJ, and the carbohydrate store (glycogen) only 2500 kJ (Stryer, 1981). Far from letting their reserves of lipids run down most human beings replenish them daily as follows:

The fatty acids are synthesized in the cytosol of the liver by the repeated addition of two-carbon units to an initial two-carbon chain that is attached to the *acyl carrier protein* (ACP). This substance, of molecular weight about 9000, has the same prosthetic group as coenzyme A (*3.11*), except that a protein replaces the iso-ATP terminal. Biosynthesis of fatty acids begins with one molecule of malonyl CoA (*3.28*) bound to the terminal –SH group of ACP, and a molecule of acetyl CoA attached to a cysteine residue in the protein of ACP. The enzyme 3-ketoacyl-ACP synthase unites these two fragments, with loss of one molecule of CO_2. Repetition of this procedure, using additional molecules of malonyl CoA, extends the chain to a maximal length of C_{16}, giving palmitic acid. This synthesis of palmitate uses 8 mol of acetyl CoA, 14 of NADPH and 7 of ATP. The malonyl CoA comes from acetyl CoA and CO_2.

The principal aliphatic acids of human adipose tissue are oleic and palmitic, present as the mixed triglycerides formed in the liver. Table 3.1 supplies some quantitative data.

Although stearic acid (C_{18}) is strongly represented in the fat of ruminants, there is little of it in human fat. Our bodies synthesize it by addition of a two-carbon fragment to palmitic acid, in the endoplasmic reticulum (Fig. 3.1). In that organelle, most of this stearic acid is dehydrogenated to oleic acid, a process in which a double bond (*cis-Δ^9*) is inserted. The linoleic acid fraction of human

Table 3.1 Human superficial fat, percentage of aliphatic acids present as triglycerides.

Acid	Number of carbon atoms	Number of double bonds	%
Oleic	18	1	48
Palmitic	16	0	23
Palmitoleic	16	1	10
Linoleic	18	2	7
Stearic	18	0	4
Myristic	14	0	4
Traces of others	—	—	4
			100

(After Heffernan, 1964)

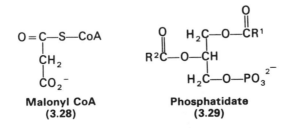

Malonyl CoA
(3.28)

Phosphatidate
(3.29)

fat, although substantial, is not synthesized in the body but accumulated from various foods (vegetable oils are very rich in it). This acid, which is used in the biosynthesis of the prostanoids (secondary messengers), is an indispensable component of our diets. The unsaturation of linoleic acid is at Δ^9 and Δ^{12}. The synthesis of fatty acids falls as the concentration of palmitoyl CoA rises in the liver cytosol.

Phosphatidate (diacylglycerol 3-phosphate) (*3.29*) is the common intermediate in hepatic syntheses of the triglycerides (neutral fats) and the phosphoglycerides such as lecithin. In *3.29* R^1 and R^2 represent oleoyl and palmitoyl, not necessarily respectively. In the synthesis of triglycerides, the phosphoryl function is replaced by a third fatty acid residue. In forming lecithin (phosphatidyl choline), the phosphoryl function of *3.29* is esterified with choline $[HO(CH_2)_2NMe_3{}^+]$, and similar esters are made from ethanolamine and serine: these three products do much to preserve the integrity of natural membranes.

Cholesterol (*3.32*), an essential controller of the fluidity of plasma membranes, particularly those in the brain, derives each of its 27 carbon atoms from acetyl CoA, three molecules of which are initially condensed to give mevalonate (*3.30*). The latter is further modified, with loss of CO_2, to 3-isopentenyl pyrophosphate (*3.31*) whose 5-carbon atom chain condenses to give the C_{30}-chain-like molecule known as squalene which, in several steps, is cyclized to cholesterol. Extra cholesterol enters the bloodstream from the diet, and is quickly transferred to the liver. Cholesterol is the precursor of all the steroid hormones, such as estradiol, progesterone, dihydrotestosterone, and cortisol. Cholesterol is also modified to

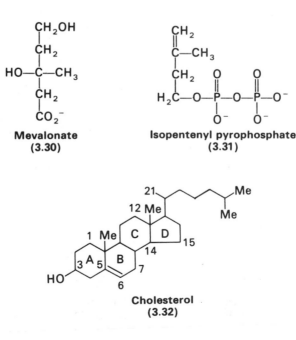

Mevalonate
(3.30)

Isopentenyl pyrophosphate
(3.31)

Cholesterol
(3.32)

form the bile salts (principally glycocholate) which emulsify dietary lipids in the jejunum (p. 16).

Proteins

Plants can synthesize all of the twenty amino acids that condense to form the majority of proteins, but human beings can make only ten of these amino acids. Although all twenty of them are necessary to make our several thousand kinds of proteins, the word 'essential' is reserved for those ten which we must obtain from our food (Table 3.2). All these essential amino acids must be present at about the same time for the synthesis of protein to take place. In many experiments, rats have been fed a diet containing all the essential amino acids but one. When the missing amino acid was fed three hours later, the rats did not grow (Lehninger, 1982, p. 765).

The human body, for the most part, makes 'nonessential' amino acids by enzymatic amination of the corresponding keto acids. Thus, pyruvate (*3.8*) is transaminated to give alanine, and oxaloacetate (*3.13*) similarly forms aspartate (*3.22*). Glutamate (*3.21*) is formed by amination of α-ketoglutarate (*3.16*). Asparagine and glutamine are synthesized from the corresponding acids. Serine, which is formed from 3-phosphoglycerate, is the precursor of both glycine and cysteine. Proline is formed from glutamate in a three-step cyclization reaction. All these syntheses are regulated allosterically, in that the committed (i.e. irreversible) step is inhibited by the *final* product.

Table 3.2 The twenty amino acids most commonly found in proteins

Synthesized in the human body	*Essential to the diet*
Alanine	Histidine
Arginine[a]	Isoleucine
Asparagine	Leucine
Aspartic acid	Lysine
Cysteine[b]	Methionine
Glutamic acid	Phenylalanine
Glutamine	Threonine
Glycine	Tryptophan
Proline	Valine
Serine	
Tyrosine[c]	

[a] The human body learns how to synthesize arginine in early childhood, but it is an 'essential' amino acid for infants.
[b] The human body synthesizes most of its requirements of cysteine from serine, but can also make it from methionine.
[c] Tyrosine, made in the human body by hydroxylating phenylalanine, cannot be formed if the latter is absent from the diet.

Proteins are synthesized on ribosomes (Fig. 3.1) in all cells. Each amino acid acylates its specific transfer ribonucleic acid (tRNA) by esterifying the 3'-hydroxyl group of the ribose moiety. This complex moves to the ribosome where it is incorporated into the growing polypeptide chain. Following the sequence: *initiation, elongation* and *termination*, the addition of amino acids to the carboxyl end of the growing peptide chain is governed by the messenger ribonucleic acid (mRNA) that has been coded (by DNA) to make the protein of the moment. As with all the other biosyntheses described in Section 3.2, a heavy consumption of ATP-stored energy is required.

Amino acids are precursors of many other kinds of biologically-active molecules. Porphyrins, such as haemoglobin and the cytochromes, are biosynthesized from glycine and succinyl CoA. The neurotransmitters, norepinephrine (noradrenaline) and dopamine, and the hormones, epinephrine (adrenaline) and thyroxine, are derived from tyrosine. Many other neurotransmitters and hormones are straightforward polypeptides.

The liver converts amino acids into the purine and pyrimidine bases of nucleic acids. The pyrimidine ring is assembled from carbamoylaspartate, carbon dioxide and ammonia, then converted to the nucleotide by 5-phosphoribosyl 1-pyrophosphate (PRPP) which is a derivative of *3.20*. Purine biosynthesis, on the other hand, starts with PRPP on whose framework the structure of hypoxanthine (purin-6-one) is built up, stepwise, from glutamate, glycine and aspartate. The deoxyribonucleotides are derived by oxidation of ribonucleotides.

Further reading

Principles of Biochemistry (Lehninger, 1982)
Biochemistry (Stryer, 1981)
Biochemistry: A Functional Approach (McGilvery and Goldstein, 1983)
Human Nutrition and Dietetics (Davidson and Passmore, 1986)
McCance and Widdowson's 'The Composition of Foods' (Paul and Southgate, 1978).

Follow-up

Using a standard biochemistry text, make a list of enzymes concerned in the metabolism of carbohydrates, starting perhaps something like this:

Hexokinase

$$\text{Glucose} + \text{ATP} \rightarrow \text{glucose 6-phosphate} + \text{ADP}$$

Phosphoglucose isomerase

Glucose 6-phosphate $\rightleftharpoons$ fructose 6-phosphate

Phosphofructokinase

Fructose 6-phosphate + ATP $\rightarrow$ Fructose 1,6-diphosphate + ADP

Fructose 1,6-diphosphatase

Fructose 1,6-diphosphate + $H_2O \rightarrow$ fructose 6-phosphate + P_i

4

Hidden dangers in
wholesome foods

Most of us believe that we know instinctively what foods are best for us, and that we shall continue to eat them enjoyably and healthily unless prevented by poverty or disaster. On the other hand, nutritionists report that a person's eating habits are acquired early in life and that they persist as a pattern characteristic of his national and social group with its fixed attitudes, traditions, prejudices and even taboos! What's more, this was found to be just as true for prosperous urban communities as for poorer agricultural ones.

Without attempting to reconcile this difference of opinion let us ask: 'Can a population be encouraged to think afresh about food, to use it in ways that will promote and maintain health?' The soundest help in this issue is to be had not from the daily papers, or brightly illustrated periodicals, but from Government publications such as the booklet *Recommended Dietary Allowances* in which the US National Research Council's Food and Nutrition Board states its aim as: 'The maintenance of good nutrition in healthy people' (NRC, 1980). This publication, which first appeared in 1943, is revised at intervals. Its compilers have adopted the World Health Organization's definition of health as 'A state of complete physical, mental and social well-being and not merely the absence of disease or infirmity'. Similar activities go on in other countries. For example, the annual reports of the British National Food Survey compare the diets of different sections of the UK population against the intakes recommended by the Department of Health and Social Security, as published in 1969. Of wider interest is the international *Handbook on Human Nutritional Requirements* (Passmore, *et al.*, 1974), compiled for the World Health Organization (WHO) and the Food and Agricultural Organization (FAO).

Admittedly such official guidance can only be general and needs modification for local conditions and for individual variability. Despite these limitations the official recommendations have proved useful in at least three ways:

1. They help a government to devise a basis for its national food policy. For example, they can define the essential food requirements of that needy fraction of the population whose meagre diet, even in affluent countries, is supplemented by public assistance;
2. They help a government to plan adequate diets for its armed forces, schools and other institutions;
3. They offer guidance to a small, but growing, fraction of the population who feel concern about traditional, carefree eating customs.

To make valid recommendations for food intake, the planners need to know the daily energy output of people in various occupations. Some well-accepted values for those whose daily work is not highly energy-demanding are set out in the upper part of Table 4.1. These figures refer to the range 20–30°C (much more energy is expended at other temperatures) and a 10% reduction is made for those over 50. Adjustments are made for those doing heavier work, e.g. 12 600 for building workers, 13 700 for steel workers, 14 400 for farmers and 15 400 each for coal miners and forestry workers (all in kJ/day). Other adjustments are made for children and mothers.

Both WHO and NRC recommend minimal daily protein intakes for men and women from infancy to adulthood. Thus for the average man of 65–70 kg, WHO recommends 37 g and NRC (always more generous) specifies 56 g. These authorities also recommend a minimal daily food energy to be met with food of the eater's choice; the NRC advises that fat should contribute no more than 35% to the dietary energy. There are also specifications for minimal amounts of various fat-soluble and water-soluble vitamins and the inorganic constituents of food.

These recommendations form part of worldwide attempts to use food more wisely. However, it is when food is used *un*wisely, we become more conscious of its essentially foreign character. With this correlation in mind, the present chapter has been constituted as follows. Section 4.1 is concerned mainly with overeating, a tendency which as early as the sixteenth century was seen as conversion of food into poison (p. 1). Section 4.2 deals with the injurious effects of unbalanced diets whether due to unreasonable enthusiasm for one single item of food, or to undernutrition because starving people have restricted choices. Section 4.3, emphasizing the large number of chemical entities naturally present in every food, notes that many of these are potential poisons whose safe dose can unknowingly be exceeded by the diner. Section 5.1 will record how, through an inborn idiosyncrasy, one man's meat can be another's poison. Section 5.2 will discuss spices and flavours (including sweeteners) as well as other much-used additives including those 'enhancers of mood': sugar, caffeine and ethanol.

Table 4.1 Estimate of minimal daily energy expended by men and women in light and heavy occupations

Activity	Hours	Man 70 kg Rate (kJ/hour)	Total kJ	Woman 58 kg Rate (kJ/hour)	Total kJ
Resting	8	284	2270	230	1850
Very light Usual seated and standing activities; sewing; ironing, painting trades; truck driving; typing; laboratory work.	12	455	5460	315	3780
Light Walking; garage work; carpentry; restaurant trades; laundering; shopping; sailing; golf.	3	840	2520	630	1890
Moderate Fast walking; weeding; plastering; loading; scrubbing floors; heavy shopping; cycling; tennis; dancing.	1	1260	1260	1010	1010
Heavy Tree felling; pick & shovel labouring; swimming; football; basketball	0	1890 to 3020	0	1510 to 2520	0
TOTAL	24	11 510 (2740 kcal)		8530 (2030 kcal)	

(Recalculated from Durnin and Passmore, 1967)

4.1 Quantitative malnutrition (overeating and undereating)

It has been noted that, when food is abundantly available and no bar exists to its consumption, there is a tendency to eat more than is compatible with good health. On the other hand, when supplies are insufficient or purchasing power is low, not enough is eaten to allow the body to fight fatigue and illness. The first of these two observations, which has some broad implications, is treated as 'overeating'. The second observation, no less important for human welfare but less germane to the subject of this book, is dealt with more briefly as 'undereating'.

Overeating

Before discussing such dangers as may exist for those who partake of good, wholesome food too liberally, it must be said that each of the three main food constituents (carbohydrates, lipids and proteins) is known to be harmful when consumed, separately, in excess (Section 4.2). Here we are concerned with what happens when all three food types are eaten in excess together, a practice which eminent health authorities state is life-shortening.

What constitutes normal life-expectancy, that is to say, the number of years available to a person between birth and death? The Old Testament in depicting this as 'threescore years and ten' (Psalms: 90-10) paints a gloomy picture of any attempted extension. Yet some humans have lived, in reasonably good health, to about 115 years, although they may have come from stock genetically favourable to longevity. In the USA average life expectancy at birth is 71 years for males and 78 years for females (Taeuber, 1983). In 1900 only a quarter of the US population survived 65 years whereas 70% now achieve at least that age. Moreover the proportion aged 80 or over has now reached 30% and is still rising (Brody, 1984). Similar trends are reported for other industrialized countries. Thus in England and Wales the expectation of life (male, at birth) was only 44 years in 1900, but had become 71 by 1983 and those aged 60 can expect to live to 77 (English Life Tables; WHO Yearbook). Citizens of Norway and Sweden add another 3 years to these figures.

Of course mere extension of life is not a worthwhile goal unless *the quality of life* is maintained in old age. Conditions that become more prevalent with ageing are: acute and chronic heart disease, cancer, blindness, deafness, diabetes, hip fracture and Alzheimer's syndrome (related to senile dementia) (Brody, 1985).

Unpleasantly as these maladies afflict those in the autumn of their lives, such illnesses incapacitate obese people much earlier. Here *obesity* is defined as the accumulation of excess triglycerides (fat). *Excess* is defined as what actuarial analysis has found to be associated with increased mortality. Thus a man is considered obese if more than 20% of his body weight consists of fat (for a woman, 30%). Women are most likely to gain extra lipid at three stages in their lives: at adolescence, after pregnancy and at the menopause. Body fat is usually measured with skinfold-calipers which pinch the fat against the restoring force of a calibrated spring. Tables convert caliper measurements to (an estimate of) the proportion of fat in the total body weight (Davidson and Passmore, 1986).

Obesity is uncommon in developing countries and common in industrialized countries. But here lies a paradox: in the latter, it is most common among the lower income groups (Macleod, 1984). Obesity can arise only when the intake of food exceeds normal physiological needs. Just how subtle its onset may be is indicated by the following. If healthy people eat one extra slice of bread a day they will probably store 200 kJ (48 kcal) of extra energy as triglycerides. After 10 years if they have maintained this habit and exercised but little, they should be burdened with 20 kg of excess lipid. Yet they could have been spared this undesirable loading by just 20 minutes of fast walking each day (Macleod, 1984; Lehninger, 1982, p. 762).

A significant proportion of fat people do not eat more than those whose weight remains normal. Yet, because these persons continue to put on weight, they really *are* overeating (Harrison, 1983). It is generally agreed that almost all obese folk are physically less active than normal people. It is hard to decide how much slowing down is the *cause*, and how much the *effect*, of their increased weight.

Apart from the burden, physical and psychological, of carrying so much extra triglyceride, the obese suffer from the principal diseases of old age several decades too soon, as follows. Some of them experience osteoarthritis of the hip arising from the extra weight carried. Gall stones and diabetes mellitus (of the mature-onset type) are much commoner in the obese than in normal people of the same age. This is also true for elevated blood-pressure which often leads to an incapacitating stroke. Such hypertension plus the extra work needed to propel an overweight body, may contribute to coronary heart disease. This ischaemia (obstruction) may start with a painful, chronic angina pectoris, or else suddenly fulminate as a myocardial infarction (occlusion) from which about 40% of those affected die within the first month. In sum, subjects who are 30% overweight incur about 30% increase in mortality, a figure which rises to 50% for those who are 40% in excess (Macleod, 1984).

The physiological and psychological factors that cause and reinforce over-eating are being vigorously investigated; so far, no fundamental principle has emerged though there have been many minor clues. Evidently, the complexities of appetite regulation are enough to make it unlikely that any single medication could produce and maintain a loss of weight, safely and pleasantly. The following factors regulate our food intake: (a) the pleasurable appeal of delicious foods as conveyed to us by our olfactory, visual, and gustatory signals, (b) the several kinds of neural and hormonal signals that arise in the gastrointestinal tract, (c) the messages relayed by food undergoing digestion, and (d) many relayed, centrally-originating messages about energy levels and the state of the stores of specific nutrients. Superimposed on these physical factors are the, often powerful, psychological urges and inhibitions that vary so greatly from person to person.

The following hormones and neurotransmitters play a role in the central regulation of appetite in the rat: β-endorphin, and norepinephrine, which seem to oppose one another but are, in turn, influenced by neuropeptide-Y, gamma-aminobutyric acid, serotonin, dopamine, dynorphin, corticotrophic-releasing factor and the calcitonin gene-related peptide. This network of influences receives peripherally-originating messages from glucagon, somatostatin, bombesin, calcitonin, cholecystokinin and some prostanoids (Morley and Levine, 1985). This is, indeed, a complex network of influences!

(*a*) *Treatment for obesity*. All who advise on obesity agree that what helps the patient most is for him to want, deeply and sincerely, to lose weight and to maintain that loss. This is because the necessarily long treatment quickly

becomes irksome to most patients. Even at the start, many of them are astonished
to learn that there is no such thing as a safe reducing pill, nor is there any known
'reducing food'. Even the anorectics (appetite-suppressing drugs) such as
dextramphetamine (the dextra isomer of *7.24*) and fenfluramine (*8.15*), act only
at the *start* of a course. Hence the need to 'eat defensively'!

The most effective treatment consists of a diet that yields only 4200 kJ
(1000 kcal) a day, consumed in only *two* daily meals. To be effective, this must be
combined with exercise, e.g. an hour's walk at 3 miles (5 km) an hour. The diet
should include adequate protein, lipid and carbohydrate. If ethanol is taken by
the patient, its energy contribution has to be subtracted from this diet. Patients
derive much help from psychological reinforcement therapy, and by belonging
to a group of fellow sufferers, such as *Weight Watchers*; these measures make the
physical treatment more interesting and bearable. For the few, often desperate,
patients whose condition does not respond to these measures, partial starvation
in hospital is considered preferable to surgery which, while often effective, carries
some risk (Macleod, 1984). Feeding patients bulky, non-nutritious material such
as methyl cellulose, has not so far proved very effective.

(*b*) *Some wider aspects of overeating.* Many industrialized countries instruct their
Department of Health to cooperate with other medical organizations in laying
down *guidelines* for the diet of the general population. These are in part aimed at
caring for disadvantaged groups, but are also concerned to reduce incidence of
coronary heart disease. Examples are: Australia (1984), Canadian Department
of National Health and Welfare (1977), Norway (1975), Swedish National Food
Administration (1981), United Kingdom (1984) and the US National Research
Council's Food and Nutrition Board (NRC, 1980). In general their recommendations are for adults to take less animal fat in the diet, to reduce the consumption
of sodium chloride and ethanol, to monitor low-density lipoprotein-cholesterol,
and to increase consumption of fruits, vegetables and cereals. These lipid
restrictions are given on p. 50.

Cancer is another pathological condition which seems to be linked to what we
eat. Epidemiologists suggest that as much as 90% of all cases of cancer may be
related to the environment (rather than to genetics, or ageing), and that about
one half of these cases are diet-related. Studies on cancer in laboratory animals
confirm the importance of diet; also substances suspected of being carcinogenic
(cancer-causing) in humans usually increase the rate of cancer occurrence in rats
and mice. However it is hard to establish such relationships in human beings
because of the difficulty of finding acceptable controls, and also because of our
much greater lifespan. At least, studies on migrants have shown significant
changes in cancer sites, incidence and mortality after adaptation to the new local
dietary pattern (Higginson and Muir, 1979; Wynder and Gori, 1977). Comparison of religious groups that have dietary restrictions has also helped.

The US National Research Council (NRC, 1982), in its report *Diet, Nutrition,
and Cancer*, found that the most apparently carcinogenic features of the nation's

diet were (a) a high fat intake, and (b) frequent consumption of salt-cured, salt-pickled or smoked foods (p. 70). They noted too that *reduction of total food intake* in laboratory animals protected them against acquiring cancer. Also, on the helpful side, they observed a lesser incidence of cancer among those who ate little fat but much fruit and vegetables. High protein diets and foods rich in cholesterol appeared to be carcinogenic.

Of the vitamins only vitamin A (or its precursor, carotene) seemed to reduce the cancer risk, and of the minerals only selenium seemed to be anti-carcinogenic. No food additive seemed to contribute significantly to the risk of human cancer. Moreover environmental contaminants, in spite of a persistently bad press, made no appreciable contribution to the risk of cancer in human beings. In similar statements on nutrition and cancer, the National Cancer Institute (US) (1979) and the American Cancer Society (1982) concurred with the above, except that they recommended increased consumption of dietary fibres. All three organizations call for reduction in the intake of ethanol, which is a suspected cause of liver cancer (usually fatal) and is linked also to oesophageal cancer. Other links between diet and cancer can be found in Sections 4.3 and 13.1.

Undereating

Gorging, so often observed when food is plentiful, does not extend uniformly through the animal kingdom. Washburn (1968) records how mice that breed in the great grain depots of Canada at first live and feed in this great wealth of food but migrate away from it into the unknown as soon as a colony of about 20 has built up.

This restraint is a far cry from *enforced undernutrition* in man, brought on by such misfortunes as: (a) severe disease of the gastrointestinal tract, and sometimes the operations carried out to correct this, (b) metabolic failure arising from hepatic or renal impairment, (c) wartime shortages, particularly in prisoner of war camps (Smith and Woodruff, 1951; Helweg *et al.*, 1952), (d) famine precipitated by natural disasters (earthquakes, flood, drought) and (e) sheer poverty.

Undernutrition is usually defined as a state where the body weight is less than 75% of normal. At first the loss of weight is rapid but it tends to stabilize as the body makes a series of adaptations. All organs, but especially the heart, become smaller and severe atrophy of the small intestine sets in. The afflicted person becomes weak and shows physical and mental apathy up to the point of death. It has been found that starvation is best treated with small, frequent feeds of milk or other easily digested food; the main problem is more administrative than medical (Davidson and Passmore 1986, p. 559).

It is generally agreed that undernutrition is the severest medical problem of developing countries. In 1945, the United Nations set up its Food and Agricultural Organization (FAO) with the comment that at least two-thirds of the World's people were ill-nourished, then, in 1948, in its Universal Declaration of Human Rights, the UN gave special prominence to good nutrition. The FAO operates through exhortation and education, policies which it implements through the governments of the affected countries. In 1948, the United Nations also established the World Health Organization (WHO), and the first of regular FAO/WHO collaborations started in 1949. This joint effort has financed many students from developing countries to study abroad for long periods; it has also sent many consultants and specialists to assist in the nutritional programmes being established by these countries.

Undernutrition in children, a still more serious problem, is measured by their failure to attain normal weight. In the developing countries, a high proportion of children under 5 suffer from protein-energy malnutrition (PEM). Of this condition there are two types. In marasmus (wasting disease) the PEM is part of a *total* food deficiency. Marasmus usually follows weaning when this has been too early or sudden. It affects mainly infants under one year whose mothers were obliged to return to the workforce without them, a situation commoner in cities than in the country. Marasmus is characterized by extreme wasting. Even when the infant is finally hospitalized and given the best of nutritional care, mortality is about 20%. For kwashiorkor, where the principal deficiency is protein only, p. 56, PEM-afflicted children are cared for by the United Nations Children's Fund (UNICEF, founded in 1946) which sends trained nurses, medicines, and food in response to matching funds from the requesting country. Thanks to UNICEF's low-cost health programmes, child mortality has been halved in the Third World since 1950, but 14 million children are still dying of malnutrition each year (UNICEF, 1987).

The severe famine that affected African countries in 1985 was monitored by the UN Office for Emergency Operations who reported that some 30 to 35 million people, at risk of dying, were saved by a massive international relief operation. This partial victory left 91 million (in Angola, Botswana, Cabo Verde, Ethiopia, Lesotho, Mozambique and Sudan) in urgent need of further help, whereas rains eventually provided harvests to Burundi, Rwanda, Senegal, and Somalia.

Progress in the scientific understanding of the pathology of starvation owes much to the help of healthy volunteers, such as the group of 32 young men who tried to live for six months on a 7700 kJ (1600 kcal) daily diet (Keys, *et al.*, 1950).

Meagre eating. When food is plentiful at mealtimes most people tend to eat until appetite has disappeared. Yet there are some diners whose intake is governed by a different maxim, such as 'Always rise from the table feeling hungry', or 'Stop eating while the pleasure of food is at its height'. These are the meagre eaters, and their numbers appear to be growing. What motivates their conduct? Are they guided by some rule instilled in childhood? or from ethical precepts? or from a logical conviction based on nutritional studies? At least we know that restriction of food intake diminishes the incidence of cancer in laboratory animals (NRC, 1982). Too much food, like too little, is detrimental to life expectancy in the rat. Wistar rats achieved maximal survival (936 days) on a daily food intake of 14 g, whereas those who ate 20 g had a mean survival of only 728 days (Everitt, Porter and Wyndham, 1982); similar results were reported by McCay, Sperling and Barnes (1943), and Masoro, et al. (1980).

It was found that undernutrition, enforced by blockade of food supplies in the Second World War, reduced incidence of cardiovascular disease (Strøm and Jensen, 1951). A similar observation has been made on prisoners (Walker, et al., 1961). We do not yet know whether meagre eaters are the healthiest and most active members of the affluent community, but we can be sure of one thing: they need a strong will!

Meagre eating is not to be confused with anorexia nervosa, a psycho-pathological condition, most often evidenced by young women from comfortable homes, who reduce their food intake until they become dangerously ill and wasted (Harrison, 1983).

Further reading

On overeating:
Energy Balance and Obesity in Man (Garrow, 1978)
Handbook on Human Nutritional Requirements (Passmore, et al., 1974)
On undereating:
Handbook on Human Nutritional Requirements (Passmore, et al., 1974)
Protein Energy Malnutrition (Alleyne, et al., 1977)
Famine (The Swedish Nutrition Foundation, 1971)
Famine in India, an Historical Survey (Passmore, 1951)
World Mortality (Lancaster, 1987)
On effect of nutrition on ageing:
Masoro, 1985 and Schneider and Reed, 1985 (reviews).

Follow-up

Ask a few people about the fashion-diets (dietary vogues or trends) that they have witnessed in their lifetimes, such as the Hay Diet, the Grapefruit Diet, the Pritikin Diet). How do these trends differ from expert advice, as indicated on p. 37.

4.2 Qualitative malnutrition (unbalanced diets)

We have just noted how eating an excess of food, no matter how wholesome and delicious, can injure the human body (Section 4.1). We now pass on to those cases where injury arises not from a total excess of food but from a relative excess of one component thus leading to an unbalanced diet.

Studies on laboratory animals

In his pioneering work, E. M. Boyd showed that each principal constituent of a human meal, if administered in sufficient amount, was lethal to laboratory animals (Boyd, 1973). These constituents were carbohydrates, lipids, proteins, water and salts. His procedure was to fast the animals overnight and the next day to feed the animals (usually albino rats) with the test material in liquid form, by gavage, i.e. by intragastric cannula (stomach tube). The results were reported in terms of LD_{50} (p. 231), namely the amount required to kill half of a statistically significant number of animals.

Water. Our discussion can conveniently begin with water; although no one would claim that it is foreign to the human body it is undoubtedly toxic in excess. Boyd found that distilled water, given to albino rats at the rate of 70 ml/kg every 20 minutes, had a LD_{50} of 470 ml/kg. Most of the animals died in coma within 2.5 hours, first exhibiting weakness, ataxia, polyuria, diarrhoea and muscular tremors. This lethal volume of water, nearly half the animal's weight, had overcome normal mechanisms for control of sodium chloride and water. The inevitably continuous diuresis eliminated more and more sodium chloride, thus preventing conduction in nerves. Water proved not to be a chronic poison: a daily dose of 20 ml/kg produced only minor and reversible toxicity after 100 days, although 120 ml/kg inhibited growth and caused dehydration of many body organs.

Healthy human beings can drink huge volumes of water which they quickly eliminate without harm. Not so for patients with acute or chronic renal disease, severe heart impairment, hepatic cirrhosis or defects of the pituitary, suprarenal or thyroid glands. Also at risk are patients who have just undergone major surgery – a procedure that liberates the pituitary's antidiuretic hormone. In such cases, even a modest intake of water produces disordered cerebral function, mental confusion and dizziness. A more severe degree of water intoxication produces convulsions, coma and death (Macleod, 1984).

Glucose. Glucose was found by Boyd to have a LD_{50} of 25.8 g/kg when dissolved in water and fed by gavage to fasted albino rats. The hypertonic nature of the solution attracted water into the gastrointestinal tract where it produced enteritis, diarrhoea and dehydration of remote organs. In addition the absorbed glucose caused stimulation (convulsions) followed by depression (hypothermic stupor) of the central nervous system. Death usually took place within 5 hours, but three times as much glucose could be tolerated when it was mixed with the diet and eaten over 24 hours.

Sucrose. Sucrose was less toxic than glucose. The LD_{50} for female rats was 27.9 g/kg, for which the human equivalent would be a child of 10 kg (22 lb) eating (and retaining) 225 g (half a pound) of candy. The rats died between 9 and 48 hours with symptoms similar to those seen with glucose. When Boyd abruptly withdrew sucrose after 100 days, in a chronic toxicity test, no withdrawal symptoms were found.

Starch. Starch was completely non-toxic (Boyd, 1973).

Vegetable oils. It was found impracticable to give doses in excess of 75 g/kg because these promptly flowed out through the anus. The cumulative LD_{50} of corn oil, given by gavage over 5 days, was 256 g/kg. Death was by respiratory failure after deep coma. Cottonseed oil gave an almost identical result (Boyd, 1973).

Proteins. Casein had an oral LD_{50} of abour 1200 g/kg when administered over 2 to 3 weeks. This spread of dose was necessitated by the physical nature of the aqueous suspension, which tended to set solid. Egg albumin behaved more dramatically: the LD_{50} was found to be 100.7 g/kg, and death occurred in about 4 hours. Those who survived recovered completely in 3 weeks. Boyd (1973) concluded that the toxic effect was mainly osmotic in origin, as with glucose and sodium chloride.

Studies on man

The remainder of this section will consider unbalanced diets as they affect man, starting with excesses and concluding with some deficiencies.

(a) Imbalance through excess of one dietary component

Carbohydrates. In many parts of the World, carbohydrates supply the main source of energy. Provided that minimal requirements of protein are present (p. 36) no adverse effects have been found.

In recent years, there has been some concern about the high proportion of carbohydrate that is, in the more prosperous nations, consumed as sucrose (synonyms: table sugar, cane sugar, beet sugar). A steep increase in the consumption of sucrose took place in the second half of the nineteenth century, then levelled off, and now seems to be declining as manufacturers use more corn syrup (glucose and dextrins) in its place.

No demonstrable hazard from the moderate consumption of sugar, other than dental caries, has been demonstrated (Federation of American Societies for Experimental Biology, 1976). In particuar, no correlation could be found with coronary heart disease, cancer or diabetes (see Davidson and Passmore, 1986). Concerning caries, the principal offenders are sticky caramels and toffees which lodge between the teeth long enough to allow resident bacteria (especially *Streptococcus mutans*) to produce that degree of acidity (pH 5) at which tooth decay starts. However sucrose eaten *with meals* is not cariogenic (Gustafssen, *et al.*, 1954).

Most dietary surveys recommend that starchy foods (e.g. bread, potato, rice) should replace part of the customarily eaten sucrose, because the latter, so highly purified, brings with it neither vitamins nor minerals. For more on sucrose see Section 5.3.

Lipids. We have seen (Section 4.1) that indiscriminate eating (i.e. of carbohydrates, lipids and proteins all together) can lead to obesity, at least in susceptible people. This state is likely to be reached sooner if the overeating was concentrated on *lipids* because these have twice the calorific value of either protein or carbohydrate (p. 8). In addition, there are strong indications that a diet rich in lipids favours development of coronary heart disease (p. 41). If true, this is a serious matter because myocardial infarction, the severest form of coronary disease, is a principal cause of death in most of the industrialized countries. To keep a fair balance, we must note that several other factors have been correlated with a tendency to coronary disease – notably physical inactivity, genetic predisposition, smoking, hypertension, diabetes and obesity – several of which seem linked to a diet rich in lipids. A sensible prophylactic measure for young people, 20–30 years of age, would be to take a test for hyperlipidaemia, particularly if they have a family history of early ischaemic heart disease.

The Japanese have comparatively few heart attacks compared to Britons or Americans. In the USA, about 40% of the daily calories have been consumed as fats, in Japan only about 14%. However, Japanese who have migrated to America and switched to the US food-eating pattern, suffer heart attacks as frequently as Americans. It seems relevant that experimental animals (about 30 species, including monkeys) develop blocked arteries when fed on a diet high in triglycerides (Lewis, 1976).

Although the role of a high triglyceride (fat) diet in *directly* promoting heart disease is not completely established, it has been shown that synthesized palmitic acid triglycerides raise the blood level of cholesterol more than those of any other common fatty acid do; oleic acid (in these experiments) did not influence cholesterol formation, and linoleic acid actually decreased it (McGandy, Hegsted and Myers, 1970). Table 4.2 lists the aliphatic acid composition of some commonly eaten fats and oils.

There is general agreement that a high level of cholesterol (*3.32*) in the blood is a direct risk factor in coronary disease. This was concluded from a randomized, double-blind study of 3806 middle-aged men, all healthy but at risk of coronary heart disease because of a high LDL (low-density lipoprotein rich in chlolesterol) blood level, which was conducted by the Lipid Research Clinic's Coronary Primary Prevention Trial (National Heart, Lung and Blood Institute, 1984). This study showed conclusively that lowering the LDL level diminished the incidence of myocardial infarction and there was a 24% reduction in deaths compared to the controls. LDL levels were best reduced by giving cholestyramine resin orally (24 g/day). Each particle of LDL, which carries the larger part of the blood's cholesterol, contains about 1500 molecules of cholesteryl linoleate within a thin shell of a specific protein. The function of these particles is to ferry cholesterol from the liver to other parts of the body where specific receptor-proteins are provided to anchor and unload this sterol (Harrison, 1983, pp. 475, 549). A high LDL blood level is thought to arise from lack of normal docking facilities (Brown, Kovanen and Goldstein, 1981).

Cholesterol is essential for the formation and maintenance of cell membranes, particularly in the central nervous system, and it is the indispensable precursor of bile salts and the whole family of steroid hormones. If the diet fails to furnish the body's requirements of cholesterol it is promptly biosynthesized (p. 34).

The pathological effects of cholesterol begin when it is deposited in blood vessels, particularly the coronary and cerebral arteries, which it lines with a

Table 4.2 The percentage composition of fatty acids in natural triglycerides (fats and oils).

Triglycerides	Saturated C_{16}	C_{18}	Unsaturated (mono-)	(poly-)	Other constituents
Beef fat (dripping)	27	13	48	4	8
Beef kidney fat (suet)	28	**27**	37	1	7
Pork fat (lard)	27	16	44	10	3
Butter	26	11	32	3	28[a]
Margarine					
vegetable	24	5	44	23	4
animal plus vegetable	16	5	47	20	12
Olive oil	12	2	73	12	1
Palm oil	42	4	43	8	3
Peanut oil	11	3	50	30	6
Corn (maize) oil	14	2	31	52	1
Cottonseed oil	23	2	22	50	3
Soya bean oil	10	4	25	59	2
Sunflowerseed oil	6	6	33	52	3
Triglycerides expressed from the flesh of:					
Beef	27	13	49	4	7
Lamb	24	**21**	41	5	**9**
Pork	27	14	47	8	4
Boiled ham	26	12	49	10	3
Chicken	27	7	47	15	9
White fish (whiting)	13	4	40	36[b]	7
Fatty fish (herring)	14	1	56	20[c]	9

[a] Butyric (3%), hexanoic (2%), decanoic (3%), dodecanoic (4%), and myristic (C_{14}) (11%);
[b] The main polyunsaturated acids are C_{20} with 4 and 5 double bonds;
[c] The main polyunsaturated acid is C_{22} with 6 double bonds.
(Figures in bold print should serve as a dietary warning.)
(From Paul and Southgate, 1978. Geographical variations are to be expected, depending on what the different animals have been fed).

plaque that becomes hardened through calcification. Flakes, detached from these plaques, tend to block the vessels by thrombosis, an event with grave consequences. We have already noted such infarcts in the heart. When vessels in the brain are similarly affected, a stroke (cerebral infarct) becomes manifest through paralysis of a limb, or loss of speech, or complete disorientation. About 30% of such patients die in the first month. When the stroke is accompanied by severe cerebral haemorrhage, the mortality rises to 80% (Matthews and Miller, 1979).

Fifteen years ago the average adult in the USA ate about 140 g of triglycerides and about 0.5 g of cholesterol each day. His meat-derived triglycerides contained nearly as much saturated (palmitic and stearic) fatty acids as unsaturated acids (oleic and linoleic). However since 1970, as the result of medical publicity, the incidence of coronary disease in the USA has fallen by one third. This result is attributed to a lowered consumption of fat-rich foods as well as the habit of taking more exercise and having blood-pressure monitored. Much less cholesterol-containing food is now eaten. Healthy young adults, who have switched from the old diet to one with a higher ratio of unsaturated triglycerides (Table 4.2), have achieved a lower LDL level in two weeks. Dietary cholesterol is highest in egg yolks and brains, and moderately high in thick cream, butter, kidneys and liver.

The National Research Council's *Recommended Dietary Allowances* (NRC, 1980) offers the following guidelines for individuals who have been overconsuming lipids. Reduce the total fat intake until it supplies no more than 35% of the dietary energy, to which polyunsaturated triglycerides should not contribute more than 10%. (There is some evidence that polyunsaturared triglycerides are harmful in excess.). Similar dietary recommendations have been made by the Royal College of Physicians, in London (1976) and by the American Heart Association (Glueck, *et al.*, 1978).

That genetic factors may help control hyperlipidaemia is suggested by the fact that many people habitually eat meals rich in fats and cholesterol without normal LDL levels being exceeded.

Intolerance to lipids is seen in the diseases steatorrhoea and sprue. The best tolerated lipids are those with some fatty acids of low molecular weight, as in butter, and the worst tolerated are those rich in stearic acid (Table 4.2).

Proteins. The American physiologist Chittenden (1909) kept himself, and several other adult males, in excellent physical and mental health on as little as 40 g of protein daily. At the other extreme of protein intake, many communities throughout the world (including the Australian stockriders) maintain excellent physique and stamina on diets containing as much as 300 g of protein a day.

A diet based largely on protein is safe only if the protein is of high nutritional quality (p. 56, Table 4.3) and the mineral intake adequate. Experimental magnesium deficiency in rats is produced quite simply by feeding a high protein diet (Bois, 1963). This lack in turn produces potassium deficiency in the rat's heart and cardiac myopathy results (Susin and Herson, 1967). In 1978 about 300 cases of illness (including 60 deaths) among young, weight-conscious women were traced to their living entirely on protein slimming solutions. This fad-diet was composed of hydrolysed collagen (gelatin). The 'crash-course' was indeed a severe one, for the participants were receiving only 300 kcal of daily energy intake, including a little carbohydrate but no lipid. They suffered myocardial degeneration; those who died did so from cardiac arrhythmia (Food and Drug Administration, 1978; Van Itallie, 1978; Bistrian, 1978; Anon. 1977).

Vitamins. The commercial extraction of vitamins, which began in the 1920s, greatly advanced a newly-evolving biochemical approach to nutrition and medicine (p. 105). Later, when the price of vitamin preparations fell because of their mass consumption, some untoward effects of overdosage began to appear. The worst offenders remain the oil-soluble vitamins A and D, which accumulate in the human body. It is now better realized that vitamins are powerfully-acting biochemicals, large excess of which must be avoided.

What constitute normal intakes of vitamins can be gleaned from the World Health Organization's *Handbook on Human Nutritional Requirements* (Passmore, *et al.*, 1974). This publication covers vitamins A and D, thiamin, riboflavin, niacin, folate, ascorbic acid and vitamin B_{12}. Suitable daily intakes are suggested for these groups: infants, children of different ages, adults, pregnant or lactating women and the aged. It is intended that the recommended allowances should be consumed in thoughtfully-chosen food rather than from pharmaceutical preparations. Alternatively, one may consult the US National Research Council's *Recommended Dietary Allowances* (NRC, 1980) which we shall refer to as *RDA*. These suggestions are on the whole more generous than those of the WHO, and cover the following extra vitamins: vitamins E and K, biotin and B_6. RDA insists that these recommended intakes should not be exceeded unless under medical supervision.

Acute toxicity has often been reported in infants given vitamin A as 25–100 mg of retinol (75 000 to 300 000 International Units). The RDA dose for infants is only 0.4 mg. About 12 hours after ingesting the overdose, infants usually become highly irritable and vomit. Smaller, chronic overdosing of infants produces enlargement of spleen and liver, bleeding lips, and peeling skin (Oliver, 1958). Adults have developed similar symptoms after taking as little as 3 mg daily for two years. Polar explorers, after a meal of polar bear's liver, which is rich in vitamin A, suffered vomiting and peeling of the entire skin of the body. For further reading on vitamin A toxicity see Mandel and Cohn (1985).

Overdosage with vitamin D has resulted in many deaths (Federation of American Societies for Experimental Biology, 1978; Chinn, 1979). The RDA for an adult is 5 μg (200 IU); continued ingestion of 1 mg daily has usually caused poisoning. This takes the form of hypercalcaemia, with fatigue, nausea and vomiting. Kidney symptoms set in quite early as calcium salts become deposited there (Davies, 1960). In children such hypercalcaemia often arrests growth and the deficit in height is seldom correctable (Parfitt, 1972). (For further reading on the toxicity of this, the most toxic of all vitamins see Haynes and Murad, 1985.)

Compared to vitamins A and D, vitamin E is relatively non-toxic. However larger doses of α-tocopherol (the main form of this vitamin) render anaemic children unresponsive to iron therapy (Melhorn and Gross, 1969). It is recommended that adults should not take large doses over a long period (NRC, 1980).

Haemolytic anaemia and other toxic symptoms followed administration of 5–10 mg of vitamin K daily to infants, and deaths are recorded for premature infants given 30 mg a day. Menadione, which lacks the side-chain in the 3-position is the most toxic form of this vitamin, but the only one that is active when bile-secretion is absent (American Academy of Pediatrics, 1981; Finkel, 1961).

As a class water-soluble vitamins are less toxic than vitamins A and D, because they are not so strongly accumulated in the body. The ready availability of such powerful but seemingly harmless chemicals ushered in the concept of orthomolecular therapy, defined as 'The provision of optimum concentrations of substances normally present in the human body' (Pauling, 1968), an incontestably worthy aim. One application of this idea has been to give unphysiologically high doses of water-soluble vitamins (also of vitamin A) to treat schizophrenia, cancer, arthritis, mental retardation in children and many other diseases and disabilities.

In their review on *megavitamin toxicity*, Alhadeff, Gualtieri and Lipton (1984) have identified five mechanisms by which high doses of water-soluble vitamins have injured human beings (their data were collected from clinical trials and from case reports). These mechanisms are (a) direct toxicity, (b) withdrawal reactions, (c) masking of concurrent diseases, (d) interference with other vitamins or drugs, and (e) increasing the absorption of more toxic oil-soluble vitamins. These reviewers conclude:

> 'The idea that even if high doses of vitamins fail to improve the patient, at least they will cause no harm, is insidious and irresponsible. It is important for physicians to be aware of the direct toxic effects produced by water-soluble vitamins, and also of the fact that large doses of these vitamins can cause harm through other mechanisms.'

The following are some of the uses and results of this form of therapy. When nicotinic acid (niacin) was prescribed (2 to 6 g daily) to reduce serum cholesterol (the RDA is only 18 mg), pruritis, desquammation and pigmented dermatoses occurred (Parsons and Flinn, 1957). More adverse symptoms include: cardiac arrhythmias (Brown and Goldstein, 1985), jaundice (Einstein, *et al.*, 1975; Winter and Boyer, 1973; Sugerman and Clark, 1974), peptic ulcer (Mosher, 1970), and acute gouty arthritis (Coronary Drug Project Research Group, 1975).

Although the RDA of pyridoxin (vitamin B_6) is only 2.2 mg daily, many members of the public take 50 mg doses for minor mental depression, also for premenstrual tension. Doses of 200 mg have been frequently prescribed to control the vomiting of pregnancy. Still larger amounts (2 to 6 g) have been prescribed for neurological illnesses, but caused severe disablement through ataxia and dysfunction of the sensory nervous system (Schaumburg, *et al.*, 1983).

The daily RDA of ascorbic acid (vitamin C) is 60 mg, but daily intakes of several grams have been used in the experimental treatment of human cancer. Careful studies have not supported this treatment, and no beneficial effect could be demonstrated (Creagan, *et al.*, 1979; Moertel, *et al.*, 1985; Wittes, 1985). Huge daily doses of several grams are often taken by members of the general public in the hope of preventing the common cold. However, in a series of three carefully controlled double-blind trials in Canada, Anderson (1977) could find no beneficial effects. Later studies again yielded negative results (Pitt and Costrine, 1979).

Because our bodies work conscientiously to destroy overdoses, withdrawal symptoms often appear when they are cut down. The classic example is provided by the widespread attacks of scurvy which broke out after the 900 day Siege of

Leningrad (1941–1944). This occurred when the citizens returned to normal well-balanced diets after the high wartime supplement of vitamin C was withdrawn (Alhadeff *et al.*, 1984). At the present time, many cases of scurvy are seen in infants who have been weaned from mothers who take excess doses of ascorbic acid, and also in adults who abruptly terminate their self-imposed megadosage (Herbert, 1975; Anderson, 1977).

There are other reasons for avoiding high doses of ascorbic acid, which interfere with the anticoagulant therapy used in preventing stroke and coronary disease (Rosenthal, 1971), impair the antibacterial action of leucocytes (Shilotri and Bhat, 1977), and destroy the body's small store of vitamin B_{12} (Herbert and Jacob, 1974). The National Research Council (NRC, 1980) advised: 'The consumption of large amounts of ascorbic acid is not recommended without medical advice'.

For further reading on ascorbic acid see Marcus and Coulston (1985).

Minerals. The WHO has *Recommended Intakes* for only two inorganic entities – calcium and iron (Passmore, *et al.*, 1974), whereas the US National Research Council (NRC, 1980) sets RDA for calcium, magnesium, iron, zinc, phosphorus and iodine, as well as provisional allowances for sodium, potassium, copper, manganese, chromium, molybdenum, selenium, fluoride and chloride.

The body of a healthy adult contains about 250 g of *sodium* (mainly as chloride) of which the greater part is extracellularly located. Natural foods contain relatively little sodium and most of this is in animal foods. Most adults ingest 5–18 g of sodium salts daily in industrialized countries. This additive comes to us from several sources. Bakers usually add about 1% of salt to their flour before baking. We consume more of it in canned meats and fish, sausages, ham, bacon, cheese, sauces and biscuits (cookies). Most housewives add salt to almost everything that they cook and the majority of diners add still more of it at the table. Sodium bicarbonate is used by the housewife in cooking vegetables and it turns up again in self-raising flour. The worldwide craving for salt is discussed by Denton (1982).

This delugeing of our meals with altogether unnatural amounts of the sodium ion would not matter much but for the fact that a significant proportion of the population responds to a high salt intake with hypertension: 20% of children are estimated to be at risk of developing hypertension later in life as a result of high salt intake (American Academy of Pediatrics, 1974). Dahl (1972) was the first to point out the association of hypertension with countries that traditionally eat a great deal of salted foods. Similar data were collected by Gleibermann (1973).

Current medical opinion is that where hypertension already exists, it can be lowered, or at least held in check, by decreasing intake of salt. Patients placed on a lowered salt diet complain, at first, of the tastelessness of their food, and exhibit listlessness and mental depression. After about three weeks the palate adjusts and there is a greater appreciation of natural food flavours. For those of us who cannot refrain from adding an electrolyte to our food at table, potassium chloride is available, attractively packed, at many supermarkets. The taste is more bitter but many people adjust to it. A word of caution though: in large doses (about 18 g) potassium becomes suddenly toxic. The first sign is usually cardiac arrhythmia, which can be fatal. The National Research Council gives this advice to adults: reduce the amount of sodium chloride added in cooking and at the meal table, and eat less of the obviously salted foods (NRC, 1980).

Because *iron* plays so important a part in the body's biochemistry, it is hard to realize how poisonous it is when in excess. To avoid this complication the human iron metabolism works in an almost sealed system whereby only 10% of the body's iron is lost each year from normal men, that is about 1 mg each day. (However women lose an additional 28 mg monthly.) Absorption from the intestine is limited by the following strategy. The duodenum, which is the principal site of iron absorption, traps the 10–25 mg of iron, which is consumed in the daily meals, in the mucosal cells which transfer a little of it to the bloodstream. When they die through senescence they shed their load of iron into the faeces (Harrison, 1983). Accidental poisoning by iron arises quite often when children swallow medicinal tablets. Within an hour vomiting sets in followed by gastrointestinal bleeding. As little as 1 g of ferrous sulfate can cause death in a child under 2 years of age. Although adults are less susceptible to iron poisoning, excess intake of over-the-counter iron supplements causes vomiting, diarrhoea and shock; and even cardiovascular collapse and death have been observed (Whitten and Brough, 1971). Excess consumption of iron (rarely possible through normal eating) interferes with the absorption of copper, zinc and manganese; deficiency of phosphate in the diet enhances the toxicity of iron (American Dietetic Association, 1978). For more on the metabolism of iron see Hillman and Finch (1985).

Although *fluoride* is an essential constituent of the human body, nature is often too sparing in supplying it. The result of this shortfall is widespread dental caries in children. Sodium fluoride, with its acute toxic dose of about 5 g (for a 70 kg man), is not a highly poisonous substance (Haynes and Murad, 1980), but deserves care in its distribution. The human body deals with potentially toxic levels of fluoride by increased urinary excretion; any excess over what can be handled in that way is deposited in the bones. Levels of 4 to 5 ppm of fluoride in the water supply are harmless (NRC, 1971; Hodge and Smith, 1965). Oral doses of 100 mg/day of sodium fluoride are being used to correct the osteoporesis of old people; in fact fluoride is the only known remedy that will rebuild lost bone (Bikle, 1983). Those elderly people who have a regular intake of fluoride are far less subject to osteoporosis fractures (Simonen and Laitinen, 1985).

A movement started in 1945 to improve the condition of childrens' teeth, by bringing the fluoride content of drinking water up to 1 ppm, found worldwide acceptance. It was advocated by the World Health Organization, the International Dental Federation, the Royal Commission on National Health Service (UK) (1979), the American Cancer Society, the American Academy for Allergy, the British Society for Allergy and Clinical Immunology, the Canadian Public Health Association and the Governments of some 40 other countries. Australia, which has 10 million of its 15 million people drinking fluoridated water has reaped great benefits from this practice (Australia, Commonwealth Department of Health, 1985).

Some concern has been expressed that water fluoridation may promote cancer, but careful comparisons made by the National Cancer Institute and by the Bureau of Epidemiology of the United States Public Health Service have found that mortality from cancer does not differ between cities with fluoridated and non-fluoridated water (Hoover, McKay anf Fraumeni, 1976; Erickson, 1978; Kinlen and Doll, 1981). No evidence could be found of teratogenic or general toxic effects resulting from the fluoridation of drinking water (Knox, Armstrong and Lancashire, 1980). Sometimes childrens' teeth show mottling as small, hard paper-white areas if the water supply has exceeded 2 ppm. Mottling occurs before the teeth erupt and is quite harmless (NRC, 1971).

So far we have been reviewing dietary constituents whose minimal essential level and toxic level lie far apart. With *selenium* the essential and toxic doses may lie closer. Whenever a high content of selenium in the soil has been reported, selenium toxicity has been observed in those who consume local crops containing about 30 ppm of selenium. The toxic constituents of this food are the amino acids selenocysteine and selenomethionine, incorporated in protein. The toxic symptoms are gastrointestinal disturbances, caries and loss of hair and nails (Bell, 1973; Liener, 1980).

Selenium is essential for the functioning of human glutathione peroxidase, an enzyme that protects the cell against oxidative damage (Hoekstra, *et al.*, 1974). From studies of selenium deprivation and toxicity in experimental animals, including livestock and primates, the National Research Council recommends that the human daily intake should lie between 0.05 and 0.2 mg (NRC, 1980). In a survey of 24 regions in China, those with high selenium in the soil had a reduced incidence of stomach cancer ($P < 0.01$) and in low selenium areas, primary liver cancer was widespread (Yu, *et al.*, 1985).

The regular eating of seaweeds rich in *iodine*, as happens in Japan, induces a type of hypothyroidism in susceptible people (Nagataki, 1974). Much commoner in the World is iodine deficiency, arising from drinking water from mountain catchments, and showing clinically as myxoedema. This is countered in many countries (such as Switzerland, the USA, Australia and New Zealand) by adding sodium iodide to the table salt (NRC, 1980).

The *phytic acid* in oatmeal and wheat bran binds and immobilizes calcium, iron and zinc. Fortunately, many people when exposed daily to phytate manage to induce the enzyme phytase. Leavened bread is subjected to phytase from the yeast in the kneading trough. Those who eat unleavened bread or oatmeal may be at risk of zinc deficiency.

(*b*) *Imbalance through lack of a dietary constituent.* Recommended dietary allowances for vitamins and minerals were discussed on p. 51. Gross deficiencies are frequently reported in the developing countries. The industrial nations also exhibit cases of deficiency but at the subclinical level. They occur principally among adolescents, the elderly, alcoholics and those who have been subjected to gastrointestinal surgery.

Deficiency of protein, when there is no lack of carbohydrate or lipid in the diet, is known as *kwashiorkor* (a word of West African origin). Frequently encountered in rural areas of developing countries, it usually arises when, after about one year on the breast, the child is weaned on to a traditional family diet, typically low in protein. (Marasmus, more of a town disease, strikes earlier, see p. 44). Kwashiorkor is characterized by oedema, apathy and failure to grow (Macleod, 1984; Davidson and Passmore, 1986).

The quality of different proteins. 'In many parts of the world today, a person may eat an abundance of what he likes from the food available to him, and not receive adequate nutrition' (Heiser, 1981). This observation applies particularly to proteins. These differ in nutritive value because they differ in their amino acid composition, and also (though this matters less) in their digestibility. These differences need to be acted upon when implementing the recommended daily protein allowances, or when assessing the protein value of an existing diet.

From knowledge of the amino acid composition of any protein, it is easy to calculate its *chemical score* (Block and Mitchell, 1946). This is done by nominating the total proteins of hen's egg as a standard and then calculating the percentage by which any essential amino acid (see Table 3.2) in the investigated protein falls below its value in the standard. Only the amino acid that shows the greatest deficit is used to provide the chemical score. Alternatively biological assays are available. The amino acids most frequently found to be limiting are lysine, tryptophan and the sulfur-containing cystine and methionine.

Table 4.3 lists the chemical scores of some typical food proteins. Milk resembles

Table 4.3 Comparative nutritive value of proteins

Foodstuff	Protein content (%)	Chemical score of protein (%)	Limiting amino acid
Whole egg	12.3	100	
Beef (lean, raw)	20	72	tryptophan
Wheat (wholemeal flour)	13	38	lysine
Rice (polished raw)	6.5	59	lysine
Maize (cornflour)	0.6	— ⎱	tryptophan +
Maize (wholemeal)	9.5	36 ⎰	lysine
Soya flour ('low fat')	45	58	cystine + methionine
Beans (haricot, raw)	21	39	cystine + methionine

(Compiled mainly from data in Paul and Southgate, 1978)

egg; most forms of flesh resemble beef. The cereals vary among one another but are uniformly poor in lysine. The beans, although deficient in the sulfur-containing amino acids, are rich in lysine and hence can give balance to a predominantly cereal diet. However, as was pointed out on p. 35, all the essential amino acids must be ingested simultaneously, or no protein will be synthesized. Man cannot store them. Archaeologists tell us that a mixture of maize and beans, called succotash, has been consumed in Mexico for at least 7000 years. Asians have many dishes that incorporate beans with rice.

Gelatin, the weight-watcher's delight, lacks cystine and tryptophan besides being low on methionine. It is better thought of as an additive than as a food.

The primary *essential fatty acid* for man is linoleic acid which is required for cellular and subcellular membranes, the transport of cholesterol and the synthesis of prostaglandins. It is abundantly present in vegetable oils (see Table 4.2). Deficiency of linoleic acid, though uncommon, is sometimes seen in intravenously-fed patients who consequently shed their skin in flakes.

4.3 Toxicants occurring naturally in food

All of man's foods consist of living creatures, some of them animal, the others vegetable. Because each of these organisms has the chemical nature best suited for its survival (Natural Selection has seen to this), the composition is far from ideal for man's requirements. Seemingly reluctant to seek alternatives, man has made the best of the situation by eating only traditionally-tested species, many of them only after special preparation.* Even so, most of his foods are complex mixtures that contain many minor constituents, any one of which could be harmful, even fatal, if consumed *in sufficient amount.*

Fortunately, those who consume a liberal mixed diet may never consume enough of these ever-present toxic constituents to suffer harm. Yet two groups of eaters are endangered, (a) the disadvantaged (whether geographically or economically) who have very few kinds of food available, and (b) the enthusiasts, who set so high a value on one particular item of food that they consume quite unreasonable amounts of it.

That many foods contain highly toxic minor constituents became more widely known in 1966 when the US National Academy of Sciences (NAS) published the book: *Toxicants Occurring Naturally in Foods,* followed by the much enlarged second edition (NAS, 1973). In Section 5.1 we shall discuss food constituents which affect only abnormally sensitive people, and Chapter 12 will deal with hazardous substances that are present in food only accidentally. The remainder of the present Section is concerned with constituents that are naturally present in wholesome foods but which can affect normal people adversely.

Just how bountifully nature bestows a whole host of chemicals on each of her

---

* However the German people survived a long blockade during the Second World War by eating fats synthesized by the Fischer-Tropsch process from coal.

species is illustrated by the common potato *Solanum tuberosum*. In this vegetable, about 150 different chemical substances had been identified by 1967. The raw, peeled potato contains water (76%), starch (20%), fibre (2%), proteins of good quality (2%), sugars (0.5%), fats (0.1%) and also potassium, calcium, magnesium, phosphorus, iron, copper, zinc, chlorine and sulfur, as well as Vitamins B_6, C, and E, thiamin, riboflavin, niacin, folic acid, pantothenic acid and biotin (Paul and Southgate, 1978). Also found were about 120 items of no known nutritional value such as the solanine alkaloids, oxalic acid, arsenic, nitrate, tannins, steroids, terpenes and phenols, as well as inhibitors of amylase, invertase and several proteases (NAS, 1973, p. 575).

Many more chemicals arise in the potato through synthesis while it is being cooked, greatly adding to the array of potentially toxic chemicals to which the diner is exposed. These volatile substances were isolated by gas-liquid chromatography and their structures were assigned from their infrared and mass spectra. The large store of carbohydrates and amino acids in potatoes provides the raw materials. In one investigation, a batch of Idaho potatoes, baked in their skins without any fat (at 205°C for 105 minutes), furnished 228 different chemicals. Of these, the principal contribution to the flavour was identified as a mixture of oxazoles, thiazoles, one furanone and several pyrazines and cyclopentapyrazines of which the last-named contributed the most pleasant and typical of the baked-potato-like aromas. Among the substances exactly identified in this analysis were 14 saturated hydrocarbons, 38 unsaturated and aromatic hydrocarbons (including 7 naphthalenes), 13 carboxylic acids, 22 alcohols, 23 aldehydes, 17 ketones, 19 esters and lactones (including 6 methyl esters), 7 ethers, 9 furans (including the typically potato-flavoured 2-methyltetrahydrofuran-3-one), 2 oxazoles, 28 pyrazines, 3 thiazoles, also 11 other nitrogen-containing, 5 other sulfur-containing and 14 chlorine-containing substances. Presumably many *non*-volatiles, which this technique could not reveal, were simultaneously synthesized (Coleman, Ho and Chang, 1981).

The toxic potentialities of this huge number of potato constituents remains, for the most part, unknown. There are hardly enough toxicologists in the World to investigate them, let alone the innumerable chemicals present in the whole of man's foods. Fortunately, the potato, which was introduced into Europe in 1570, has been eaten in Peru for about 4000 years (Heiser, 1981). Hence it has undergone a long period of biological testing in man, mostly with favourable results.

However, from time to time, people become poisoned from eating potatoes. This occurs when the normal content of glyco-alkaloids has increased through sprouting, bruising or exposure to light (greening). In such cases the amounts of these alkaloids that the body can normally detoxify has been exceeded. Solanine (*4.1b*), the most abundant of these alkaloids, is normally present in the ratio 3–6 mg per 100 g. Thus, a person eating 0.45 kg (1 lb) of potatoes daily would consume about 8 g of this substance annually, and would suffer no symptoms. Solanine, although not destroyed by cooking, is rapidly eliminated in the urine,

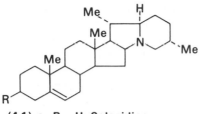

(4.1) a. R = H: Solanidine
b. R = Rhamnosyl-galactosyl-glucosyl: Solanine

partly as solanidine (*4.1a*). Severe toxic symptoms appear when growing (or storing) conditions increase the solanine content of potatoes to about 40 mg per 100 g. Diarrhoea sets in, with difficulties in breathing leading to coma (NAS, 1973; Roberts, 1981). Death has followed a higher intake (Willimot, 1933).

These results exemplify the difference between toxicity and hazard. The toxicity of a natural food constituent is its ability to produce injury when tested alone; but the hazard is its ability to produce injury under the circumstances of its human exposure, namely eating food that contains it. The following three factors help to restrain the hazard of toxic food constituents (Coon, in NAS, 1973, p. 575).

1. The natural concentration of the toxicant is often so low that the body's ability to detoxify or eliminate it is not exceeded. To obtain benefit from this factor, though, the food must not be eaten in excess, nor altered by storage or by preparation in an unusual way.
2. The thousands of chemicals, which are presented to our bodies by the natural foods that we eat, are not necessarily additive in their toxicity; in fact their toxicities are likely to be spread over many different receptors (see p. 171 for receptors).
3. Some toxic constituents of food are mutually antagonistic in their physiological action. Thus a parasympathetic agonist (such as solanine) could be countered by a parasympathetic antagonist or a sympathetic agonist. The toxic effects of cadmium, moreover, can be offset by zinc, and those of manganese by iron. Copper and molybdenum are also mutual antagonists. The known toxic effects of the oil-soluble vitamins, when taken singly (p. 51), are lessened if they are taken together.

What we have observed in a typical vegetable (potato) has also been encountered in fruits. Let us consider the pineapple which has been cultivated in South America for about 6000 years (Heiser, 1981): Often considered a luxury food in colder climes, this fruit is an important nutritional item in many warmer ones. The raw flesh contains water (84%), sugars (12%), fibre (1%), protein (0.5%), potassium, calcium, magnesium, phosphorus, carotene, pyridoxin, niacin, folic acid, pantothenic acid and about half as much vitamin C, weight for weight, as oranges (Paul and Southgate, 1978). Also present are bromelain (a powerful protease), 4-allylphenol, citric, malic, coumaric and ferulic acids.

Näf-Müller and Willhalm (1971), by using gas chromatography and mass spectrography, identified 59 volatile aliphatic substances of which 32 were esters, 10 alcohols, 6 aldehydes or ketones, 6 lactones whereas 5 contained sulfur. As with the potato, the toxicity of most of these substances is unknown, except that 19 of the esters were methyl esters. Actually 13 of these esters had been noted by Flath and Forrey (1970), moreover Connell (1964) had isolated free methanol. Although none of these authors quoted the proportions for any constituent, it is disquieting that such a fruit, of which many people eat about 250 g daily, is so rich in methanol and its easily-hydrolysed esters.

As little as 4 ml of methanol has brought about permanent blindness in man (Ritchie, 1985). The recommended maximal concentration in food is 2 ppm (Ministry of Agriculture, Fisheries and Food, 1978), but pineapple almost certainly exceeds that. We can conclude that, as with the potato, a hazard exists but toxicity is not found when no more of the food is consumed than the body can eliminate or detoxify.

The onion exemplifies a concept, outlined on p. 10, that plants survive best if they can repel their predators. This bulb is well known for liberating a tear-provoking (lachrimatory) substance when bruised. Carson and Wong (1961) isolated 16 sulfur-containing substances from the onion, but found that the lachrimatory substance had too short a half-life to permit identification.

In roasting coffee beans, before grinding them, several hundreds of new compounds are generated (see p. 95).

Nitrate-accumulating plants

Because it improves productivity farmers take pride in increasing the nitrogen content of their soil. However, when the weather becomes dry, sodium nitrate starts to accumulate. The most avid absorber of nitrate seems to be spinach, followed closely by beets, cabbage, carrots, celery, lettuce and radishes. In such a season, the local drinking water (particularly well water) is likely to have a higher nitrate content. Adults are not greatly at risk because, when potassium nitrate was formerly prescribed as a diuretic (e.g. in dropsy: 1 g/day), the side-effects were mainly physical weakness and mental inertia*. A lethal dose was in the region of 15 g.

However, infants do not tolerate nitrate well for, if less than 4 months old, they have little acidity to combat bacterial growth in the stomach. As a consequence, nitrate-reducing bacteria multiply there and produce nitrite which leads to methaemoglobinaemia which produces distress and weakness, and many have

---

* Mothers in the English-speaking countries would often coax their children to eat large amounts of spinach, in the period 1935–1960, during which time this source of nitrate largely replaced mercury as a quieting aid (from 'teething troubles' onwards). Paediatricians now discountenance both practices.

died (Swann, 1975). The safe upper limit for nitrate in drinking water for infants has been set at 20 ppm (WHO, 1974). Methaemoglobinaemia is also common following bacterial spoilage of cooked babys' foods made from nitrate-rich vegetables (Hölscher and Natzschka, 1964). For a 70 kg man, 28 mg of nitrite has been set as the highest acceptable daily intake in food and water (FAO/WHO, 1980).

A comparison made between (a) museum specimens of vegetables canned at the beginning of this century (vegetables grown in fields fertilized with animal manures) and (b) contemporary samples (from fields improved with refined fertilizers) showed the same average content of nitrate (Jackson, Steel and Boswell, 1967).

Toxic proteins in common foods

The plant *lectins* (also known as haemagglutinins) are glycoproteins that have a strong affinity for carbohydrates. Although they can cause clumping of red blood cells, the nutritional damage results from their strong affinity for the cells that line the gastrointestinal tract. This union prevents absorption of carbohydrates, lipids and amino acids, so that starvation, wasting and even death occur. Whereas a few of the lectins seem to be harmless (such as those in peas and lentils), many are highly toxic (such as those in soya and kidney beans). The lectin from castor-oil seeds (*Ricinus communis*, Euphorbiaceae) is one of the most poisonous of known substances. The minimal lethal dose for mice is 10^{-8} g per gram body weight. Fortunately lectins are destroyed by cooking. Although they occur in potatoes and cereals, the ones that have been most studied were isolated from the Leguminosae (legume family: beans, peas and lentils) because of the many toxic lectins extracted from beans.

The lectin in soya beans (*Glycine max*, also called *Soja hispida*) inhibits the growth of chicks and rats unless the beans are first heated. This lectin is seldom fatal because some is hydrolysed by pepsin in the stomach. The lectin of *Phaseolus vulgaris* is more dangerous because it is not readily digested by pepsin. This bean has many cultivars, known variously as kidney bean, haricot bean, black bean, white bean, navy bean and wax bean; it is eaten all over the world and provides English-speaking countries with the baked 'Boston' bean. The whole green pod is often eaten as 'French' or 'snap' beans. In spite of its lengthy association with the human diet, many people are poisoned each year by *P. vulgaris*, eating it raw or incompletely cooked. The symptoms are diarrhoea, wasting and occasionally death.

Field beans (hyacinth beans, *Dolichos lablab*), which are much eaten in India, Africa and parts of South America, have a lethal but heat-sensitive lectin. Lima beans (*Phaseolus lunatus*) have a lectin that inhibits growth in rats but does not kill them. Greater danger lies in the cyanide released by these beans (p. 65).

Most lectins have a molecular weight of about 100 000. They are easily purified by affinity chromatography on a polysaccharide column (e.g. Sepharose). For more on lectins, see Jaffé (1973, 1980).

The *protease inhibitors* form a distinct class of plant toxins, which occur in the seeds of grains and legumes and also in edible roots. Two inhibitors from soya beans have been sequenced. The major one is inactivated by heat, has a molecular weight of about 20 000, and possesses very few disulfide bonds. The other inhibitor (MW about 8000) is rich in these bonds and, consequently, less heat sensitive; moreover it inhibits chymotrypsin as well as trypsin. Rats and chicks thrive poorly on unheated soya meal, but do very well if it is first cooked; the same responses were obtained with the isolated inhibitor. The pathology of these inhibitors seems to rest not so much on protein starvation as on the pancreatitis that they cause, at least in chicks and rats. Such inflammation does not occur in other laboratory mammals so that man may not be at risk. To be on the safe side, all 'Infants' Formula' made from soya beans, which is used for children who cannot tolerate cows' milk, is legally required to be heat-treated in most of the industrialized countries.

Similar trypsin and chymotrypsin inhibitors occur in *Arachis hypogea* (the peanut), *Vicia faba*, *Phaseolus lunatus*, *vulgaris*, and *aureus*, and in *Vigna sinensis* (the black-eyed pea). Protease inhibitors in raw potato tubers account for 20% of the protein. For further reading on trypsin inhibitors see Liener (1980).

A protein, *avidin*, in hens' eggs, rapidly and specifically inactivates the vitamin, biotin. Biotin deficiency has been produced in volunteers and occurs in patients on diets in which raw eggs preponderate. The symptoms are sleepiness, nausea and severe, peeling dermatitis (Davidson and Passmore, 1986). Avidin is inactivated by cooking.

Toxic peptides from bacteria and fungi

Cyanobacteria (once known as 'blue-green algae') often bloom over the surface of reservoirs. One genus, *Microcystis*, exudes highly toxic peptides of MW about 1200 into drinking water and this has caused many human deaths (a blood-engorged liver at autopsy is diagnostic). The toxins are pentapeptides with three invariant D-amino acids (alanine, glutamic acid and methylaspartic acid), and two variant L-amino acids. (See also Carmichael and Mahmood, 1984.)

Of the several hundred species of mushroom consumed by man, about 100 have caused food poisoning but only 12 species are lethal. One of the commonest and most dangerous is *Amanita phalloides* whose toxic octapeptides produce painful symptoms about 10 hours after consumption. This toxic action is exerted by inhibition of RNA polymerase in the nuclei of liver cells. A single mushroom has been known to kill a man (Jaffé, 1973).

Toxic amino acids

The 20 amino acids from which mammalian proteins are constructed (Table 3.2) are usually innocuous, even in much larger doses than would be liberated from the daily intake of protein. Thus glutamate has shown no serious side effects when given orally in doses of up to 45 g daily, for 10 weeks, in attempts (apparently unsuccessful) to treat mental retardation or petit mal epilepsy. However diners in Chinese restaurants in the USA, who sometimes experience a burning or numbing sensation in the back of the neck, particularly if much ethanol has been taken, attribute this to glutamate used too freely for seasoning. For more on the results of ingesting large doses of the dietary amino acids see Harper (1973). For an inborn sensitivity to phenylalanine see p. 76.

Some illnesses are caused by amino acids that form no part of the proteins commonly eaten by man. A particularly troublesome example is lathyrism which can follow eating the seeds of *Lathyrus sativus* (chickling vetch, or chick-pea) as is done by large populations in Algeria and India. Lathyrism is characterized by an irreversible paralysis of the legs brought about by degeneration of the spinal cord. The seeds are used in India to make unleavened bread (chapatis); these cause no harm when used to supplement an otherwise adequate diet. However, in famine years following prolonged drought, whole populations are obliged to exist mainly on this legume, which survives protracted aridity better than any other available food plant. For these people the choice between death by starvation or lifelong incapacitation thanks to lathyrism is indeed a grim one. Research is under way to find a method for detoxifying *Lathyrus* seeds without loss of its rich content of the B vitamins, or of its breadmaking properties. The principal toxic agent is β-N-oxalyl-L-α,β-diaminopropionic acid which inhibits binding of the neurotransmitter, glutamate, to its receptor. For further reading on lathyrism, see Bell (1973) and Padmanabam (1980).

For other amino acids occurring in foods and toxic to man, e.g. mimosine, djenkolic acid, and dihydroxyphenylalanine, see Liener (1980, p. 436).

In praise of beans

We have seen that most legumes contain two poisonous principles, lectins and protease inhibitors. Moreover several much-eaten members of the bean family exhibit other forms of people-unfriendliness. Apart from lathyrism (p. 63), they can inflict cyanide poisoning (p. 67), favism (p. 74) and polysaccharide colic (p. 67). Until he learnt how to circumvent these hazards, beans simply spelt 'bad news' to early man.

Fortunately there is another side to this story. In our World which is so short of food (p. 43) a large botanical family, the Leguminosae, has many members that bear highly nutritive crops in very different soils and climates. Those who cultivate them have, for the most part, learnt how to detoxify them. Hence beans are being cultivated in almost every part of the world and many millions of people depend heavily upon, and have no equivalent alternative to, this source of nourishment. In Asia, beans make a huge contribution to the diet, replacing much of the cereal load consumed in European diets. Compared to cereals, legumes have a higher protein content, and the protein is of better quality (p. 56), being rich in the lysine that cereals lack. Provided they are eaten in the same meal, a combination of beans and cereals present a balance of amino acids as nutritive as that furnished by animal protein. Legumes are also an excellent source of the B group of vitamins and, if eaten while sprouting, of vitamin C as well (Davidson and Passmore, 1986, p. 327).

Cyanogenetic glycosides

Traces of hydrogen cyanide are steadily produced in the human body, particularly by polymorphonuclear leucocytes during their phagocytosis of bacteria (Vennesland, *et al.*, 1981). As this cyanide escapes from the white cells, it is detoxified to thiocyanate (which is itself toxic in higher concentrations). This detoxification mechanism is in any case only a limited safeguard, because as little as 140 mg of HCN has often proved fatal to human beings. Death follows addition of hydrogen cyanide to the iron atom of cytochrome oxidase which can no longer take up atmospheric oxygen. This causes local suffocation in the tissues, of which the brain is an early victim (see also, p. 242).

The cyanogenetic glycosides that present the greatest hazard in human food are amygdalin and linamarin. They are both β-glycosides, and hence are not substrates for the α-glycosidase (amylase) of the human duodenum. Yet in the plant they are separated from their hydrolysing enzyme by only a thin membrane which mastication, or other form of bruising, rapidly bursts. *Amygdalin* is the gentiobioside of mandelonitrile (*4.2*). Intestinal bacteria rapidly hydrolyse amygdalin to hydrogen cyanide, benzaldehyde and gentiobiose. Linamarin, the *O*-glucoside of 2-hydroxyisobutyronitrile (*4.3*), is similarly hydrolysed to hydrogen cyanide and acetone. Whereas benzaldehyde and acetone are relatively harmless, hydrogen cyanide is lethal in small doses (see Section 11.1 for its pharmacology).

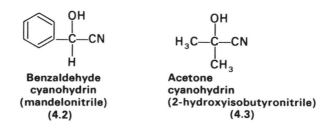

Benzaldehyde cyanohydrin (mandelonitrile) (4.2)   **Acetone cyanohydrin (2-hydroxyisobutyronitrile)** (4.3)

Amygdalin is present in the kernels of the seeds ('stones' or 'pits') that occupy the core of many fruits belonging to the Rosaceae, notably almonds, apricots, peaches, plums and cherries. Bitter almonds, the original source of amygdalin, are now rarely grown; their volatile oil, known as essence of almond (actually benzaldehyde contaminated with hydrogen cyanide) has been replaced by pure benzaldehyde made by oxidizing toluene. The sweet almond, widely eaten as a nut, lacks amygdalin but is rich in β-glycosidase which can rapidly hydrolyse this glycoside. Many children who have cracked apricot stones and eaten the kernels have died (Herbert, 1979). However, there is a well-established industry that obtains apricot stones from the canneries, frees the kernels from amygdalin, and markets the product as an economical replacement for almond meal in confectionary (e.g. marzipan) and pastrymaking.

Amygdalin, under the name 'laetrile', was sold to cancer patients in the 1960s and 1970s by some advocates of 'alternative medicine'. The medical profession protested, the US Food and Drug Administration legislated against it, but public opinion remained divided. Finally a US Senate subcommittee conducted hearings (US. Senate, 1977), which ended by condemning treatment with laetrile. Ernst Krebs, the principal source and advocate of laetrile, was brought to Court and convicted of gross fraud (People of the State of California, 1977; Herbert, 1979).

Curiously enough a strong public demand for laetrile therapy persisted. Some terminally ill cancer patients, to whom orthodox medicine no longer held out hope, unsuccessfully sought (in a class action: Rutherford v. United States (1978) in the US Supreme Court) a *legal right* to be treated with laetrile. Finally, the US National Cancer Institute, supported by the Food and Drug Administration, conducted a clinical trial on 178 cancer patients who had asked for this form of treatment. Unhappily nothing beneficial came to light, whereas much could have been done for these patients at the time treatment began. The trial led to this official statement: 'Amygdalin (laetrile) is a toxic drug that is not effective in cancer treatment' (Moertel, *et al.*, 1982).

Some observers see the attempt of the terminally ill to decriminalize laetrile as a move to legalize euthanasia (defined on p. 220). One patient for example, in the report of Herbert (1979), was taking apricot meal (a rich source of β-glycosidase) with her 'laetrile', a procedure certain to accelerate hydrogen cyanide poisoning.

Linamarin is associated with greater danger, because it is abundantly present in some of the most used foods of the developing nations. It presents a hazard in lima beans (*Phaseolus lunatus*), and in cassava root (*Manihot esculenta*) which is made into tapioca, manioc and yuca. The lima bean, archeologists tell us, was being eaten in Peru 8000 or more years ago. How one admires the tenacity with which these early farmers must have learnt how to prepare this initially poisonous food safely! Many lives must have been lost in the process. The bound HCN content of different cultivars varies from 10 (the white beans marketed in the USA), through 200 (the white beans eaten in Burma), to 300 (black beans eaten in Puerto Rico), all expressed as mg per 100 g of bean. Fatalities from mis-preparation of the food are still encountered. Yet when the beans are soaked overnight so that the enzyme can hydrolyse the glucoside, and then boiled to remove the hydrogen cyanide, they are quite safe, and they continue to provide excellent nutrition in many countries.

The root of the cassava plant is grated, soaked in water, then allowed to ferment for several days. The mass is drained, dried, and pounded to a flour which can be either baked as bread or boiled. Without such long and careful processing, cassava is acutely toxic. Some ways of preparing cassava in Nigeria seem not to remove all the HCN which is credited with causing a chronic form of poisoning known as tropical ataxic neuropathy. The afflicted, who have difficulty in walking, have higher levels of plasma cyanide and thiocyanate than control patients. Related neuropathies, sometimes leading to blindness, have been reported from areas in West Africa, the West Indies and Malaya where cassava forms a major part of the diet. In spite of its hazardous nature, cassava is a starchy food of enormous economic importance: it is said to meet some 10% of the World's caloric requirements.

For further reading on cyanogenetic glycoside poisoning see Conn (1973) and Montgomery (1980); for the behaviour of the cyanide anion in biology, see Vennesland, *et al.* (1981).

The *cycads* e.g. *Zamia* are surviving members of an ancient division of the Gymnosperms found in tropical and subtropical regions. Their cones produce a starchy food (p. 11) which is eaten in the Pacific Ocean area. All of its users know how to remove the toxic agent, methylazoxymethanol (*2.1*) present as its glycoside, cycasin. The aglycone produces acute jaundice and a partial but permanent paralysis in man, whereas in rats and guinea pigs it is a carcinogen. For further reading see Wogan and Busby (1980) and Miller (1973).

Sulfur-containing toxicants

Many edible members of the Cruciferae contain glucosinolates of the type (*4.4*), in which R is usually allyl or other unsaturated aliphatic group. Significant amounts of these substances can be consumed by eating large amounts of cabbage, broccoli, cauliflower, sprouts, mustard or horseradish. These glucosinolates become enzymatically hydrolysed, during preparation for the table, or within the stomach, to give glucose, sulfuric acid and an isothiocyanate, such as allyl isothiocyanate from cabbage ($H_2C=CH-CH_2-N=C=S$). The thiocyanate ion ($N\equiv C-S^-$), formed by hydrolysis of these isothiocyanates, is a goitrogen that causes hypothyroidism by preventing the thyroid gland from taking up the iodide ion. This is a simple matter of anion competition. Most of the goitrogenic work has been carried out on rabbits but, in the human, goitre has been traced to consumption of excessive amounts of cabbage (Kelly and Snedden, 1960). It is true that cruciferous vegetables have a long record of safety when eaten in moderation. However, those enthusiasts for shredded raw cabbage (coleslaw), who take large helpings of this dish with every meal (whether as a reducing diet or to prevent colonic cancer) may be at some risk.

When R in (*4.4*) is hydroxybutenyl, as in turnips and Chinese cabbage, the isothiocyanate product becomes isomerized to goitrin (*4.5*) which is 5-vinyloxazolidine-2-thione. This is a more potent goitrogen, which functions differently, namely by preventing iodination of the precursor of thyroxine to give the thyroid hormones.

For further reading on toxic glucosinolates see Tookey, Van Etten and Daxenbichler (1980), Van Etten and Wolff (1973).

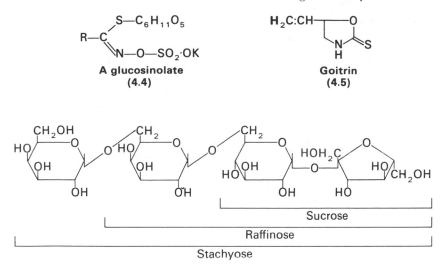

Fig. 4.1 Oligosaccharides present in beans that produce flatus (from Liener, 1980).

Bean-induced colic

Several varieties of bean (e.g. navy, lima, boston-baked) contain a tetrasaccharide (stachyose) and a trisaccharide (raffinose) made up of galactose, glucose and fructose units but non-assimilable by man (Fig. 4.1). Unfortunately many people harbour anaerobic bacteria in the colon which attack these oligosaccharides and release uncomfortable volumes of hydrogen and methane. This situation usually leads to much flatus and agonizing cramps (Patwardhan and White, 1973; Liener, 1980).

Tannins

Tannins are polyphenolic substances of high molecular weight which are found in plants. The core of the tannin molecule is a polymerized polyhydroxyflavan (an oxygen heterocycle). The single-dose (oral) acute toxicity (LD_{50}) is high (about 2 g/kg), which is as well because many people consume about 1 g daily in tea, coffee, cocoa and other vegetable products such as the hulls of nuts. Being protein precipitants, tannins affect nutrition of those on low protein diets. More disturbing is the high incidence of oesophageal cancer in the Transkei region of South Africa whose inhabitants consume much sorghum (a grain) of which the high content of tannin produces chronic irritation of the throat (Singleton and Kratzer, 1973). Both physical injury (e.g. scalding) and zinc deficiency (Newberne, 1985) contribute to the onset of this malignancy.

Toxic seafoods

The steady increase in the World population, now well over 4000 million people, exerts pressure to harvest more of the wealth of protein that is so abundantly present in fish and shellfish. However, some marine foods present a dietary hazard. Most of the poisoning that results from eating seafood arises from bacteriological contamination (Section 12.2). Usually, seafood that is intrinsically poisonous is not sent to market, or the offending organs are first removed (Ragelis, 1984). An example is provided by puffer fish (various species of *Fugu*) which is eaten in Japan and China as a special delicacy. The poison, tetrodotoxin, is present in the ovaries, liver, intestines, and skin, all skilfully removed by trained staff. Tetrodotoxin (*4.6*) has a cage-like perhydroquinazoline molecule from which a guanidinium ion substituent protrudes like a tongue. By blocking sodium ion channels, this toxin prevents generation of transmission in both nerve and muscle. However, transmission at synapses is unaffected, so that those who die do so by purely peripheral intoxication, usually by respiratory paralysis. In fact, tetrodotoxin is one of the most powerful of all known poisons, having a LD_{50} (mouse) of only 12 ng/kg.

Succulent bivalves, such as clams, mussels, and scallops, have often become poisonous by feeding on certain species of dinoflagellates (e.g. *Gonyaulax*). These single celled organisms, floating in the marine plankton, multiply from time to time to such an extent that the colour of the sea is changed. Such 'red tides' occur off the western as well as the eastern seaboards of Canada and the United States. The poison is a perhydropurine, saxitoxin (*4.7*), which, although it is non-toxic to the mollusc, affects man in the same way as tetrodotoxin (the lethal dose for man is about 1 mg). Neither toxin is altered by cooking. Fortunately, not all red tide-forming dinoflagellates are toxic.

The malady known as ciguatera occurs in the West Indies following eating of barracuda and other species of fish that are either bottom dwellers or predators of these. Fish that are normally safe to eat can acquire this poison after coral reefs are destroyed either by storms or dredging. The nature of the toxin is unknown. Symptoms in man are both muscular and neurological, with cramps, prostration, visual disturbances and convulsions. Several deaths have been reported.

Oysters in Hamana Bay (Japan) caused many deaths from liver poisoning in

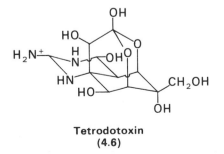

Tetrodotoxin
(4.6)

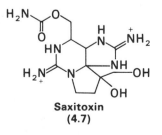

Saxitoxin
(4.7)

1942 which were traced to this mollusc's feeding on toxic dinoflagellates. The red whelk (*Neptunea antiqua*) in Japan produces a poison (apparently a simple aliphatic amine) in its salivary gland, and photophobia and vomiting in man have been traced to this.

For further reading on toxic seafoods see Schantz (1973) and Ragelis (1984).

Roasting and toasting

We have had occasion to note the considerable gains in health and nutrition achieved by man as soon as he began to cook his food (p. 10). There were also some disadvantages, such as loss of the more labile vitamins. Perhaps the most ominous aspect of cooking is that it generates so many chemical substances, none of which were present in the raw material. A skilled organic chemist would indeed be proud to synthesize one new compound each week; yet the cook working in the kitchen for an hour is bound to generate several hundred (p. 58), most of them of unknown toxicity.

Perhaps the greatest area of concern over the effect of cooking on our health, has been the detection of polycyclic aromatic hydrocarbons in roasted, and smoked, foods. The first link between cancer and the products of combustion was made in 1775 when Pott traced the frequent occurrence of scrotal cancer in young chimney-sweeps to their contact with tar and soot (these lads were commonly stripped of their clothes and impelled up the flue). A century and a half passed before the first carcinogen was isolated from tar. It turned out to be benzo[a]pyrene (*7.31*) of which the merest trace produced dermal tumours when painted on shaved mice (Cook, Hewett, and Hieger, 1933). Also, when injected into hamsters, it produced respiratory tract tumours (Feron, 1972). However it proved not to be orally active because, when fed to mice in doses of 40 μg/day, no gastrointestinal cancer developed (Neal and Rigdon, 1967). This dose exceeds any relative human intake. Summarizing the evidence, Clayson (1981) wrote: 'There is no direct evidence that benzo[a]pyrene itself is carcinogenic in man'.

This statement does not exclude the possibility that other products of incomplete combustion may be hazardous. Polycyclic aromatic hydrocarbons (PAH), of which about 100 have been identified in treated food (Fazio, 1984), are defined as molecules with three or more fused benzene rings, with or without substituents. Only a minority of them are known to be carcinogenic; the favouring factor is a 'bay region', e.g. the recess between positions 10 and 11 in formula *7.31*. Because benzo[a]pyrene is highly fluorescent the earlier workers found it the easiest PAH to investigate. However, improved instrumentation, particularly gas chromatography (capillary), if followed by mass spectrography, can now provide the resolving power to deal with the highly complex PAH mixtures that occur in foods (Fazio, 1984).

Polycyclic aromatic hydrocarbons are generated by man through his operation of vehicles, industrial combustion, home heating, garbage disposal, asphalt paving and cigarette smoking. However nature is not resting:

'The existence of a natural background concentration of polyaromatic hydrocarbons has now been well established. It consists of PAH synthesized on a worldwide scale by plants and microorganisms on land and in the water, and formed during open burning of forests and prairies not ignited by man. Volcanic activity is an additional source' (Hancock, Applegate and Dodd, 1970).

Crops grown close to cities show some but not much extra contamination (Miller, 1973; Fazio, 1984). The significance of this intake for man, in the plant-derived portion of his diet, is unknown; its proportion can vary from 3–25 parts per billion (ppb). This ratio should be compared with barbecued beef (3), grilled (broiled) steak (1) (but charcoal-grilled steak (8)), smoked fish (1), smoked ham (3) and coffee (1), all in ppb. These figures were extracted from a table in which they are compared with those for 1,2-benzanthracene (*4.8*), a feebly carcinogenic but widely distributed PAH (Grasso, 1983).

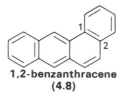

1,2-benzanthracene
(4.8)

Grasso continues: 'Several epidemiological studies have been made in an attempt to correlate consumption of grilled or roasted fish or meat with an increased incidence of cancer of the stomach, but no firm evidence in this direction has been produced so far', a statement supported by the work of Masuda, Mori and Kurastune (1966).

Also, rats fed on charcoal-grilled beef were no more subject to gastrointestinal tumours than controls fed raw beef or soya bean meal (Visek and Clinton, 1985). Neither prospective nor retrospective studies have given any indication yet that the usual charring and smoking of food makes any contribution to human cancer. However intensely smoked fish and meat, with blackened exterior, remain under a cloud of suspicion (Grasso, 1983).

Completely different chemical processes occur when the food that is being singed has a high carbohydrate content. The golden-brown crust of freshly baked bread is widely appreciated. The browning owes its formation to the Maillard reaction between the aldehyde group of carbohydrates and the terminal amino-group of lysine (*4.9*). First, an azomethine (–CH=N–) linkage is formed, then the product undergoes an Amadori rearrangement to give a N-substituted 1-amino-2-ketose (a 'pre-melanoidin'). The latter polymerizes to brown products known as melanoidins. Because the human body cannot synthesize lysine (see Table 3.2) those people who are on a meagre diet may suffer deprivation. Thus 10–15% of available lysine is lost during the baking of bread, and much more on toasting it. The roller-drying of skim milk locks up 40% of the lysine (Davidson and Passmore, 1986, p. 233).

The pre-melanoidins (but not the melanoidins) are toxic to rats, causing hypertrophy of the caecum and (in females) a reduced yield from pregnancy. No comparable human pathology has been reported. For more on the Maillard reaction see Yannai (1980). Carbohydrates, if heated in the absence of nitrogenous material, still turn brown, but through the process called 'caramelization'.

Frying

There are two principal ways in which oils and fats used for frying can undergo deterioration. (a) When exposed to air for many weeks (even without being heated) they may take up oxygen and acquire the odour described as *rancid*. (b) When used for frying, day after day without being replaced, they thicken and acquire a different kind of unsavoury odour.

Proper understanding of what occurs in the autoxidation of unsaturated fats (rancidification) began with the studies of Farmer, *et al.* (1942). First a molecule of oxygen becomes attached to a carbon atom that is situated next to a double bond; this reaction gives a peroxide free radical (*4.10*). This intermediate abstracts a hydrogen atom from a methylene group adjacent to a double bond in *another* molecule, thus forming a new free radical which promptly reacts with atmospheric oxygen. This chain reaction, of which the difficult first step is initiated by iron, continues easily by self-propagation. No dimerization takes place and no double bond is lost. Contrary to early hypotheses, no epoxides or cyclic peroxides are formed. Ultraviolet light can accelerate the chain reaction but it can be prevented by antioxidants. These may be present naturally, as tocopherol is in many vegetable oils, and as a sterol (avenasterol) in olive oil; or they may be added by the suppliers. Animal fats become rancid faster than vegetable oils. The degree of unsaturation increases susceptibility: linoleate oils oxidize about ten times faster than oleate oils under comparable conditions.

The objectionable odours of rancid lipids arise not from the peroxides but from secondary oxidation products that these generate. The toxicity of rancid fats was found to correlate better with the concentration of peroxides than with any other constituent. This toxicity is characterized by intestinal damage followed by loss

$$H_2N-CH_2$$
$$|$$
$$(CH_2)_3$$
$$|$$
$$H_2N-CH-CO_2H$$
Lysine
(4.9)

$$-C-CH=CH-$$
$$|$$
$$O-O$$
Peroxy radical
(4.10)

$$(CH_2)_x-CO_2H$$
$$(CH_2)_y-CO_2H$$
'Cyclic monomer'
(x + y = 10)
(4.11)

of weight and early death. Lipids that have become only slightly rancid do no harm to laboratory animals. For human beings, rancid food is not considered to be a hazard because it is usually rejected by the customer.

Turning to the deterioration of lipids by *heating*, it should be noted that commercial frying is usually conducted at about 180°C, in deep, thermostatted baths. Home frying, on the other hand, is performed more haphazardly, often in shallow pans whose temperature varies widely and may reach 250°C in places: at that temperature triglycerides decompose rapidly. In commercial frying the raw food (e.g. potatoes, fish, shrimps, chicken, doughnuts) supplies a steady source of water vapour, some of which forms a blanket of steam over the surface of the oil, providing a barrier to access of oxygen. As fresh, moist materials are added to the bath, sudden spurts of water vapour perform steam distillations that remove the more volatile decomposition products (e.g. heptaldehyde) formed in the preceding batch.

Repeated use of the same bath, day after day, generates two types of altered lipids: (a) viscous dimers, which have proved to be non-toxic to experimental animals, and (b) what are termed 'cyclic monomers' of the type *4.11**. The latter are considered to be the toxic components (Artman and Smith, 1972; Meltzer, *et al.*, 1981).

Human beings exert a beneficial influence on frying procedures by simply refusing to eat ill-tasting products. In the USA, the 'Fast Food' eating houses and takeaway outlets, which cater for the needs of a large section of the population, has been led to standardize on lightly hydrogenated cooking oils that lack triply-unsaturated (and are low in doubly-unsaturated) components. These 'short-enings' provide baths that deteriorate only slowly. Sponsored by the US Department of Agriculture, a recent survey of used oil from Fast Food outlets in Illinois and California found the content of cyclic monomers to be acceptably low (0.1–0.5%). These results were compared to those obtained on specimens flown in from street vendors in Egypt and Israel who were cooking vegetable patties (falafel) in open-air stands (0.2–0.8%) (Frankel, *et al.*, 1984), also acceptably low.

A large literature exists in which it has been shown that fats and oils, after use for frying under commercial or domestic conditions, cause no harm to rats or dogs, compared to control animals fed on unheated lipids. However, by the use of unusually high temperatures, or forced oxygenation, or simply by using rats on a low protein diet, indisputable harm (diarrhoea, wasting, hepatomegaly) has been demonstrated. In an example intermediate between these extremes cottonseed oil was heated at 182°C for 8 hours a day, for 6 days. The product, in which 136 new compounds were detected, and over 50 of them identified, was found to depress the growth of rats (Artman and Smith, 1972).

---

* One carboxy group in *4.11* has been generated by hydrolysis, the other by a terminal oxidation that did not occur in the laboratory when *pure* chemicals were used.

Investigation of the thermal decomposition of lipids is clearly only in its infancy. An early concern over malondialdehyde seems to have been laid to rest, whereas one that involves the oxidation products of cholesterol (from animal fats) has not yet had time to state its case (Addis, Csallany and Kindom, 1983).

In the absence of prospective and retrospective studies (p. 288) on contrasted groups of people (of whom some never, whereas others often, consume fried foods), it is reasonable to assume that the traditional and widespread custom of including fried food in the diet is, in moderation, safe. Admittedly this practice is not altogether free from suspicion, but it is not likely to be surrendered unless evidence of a grave hazard is brought to light. For further reading see Mattson (1973); Yannai (1980).

Further reading

Toxicants Occurring Naturally in Foods (NAS, 1973)
Toxic Constituents of Plant Foodstuffs (Liener, 1980)
Food Safety (Roberts, 1981)
For supplementary reading:
Toxic Hazards in Food (Conning and Lansdown, 1983)
Xenobiotics in Foods and Feeds (Finley and Schwass, 1983)
Xenobiotic Metabolism: Nutritional Effects (Finley and Schwass, 1985).

Follow-up

Compare and contrast the problems created by inclusion of additives (Section 5.2) in manufactured foods with (a) the prolific and random inclusion, by nature, of many chemical substances in natural foods, and (b) the prolific and random multiplication of foreign substances effected by the everyday preparation of family meals.

5

Special aspects of wholesome foods

5.1 Inborn sensitivity to a particular food

Dining in company can be one of the most delightful of social experiences, while making its due contribution to both nutrition and sensory satisfaction. In fact, the onward sweep of the culinary arts and crafts has helped to produce meals that are not too demanding to prepare and yet have a splendid palatability. Yet for many people, indeed for quite a significant fraction of the population, an invitation to dine creates pangs of anxiety: Will the food be compatible with the guest's non-average genetic or immune systems? Or will it lead to long hours of suffering? An investigation into the background of this dilemma can usefully be divided into (a) the inborn lack of an enzyme or other essential body chemical, and (b) the creation of an immunological error, expressed as an allergy.

Lack of an enzyme or receptor

The temporarily incapacitating illness known as favism, characterized by severe haemolysis and haemoglobinuria, often strikes hard when broad beans (*Vicia faba*) are eaten by genetically predisposed persons. The victims have an almost complete lack of the enzyme glucose-6-phosphate dehydrogenase (G6PD) in their erythrocytes. Lack of G6PD is one of the commonest of all inborn errors of metabolism and affects an estimated 100 million people throughout the world. It arises from an incompletely dominant gene on the X-chromosome. Although unevenly distributed this deficiency is particularly common among many of the nations who live on the Mediterranean shores. Outbreaks of favism have been frequent in Sardinia, Sicily, Cyprus, Rhodes, Algeria and also in China, yet fairly uncommon in many other countries where broad beans are eaten.

A precipitating factor is the pyrimidine glucoside vicine (*5.1a*) which occurs in the beans. This is harmless until hydrolysed to its aglycone, divicine (*5.1b*). The latter sustains a free radical type of oxidation of glutathione, a substance that normally protects erythrocytes from haemolysis. When present, G6PD generates NADPH which protects the glutathione. When absent, divicine breaks down a precarious equilibrium in the red cell deprived of this enzyme.

Another, unknown, factor has to be postulated to explain the capriciousness of the outbreaks of favism. For further reading see Patwardhan and White (1973); Mager, Chevion and Glaser (1980).

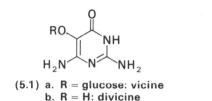

(5.1) a. R = glucose: vicine
      b. R = H: divicine

Histamine
(5.2)

(5.3) a. R = H: phenylethylamine
      b. R = OH: tyramine

Enthusiasm to rush great consignments of milk products to famine-stricken countries could be tempered by the knowledge that many adults cannot tolerate even as little as half a litre of milk because of the 25 g of lactose contained in it. The enzyme *lactase* becomes deleted in late childhood by many Africans and East Asians and it cannot be re-induced in the adult. Failure of the jejunal cells to produce this enzyme allows lactose to pass unchanged into the colon where it is bacterially decomposed, giving rise to bloating, colic, flatus and a frothy diarrhoea. In most Caucasians and in those African tribes that maintain dairy herds the enzyme persists throughout life.

Congenital lactase deficiency is also known but is rare; congenital deficiency of other disaccharidases is rarer. The inborn inability to metabolize galactose is also rare, but serious because it leads to cataract formation. For further reading on sensitivity to particular carbohydrates see Patwardhan and White (1973).

A genetically-based inability to deal with the *pressor amines* creates much physical distress for many people. Normally these amines, which arise in the gut by bacterial decarboxylation of the corresponding amino acids (histamine, phenylalanine, tyrosine), are destroyed by the widely-present enzyme mono-amine oxidase. This enzyme is insufficiently provided in certain individuals. Excessive absorption of histamine (*5.2*) can produce a sudden fall in blood pressure (accompanied by fainting), whereas phenylethylamine (*5.3a*) and tyramine (5.3b) drastically raise it. Tyramine is present in many fermented foods such as yeast extract, pickled herring, cheeses, sauerkraut, beer and wine; it is also present in orange, banana, avocado, broad beans and liver. Phenylethylamine and histamine occur in chocolate. Decomposing fish, even before it acquires a perceptible taint, has often undergone bacterial decomposition with liberation of much histamine from the free histidine that is abundantly present in fish muscle. When the concentration is high, quite normal adults become ill. Patients receiving drugs that are monoamine oxidase inhibitors, for the treatment of mental depression, suffer hypertensive crises when they consume tyramine-containing food, and many have died while help was being summoned. For more on the pressor amines see Lovenberg (1973).

There are more than 50 known conditions, most of them very rare, where an enzyme responsible for metabolism of a particular amino acid is congenitally lacking; about 15 of these have been more or less successfully treated with a diet in which the amount of this amino acid is reduced. Of these disorders, phenylketonuria is the only one where many patients have been successfully treated through more than two decades. In this complaint, a genetically-based deficiency of phenylalanine hydroxylase, phenylalanine builds up in excess – a condition that leads to irreversible brain damage unless treatment is begun promptly. Paediatricians require that *all* infants be examined for this defect no later than the second week of life. The condition is widely distributed among Caucasian people; for example in Scotland it is found in one of each 8000 births. The restrictive diet can usually be abandoned at eight years of age (Harrison, 1983, p. 503).

Six other genetic defects lead to failure to handle some part of the ornithine cycle; other defects limit utilization of one of the following: methionine, lysine, histidine, branched chain amino acids or propionyl CoA (Nyhan, 1974). Several other ailments in the newborn have been identified as inherited disabilities to handle one or other vitamin; when this is supplied in slight excess, the mass action law often operates to benefit the infant who can later dispense with this prop.

In yet another gene-based deficiency, which affects one child in 500, cells which require cholesterol fail to produce the receptors to bind the LDL particles which ferry cholesterol in the bloodstream (p. 48) (Goldstein, Kite and Brown, 1983). Such children, particularly if homozygous, usually display coronary atherosclerosis by age ten, followed by death from myocardial infarction before age 20 (Harrison, 1983, p. 553).

For more on inborn errors of metabolism see Davidson and Passmore, 1986, pp. 346–51.

In prosperous communities, people who are both middle-aged and sedentary are prone to develop three metabolic disorders which can occur separately or in combination, and are often accompanied by obesity. The adverse states are diabetes, gout and hyperlipidaemia, which are denoted by abnormally high blood concentrations of glucose, uric acid and lipids respectively. A genetic factor has been demonstrated in each case, but their manifestation is accelerated by a rich diet. For further information see Davidson and Passmore (1986).

Intolerance to sodium chloride, apparently genetically-based and leading to increased blood-pressure, was referred to on p. 53.

Allergies

That certain wholesome foods can distress a small proportion of the population has long been known. As far back as the fifth century BC Hippocrates was describing the urticaria and gastric disturbance that he observed when susceptible people drank cows' milk. Today we define food allergy as any unpleasant reproducible response to a particular food when this is consumed in amounts that evoke no symptom in normal people. This adverse reaction is usually 'all-or-nothing' rather than proportional to the amount of the offending food consumed.

Allergic reactions depend on the union of an allergen, present in the food, with an immunoglobulin (antibody) in the victim. This is not the ordinary, infection-fighting immunoglobulin (IgG) that circulates in the blood, but a special one known as IgE which is located on the membranes of cells, particularly the mast cells*. This combination initiates a cascade of phosphorylations which sensitize these cells to further increments of the allergen. As a result, the mast cells rupture, and discharge their content of histamine and leucotrienes. Some individuals have a more plentiful stock of IgE than others, a tendency that is often inherited, although not necessarily directed toward the item of food that plagued the parent. The speed of the reaction, after consuming the sensitizing food, can vary from a few minutes to several days. Serum taken from a person undergoing an allergenic attack can raise a wheal in the skin of a normal volunteer.

The prevalence of food allergies is greatest in infancy, doubtless because of the immaturity of the baby's immune system. Most food allergies disappear spontaneously by the age of five but they may then (or much later) be replaced by allergy to pollen, dust or animal dander. The list of substances known to cause a food allergy is very large. In infants, milk, eggs and wheat proteins are the commonest, because these nutrients figure prominently in their diet. Infants who cannot tolerate cows' milk usually thrive on goats' milk. At any time after being weaned, a human being may develop allergies to one or more of the following: red meat, poultry, eggs, fish, crustaceans, molluscs, tomatoes, carrots, bananas, oranges, pineapple, strawberries, nuts, chocolate and countless other normally harmless foods. The allergen is either a protein or (less often) a substance that can become covalently bound to a protein.

The manifestations of food allergy may take any of the following forms: urticaria (nettle rash), asthma, abdominal cramps, vomiting or diarrhoea. In a few severe cases anaphylactic shock sets in with a catastrophic fall in blood

---

* Mast (from the German for *well-fed*) cells occur near the exterior of many human tissues. Their normal function is not well understood.

pressure, collapse, and sometimes death. This condition was often encountered when intravenous feeding made use of protein hydrolysates, but it is much rarer now that purified amino acids have replaced these.

Identification of the food that provokes the allergy can prove difficult. The patient often has a special liking for the food that so affects him and is reluctant to denounce it. Elimination diets, though tedious, are most informative, skin tests less. Treatment consists of eliminating the provoking food, at least for several years. It should be noted that many items (e.g. tomatoes) that are allergenic when taken raw, lose this property when cooked. Desensitization, by administering ever-increasing quantities of the offending food, has seldom proved effective. The patient can usually be helped through an attack with oral ephedrine (but not after 2 pm, as it may produce insomnia) or antihistaminics (those which cause sleepiness must be avoided by drivers). These two types of drugs are also effective for the inhalation-provoked allergies if rhinitis is the main symptom, whereas asthma is better handled with β-adrenergic agonists (e.g. terbutaline) or inhaled corticosteroids (e.g. beclomethasone), or a prophylactic such as sodium cromoglycate.

Much has still to be learnt about the allergenic process and a great deal of research funding is being directed towards it. Some authorities think that about 20% of all people suffer from an allergy at some period in their lives; this figure includes those susceptible to hay fever and other inhalation allergies including most cases of asthma.

Contrary to a popular belief, there is no indication that allergenic cases are on the increase. The basis for this belief seems to be that, in the past, speech was less exact. Thus earlier in this century people would say 'I like oysters but they don't like me'. Still earlier (according to a familiar rhyme) 'Jack Sprat would eat no fat, his wife would eat no lean' and, in the first century BC, Lucretius wrote 'Quod ali cibus est, aliis fiat acre venenum' (one man's meat is another man's poison). The true immunological basis of these happenings had escaped them all!

Coeliac disease (from the Greek *koilia* a cavity) is a malabsorption condition in children which sometimes persists into adult life. It is usually manifested by sensitivity to one of the constituent proteins of the gluten fraction of wheat and, in severe cases, to that of rye and barley also, whereas oats and polished rice are often well tolerated. Such persons suffer from diarrhoea, an irritable colon and malnutrition. Its prevalence for Caucasians has been put at 1 in 2000. On the other hand it is most uncommon in Africa. Such patients do well on a wheat-free diet, difficult though this is to maintain under usual working and social conditions. Coeliac disease, which tends to run in families, resembles an allergy but there seems also to be an inherited defect of the jejunum, namely too few villi. This defect prevents adequate absorption. Baker's eczema and baker's asthma, two well-known occupational diseases, are related to coeliac disease.

To learn how to cure an allergy is still one of medicine's most daunting problems, all the more forbidding if one adds in the autoimmune diseases such as arthritis and myasthenia which may be viewed as allergy to self. For further reading on allergy see Lessof (1984); Perlman (1980).

5.2 Enhancing the enjoyment of meals: herbs, spices and other additives

When we feel the promptings of hunger how easily we could deal with them by suddenly gulping some food, much as one refuels a car! However, to do so would fly in the face of one of man's oldest traditions. We have noted (Section 2.1) how keenly the nomadic tribes garnish their food with small additions of whatever is seasonable and decorative. This instinct finds expression in some of the most cherished dishes of our times. Thus, Vienna schnitzel (veal) always comes to table with its slice of lemon, roast lamb (in Australia) with garden mint, grilled steak (in Paris) with a spray of watercress and Canton duck with orange. These additions have no nutritive value, but their presence makes a familiar dish at once more attractive-looking and appetizing. There will be occasion, a little further on, to say much more about the strongly-entrenched custom of adding extraneous materials to food, before, during and after it is cooked, always with the aim of making the product more palatable.

How safe are additives?

The word 'additive' often gets a bad press, as though something sinister and inimical to good health surrounded these food-improvers. Yet the majority of food additives are flavouring agents of natural origin which, by improving the taste of food and bringing variety to disguise a considerable degree of monotony, might well receive a little praise. Medical statistics show that most people who fall ill with food poisoning owe this, not to any additive, but to bacterial contamination.

It is true that from time to time some undesirable additives are brought to light. An example is the attempt in North America to stabilize the foam on beer by adding cobaltous sulfate, a substance not toxic in itself but, as it turned out, one that caused cardiac damage in those who consumed it in large amounts of ethanol. The use of this additive was promptly terminated by the health authorities, in their steady watch for possibly injurious practices (Conning and Lansdown, 1983, p. 5).

Consumer protection

The consumer is protected in two ways against possible ill effects from commercial additives: at the national level by Pure Food Acts and their implementation through the courts, and at the international level by the Joint Expert Committee on Food Additives, operated by the Food and Agricultural Organization and the World Health Organization (FAO/WHO) (see p. 43 for the origins and locations of these bodies). The Joint Committee's annual reports of acceptance, rejection and permitted limits of additives have earned wide respect. A selection of their findings is in Table 5.1.

The umbrella of protection that shelters today's consumer began with the *Sale*

Table 5.1 Food additives: acceptable daily intake (ADI) for man (in mg/kg body weight)

Class	ADI	FAO/WHO Report No.	Date	WHO Technical Report series
Natural colourants				
Canthaxanthone	25.0	18	1974	557
Caramel	100.0	24	1980	653
Carmines	5.0	26	1982	683
β-Carotene	5.0	18	1974	557
Chlorophyll copper complex	15.0	22	1978	631
Curcumin	0.1	26	1982	683
Indigotin	5.0	18	1974	557
Turmeric	2.5	26	1982	683
Synthetic colourants				
Allura red	7.0	25	1981	669
Amaranth	0.5	28	1984	710
Azorubine	4.0	27	1983	696
Brilliant black RN	1.0	25	1981	669
Brown HT	1.5	28	1984	710
Erythrosine	1.25	28	1984	710
Fast green FCF	12.5	25	1981	669
Ponceau 4R	4.0	27	1983	696
Quinoline yellow	10.0	28	1984	710
Red 2G	0.1	25	1981	669
Sunset yellow	2.5	26	1982	683
Sweeteners				
Acesulfame	9.0	27	1983	696
Aspartame	40.0	25	1981	669
Cyclamates (Na, Ca)	11.0	26	1982	683
Mannitol	50.0	20	1976	599

(Sorbitol, lactitol and xylitol are classed as 'safe as commonly used'. Saccharin was temporarily accepted at 2.5 mg/kg in 28th Report)

Class	ADI	FAO/WHO Report No.	Date	WHO Technical Report series
Other flavourings				
Anethole	2.5	28	1984	710
Benzyl acetate	5.0	27	1983	696
Carvone	1.0	27	1983	696
Cinnamaldehyde	0.7	25	1981	669
Citral	0.5	23	1980	648
Eugenol	2.5	26	1982	683
Glutamates, additional to protein	120.0	25	1981	669
Ionones	0.1	28	1984	710
Linalool	0.5	23	1980	648
Menthol	0.2	20	1976	599
Methyl anthranilate	1.5	23	1980	648
Methyl N-methylanthranilate	0.2	23	1980	648
Nonanal	0.1	28	1984	710
Octanal	0.1	28	1984	710
Ethyl methylphenylglycidate	0.5	28	1984	710

Table 5.1   *(Contd.)*

Class	ADI	FAO/WHO Report No.	Date	WHO Technical Report series
Antioxidants				
Alkyl gallates (dodecyl, propyl, octyl)	0.2	24	1980	653
Anoxomer	8.0	28	1984	710
Butylated hydroxyanisole	0.5	27	1983	696
Butylated hydroxytoluene	0.5	27	1983	696
2-*tert*-Butylhydroquinone	0.75	19	1975	576
Other preservatives				
Benzoates (Na^+,Ca^{2+})	5.0	27	1983	696
p-Hydroxybenzoate esters (ethyl, methyl, propyl)	10.0	17	1974	539
Nitrites	0.4	23	1980	648
Metabisulfites (Na^+, Ca^{2+})	0.7	27	1983	696
Emulsifiers				
Sorbitan monolaureate	25.0	26	1982	683
Sorbitan monooleate	25.0	26	1982	683
Stearates of polyoxyethylene and of propylene glycol	25.0	17	1974	539
Sucrose esters	2.5	20	1976	599
Thickeners				
Ethyl cellulose	25.0	26	1982	683
Ethyl hydroxyethylcellulose	25.0	27	1983	696
Karaya gum	20.0	27	1983	696
Methyl cellulose	25.0	17	1974	539
Polyvinylpyrrolidone	25.0	27	1983	696

(Gum arabic, carob (locust) gum, pectins, and modified starches are classed as 'safe as commonly used'. Tragacanth is still under consideration).

Bleach (for flour)				
Potassium bromate (temporarily accepted)	—	27	1983	696

This table was compiled from the Reports of the Joint FAO/WHO Expert Committee on Food Additives, published by WHO in Geneva (Switzerland). For accidental additives (contaminants) introduced into foods see Section 12.

of Food and Drugs Act, passed in 1875 by the British Parliament. Thus began a worldwide struggle to free life-sustaining substances from the adulteration that was already rife in Classical Antiquity, hence the advice 'Caveat emptor' ('Let the buyer beware'). Two features ensured the success of this legislation, (a) the recent advances in chemical analysis, and (b) allocation of enforcement to local government authorities supported by teams of inspectors. The truly appalling state of affairs that this Act began to remedy can be visualized from an early nineteenth century account (Accum, 1820). There was widespread adulteration of bread, beer, wine, liquors, tea, coffee, cream, confectionery, vinegar, mustard, pepper, cheese, olive oil and pickles. Accum chronicles the frequent presence in food of lead, copper and mercury. The widespread occurrence of arsenic was not revealed until later in the century when methods for measuring it were discovered. Experience with this Act led to the stricter Food and Drugs Acts of 1938 and 1955, followed by the *Medicines Act* of 1968 and the *Foods Act* of 1984. This act is amplified by Regulations made under the Act, e.g. the Condensed and Dried Milk Regulations. The Act established the Foods Advisory Committee (1985) to collect and assess data and opinions from all affected parties. In turn, the Committee advises the Ministry of Agriculture, Fisheries and Food and the Department of Health and Social Security, who jointly draft the Regulations.

The pioneer act of 1875 eventually gave rise to parallel legislation in other countries. In the USA federal protection was made available for the first time by the *Food and Drugs Act* of 1906, which was replaced in 1938 by the more stringent *Federal Food, Drug and Cosmetic Act*. The latter set up a Food and Drug Administration (FDA), responsible to the Department of Health, Education and Welfare for the protection of public health. In 1958, the Food Additives Amendment put an onus on the manufacturer to prove the safety of all new additives before FDA can give a clearance. Once cleared, additives are entered on the GRAS (generally regarded as safe) list. If new evidence suggests that an entered substance may not be safe, it is removed (as happened to saccharin, the cyclamates and amaranth) although it may be restored if more searching tests establish its safety.

Many other countries have built up similar organizations to safeguard the wholesomeness of food. The overall picture, for the industrialized nations, is well put by Davidson and Passmore, 1986, p. 257:

'Consumers in the industrialized countries are protected by complicated systems involving government, manufacturers, advertisers and the media, and operating through statutory regulations and voluntary codes of practice . . . Consumers may be assured that the system protects them adequately against hazards to health which may arise from chemicals added to foods and from loss of nutrients in foods as a result of processing . . . It still remains true that the most frequent hazards to health arise not from additives or from processing but from poor hygiene and its associated microbiological risks, which can arise in shops, in restaurants, cafés and canteens in institutions and, all too frequently, in the home.'

Herbs and spices

Less conspicuous than the lemon, mint and watercress which illustrated our opening paragraph are the herbs and spices which add a still wider range of flavourings to our meals. With their assistance a single staple food can appear, day after day, in new and appetizing guises.

Herbs tend to be leafy products from temperate climes. Examples are thyme, basil, sage, origanum (marjoram), mint, parsley, rosemary. A few though are of subterranean origin: horseradish, garlic, onion. Spices tend to be of harder texture (seeds, bark, roots or dried fruits) and usually hail from the tropics. Typical spices are pepper, nutmeg, clove, cinnamon, coriander, caraway, cummin, turmeric, cardamon, chillies, ginger and vanilla. The various kinds of mustard are extracted from seeds whose pungent principles are glucosinolates (*4.4*). They are grown in both temperate and tropical zones and have an annual production of about 300 000 tonnes.

Many herbs and spices are carminative; just as they exert a tingling effect on the tongue, so do they stimulate the proximal portions of the gastrointestinal tract, thus helping to 'bring up wind'. They also promote peristalsis, a property that aids digestion. Where refrigeration is not available, spices help to preserve meat against bacterial spoilage.

Instead of using herbs and spices in this way (i.e. as gross plant material), an alternative approach has been to prepare an extract that contains and concentrates all of the aromatic substances for which these additives were valued. This refinement has produced such useful products as the essences of lemon, orange and vanilla, the tincture of capsicum, and the oils of clove, cinnamon, dill, aniseed and peppermint. When it was found that many essences depended for their aroma on a single constituent, it proved advantageous to have this in isolation, e.g. vanillin (*5.4*), from vanilla pods, cinnamic aldehyde from cinnamon bark, eugenol from clove buds, and anethole from fennel and aniseed. A further advance was to synthesize these fairly simple derivatives of benzene, thus ensuring an uninterrupted supply as well as a standard product of high purity. Thus very little vanilla flavouring now comes from the uncommon orchid, *Vanilla planifolia*, because it is more readily available by direct synthesis of vanillin.

Many of the most characteristic flavours of foods are present in only minute proportions. Thus, the total volatile odourants of a tomato measure only 3–5 ppm, and those of a banana 12–18 ppm. For a few, particularly powerful odourants, the nose can detect as little as 10^{-19} mol, which exceeds current analytical sensitivity (Lawrence, 1984). Many flavours that are delightful in low concentration can be obnoxious when dispensed with a heavy hand. Thus the oils of orange and peppermint, when suitably diluted, add character and interest to liqueurs and candies. But when the concentration is raised they become unbearable irritants of the gastrointestinal tract. The carminative dose lies between these extremes.

It does not follow that because a flavouring has its origin in nature it is free from harm to humans. In the past coumarin (*5.5*), from either tonka beans or sweet clover, was a close contender to vanillin for flavouring chocolate. However by the middle of the present century coumarin became banned from human food following observation of hepatoxicity in rats (Food Standards Committee, 1965). Again, large doses of apiole (*5.6*), the characteristic flavouring principle of parsley, have caused haemolytic anaemia, thrombocytopenia purpurea, neph-rosis and hepatic dysfunction (Lowenstein and Ballew, 1958). This is not a caution against the use of parsley as a garnish, but a warning against excess.

Nutmeg, whose active principle is myristicin (*5.7a*), is a deservedly popular spice. However in small excess myristicin induces stupor and (if intake is continued) some hallucination. In the English-speaking countries it was formerly used as a topping for two items of food much loved by children: junket (coagulated milk) and malted milk (a long drink). From about the middle of this century medical advice discouraged use of this seemingly innocent quieting agent (cf. spinach, p. 60). A related substance, safrole (*5.7b*), occurs in many essential oils that have been used in flavouring: star anise oil, oil of camphor, cinnamon leaf oil, oil of mace, California bay laurel oil and in ginger. It is the main constituent of sassafras oil, which was frequently used to flavour soft drinks. However since the 1960s safrole has come under a ban because it causes liver cancer in rats. The actual carcinogen seems to be a metabolic product: 1′-hydroxysafrole (*5.8*) or its 2′,3′-oxide (*5.9*) (Wislocki, *et al.*, 1977).

Another banned natural flavouring is thujone (*5.10*), the main constituent of a once-popular, stupefying (in excess, convulsing) drink known as absinth which was made from *Artemesia absintha* (wormwood).

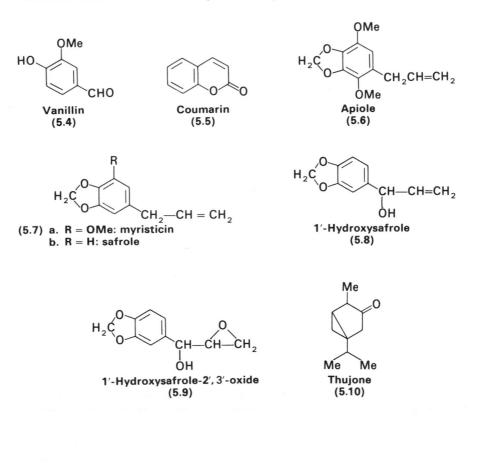

Vanillin
(5.4)

Coumarin
(5.5)

Apiole
(5.6)

(5.7) a. R = OMe: myristicin
b. R = H: safrole

1′-Hydroxysafrole
(5.8)

1′-Hydroxysafrole-2′, 3′-oxide
(5.9)

Thujone
(5.10)

Salt

Common salt has been widely used to preserve meat and fish for at least the last 3000 years. In proportion as refrigeration became available in the industrialized countries, the need for salting disappeared, but the taste for salted food remained! The connexion between salt intake and hypertension was discussed on p. 53.

Are additives really necessary?

Most diners think so! Often within their reach you will observe salt, pepper, vinegar, mustard, sugar and a couple of sauces. Purists say 'These should be in the cooking', but that policy hardly allows for individual preferences.

The leisured cook works in the kitchen with a wider range of additives than this, and can display much skill in turning each initially insipid dish into one that earns the family's plaudits. In the English-speaking countries not only the diners' favourites listed above are ready to be added, to taste, but also yeast, chicken or beef extracts, lemon juice, mushroom sauce, grated cheese, onion, garlic and many of the herbs and spices listed on p. 82. Dishes can also be extended with thickeners such as flour, cornflour, gelatin and agar. Apart from all these additives, there are the hundreds of new chemical substances introduced by the act of cooking (p. 58). Cooks in other countries work to different, but equally long, lists of additives.

Unhappily all domestic cooks are not leisured. Economic or social pressures make many depend, at least in part, on convenience foods, factory-prepared in large batches. The factory chefs have access to a wider range of additives, most of them flavourings of natural origin*. In our crowded world, there is no longer enough prime quality food to go around, not even in the better-off nations. Additives help people consume with pleasure that large fraction of the crop that would otherwise be rejected as spoilt, insipid or even unpalatable. Without additives a large percentage of our food would seem tasteless, odourless, discoloured or simply under-ripe, and it would spoil fast. The following are the principal kinds of additives needed in food processing: Flavouring agents (mainly), colourings, emulsifiers and thickeners, preservatives against oxidation or the attacks of moulds and bacteria.

Colourants

Investigative and legislative control of the substances used for colouring foods is strongly enforced in the industrialized countries. In addition carcinogenicity testing in rats is regularly performed by the British Industrial Biological Research Association and the US Food and Drugs Administration.

---

* The legally-imposed labelling 'artificially flavoured' means that a flavouring (almost always one of natural origin) has been added to the food; it does not mean that an artificial flavour has been added.

Let us now review the FAO/WHO lists of permitted food colourants, assembled in Table 5.1. It is evident that those manufacturers who wish to label their products: 'Only natural colourants used' must work from a very short list, because many of nature's glowing and appetizing colours have little permanence outside the living cell. Chlorophyll, which looks perfectly appealing in a lettuce leaf, when isolated turns out to be pale, waxy and of curious odour. These problems disappear when its colour is intensified by complexation with copper (restaurateurs have long practised the art of popping a copper coin into the boiling greens); but is it then a natural colourant (although a harmless one)?

A workable number of synthetic colourants are available (Table 5.1), all of them certified as harmless. The safety, at least for rats, of the traditional red colourant amaranth was queried in Russia, where great care is accorded all that is krasnii (Shtenberg and Gavrilenko, 1970). It was removed from the FAO/WHO lists for a thorough investigation. However this showed that it posed no threat to humans, and hence it was restored to the lists (Lansdown, 1983). The yellow dye tartrazine was excluded from the FAO/WHO lists because, in a small fraction of the human population, it provoked urticaria, asthma or intestinal spasm. As with intolerance to benzoate and salicylate, this is not an allergic phenomenon because it is unrelated to serum IgE (Conning and Lansdown, 1983, pp. 57–61). Hyperactive children, claimed by Feingold (1975) to grow steadily calmer on a diet that excluded artificial colourants, flavours, and salicylates, were found to exhibit an equal response to placebos (defined on p. 154) (Conning and Lansdown, 1983, p. 12; Anon., 1979).

Sweeteners

No other additives seem to have created so much controversy, both scientific and public, as the artificial (non-nutritive) sweeteners. Briefly their history is that saccharin (*5.11*) was introduced about 90 years ago so that diabetics could enjoy a sweet taste in their food from which sugars were necessarily excluded. In spite of early concern that saccharin might have some long-term toxic effect, none was found. In the 1930s sodium cyclamate (*5.12*) was introduced as an alternative. Although less than half as sweet as saccharin (but many times sweeter than sucrose), sodium and calcium cyclamate showed two advantages: they lacked the bitter aftertaste of saccharin and they were not destroyed by heat so that diabetics could now enjoy sweet cooked foods for the first time.

In the 1950s, another use was found for these sweeteners: they were adopted by dieters struggling with their obesity. Hence many 'low calorie' drinks appeared on the market and found ready acceptance; sales of sucrose began to suffer.

In 1970, much concern was generated by a paper which found that mixture of saccharin and sodium cyclamate produced a high incidence of bladder tumours in rats (Price, *et al.*, 1970). However, it was found that sodium cyclamate on its own had no long-term effect on rats (Brantom, Gaunt and Grasso, 1973). By 1979 it was established that saccharin on its own, in doses equivalent to 700 times the usual human intake, could produce cancer of the bladder in rats (Chowaniec and Hicks, 1979). Further, when rats were exposed to saccharin *in utero* and then throughout their lives, the likelihood of developing bladder tumours was greater than in controls (IARC, 1980). These results led to the banning of saccharin in Canada, and to impassioned debates (but no banning) in the USA and Great Britain. Meanwhile, but none too logically, cyclamates were banned in both these countries.

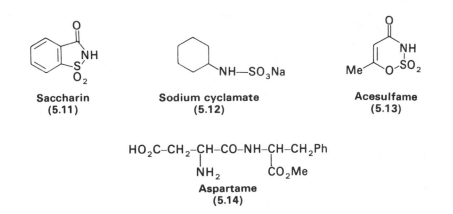

Saccharin	**Sodium cyclamate**	**Acesulfame**
(5.11)	**(5.12)**	**(5.13)**

$$HO_2C-CH_2-CH-CO-NH-CH-CH_2Ph$$

Aspartame
(5.14)

There is a well-recognized uncertainty in extrapolating to human beings from results obtained in rats (p. 288), particularly results obtained with such gross overdoses. Fortunately, the suspected substances had been in use by a great many people for many years; hence it was possible to settle the issue by epidemiological studies of the retrospective type (p. 288). A study of 3010 patients with bladder cancer and of 5783 healthy people revealed that the relative risk of developing bladder cancer was similar in users and non-users of these two artificial sweeteners (National Cancer Institute, 1979; Hoover and Strasser, 1980). Two similar studies confirmed that people are at no risk from these sweeteners (Morrison and Buring, 1980; Wynder and Stellman, 1980). The current position is that the cyclamates, after careful consideration of all evidence, have been restored to the FAO/WHO list of permitted additives, and saccharin is provisionally accepted (Table 5.1). For further reading on these sweeteners see Roberts (1981, pp. 264–70); Grasso (1983).

Meanwhile aspartame (*5.14*), which is a methyl ether of the dipeptide aspartylphenylalanine and is said to be 200 times sweeter than sucrose, was authorized for public use by regulatory bodies in most of the industrialized countries. Aspartame survives neither acidity nor cooking, two deficiencies that limit its use. Acesulfame (*5.13*), whose structure resembles that of saccharin, is accepted by the FAO/WHO Additives Committee. Among sweeteners likely to gain acceptance are the polychlorodeoxysucroses, up to 2200 times sweeter than sucrose and stable to heat (Hough, 1985). The plant glycoside, stevioside, 300 times sweeter than sucrose, is also attracting attention.

Non-nutritive sweeteners are seen as competitors of sucrose by growers and refiners of that disaccharide. Sugar cane has been cultivated in SE Asia for more than 2000 years (Heiser, 1981). The consumption of sucrose in England and North America increased enormously during the Industrial Revolution but has fallen steadily since 1958. Whether derived from cane or from the more recently introduced beet, white crystalline sucrose is the purest food available anywhere in the world and, if consumed in moderation, causes no harm to man (p. 47). A sugar lobby exists to point out disadvantages in the rival products and to persuade consumers to eat more sugar. Sugar farmers face losses from several sources: from dentists' warnings against caries (p. 47), from Government-level health advice to consume less sugar and more starch (p. 47), and from the replacement of sugar by artificial sweeteners (in dentifrices and by 'weight-watchers').

These weight-watchers claim that in the absence of these sweeteners they would lose one quarter of their taste-pleasures, because physiology has shown that we have only four tastes – salt, bitter, sour and sweet. Actually, they have even more at stake, because much pleasure depends on interplay between the four variables, a richness that is greatly diminished when one of them is missing.

Other flavourings

Looking in Table 5.1, we see that every item has a natural origin, such as eugenol from oil of cloves. This is indeed a conservative choice. Information on what substances give the various fruits, vegetables and other foods their characteristic flavours may be found in *'Fenaroli's Handbook of Flavor Ingredients'* (Furia and Bellanca, 1975) and in such periodicals as the *Journal of Food Science* and the *Journal of the American Oil Chemists Society*.

Of the meat- and yeast-like flavours, glutamic acid (as its monosodium salt MSG) has captured most public attention. Its over-consumption can lead to unpleasant, though harmless, symptoms (p. 63). The FAO/WHO Expert Committee has determined that 8.4 g (in addition to what he receives from digestion of his dietary protein) daily is harmless for a 70 kg man. The US Code of Federal Regulations (1979) recognizes MSG as a harmless condiment along with pepper, salt and vinegar. The former practice of including MSG in infants' foods was discontinued after representations from the US FDA concerning possible brain damage before the protective membranes have been formed at about 6 months (Federation of American Societies for Experimental Biology, 1978b). Disodium inosate and disodium guanylate are used as yeast-like flavours. For further reading on MSG see Davidson and Passmore, 1986, p. 250; Roberts, 1981, pp. 97, 248–9; Conning and Lansdown, 1983, pp. 11, 98.

Antioxidants

Fats and foods rich in lipids deteriorate on storage because of chain reactions (p. 71). These reactions can be inhibited by adding very small proportions of such antioxidants as 'butylated hydroxytoluene' (*5.15*), butylated hydroxyanisole or propyl gallate (*5.16*). These prevent the oxidation of lipids that leads to rancidity and other unacceptable flavours, and to the destruction of linolenic acid and the oil-soluble vitamins. FDA regulations limit the total of antioxidants to 0.02% for fats. These antioxidants are classified as GRAS (Generally Regarded as Safe) by FDA, and have also been cleared by the Carcinogenesis Program of the US National Cancer Institute. Some fats and oils are self-preserving through their content of tocopherols or steroids.

Ascorbic acid is much used as an additive to prevent oxidative browning in the processing of fruits and vegetables. The annual production of this vitamin is 40 million pounds (18 000 tonnes), and is valued at $400 million; canning accounts for a high proportion of this output.

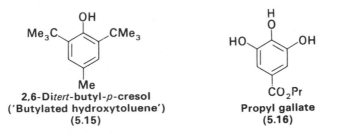

2,6-Di*tert*-butyl-*p*-cresol
('Butylated hydroxytoluene')
(5.15)

Propyl gallate
(5.16)

Other preservatives

Through the centuries, effective use has been made of the food-preserving effects of salt, saltpetre (KNO_3), acetic acid (as vinegar), boric acid and sulfur dioxide (as such or as sodium metabisulfite). Of these, only boric acid has been completely dropped (it has caused death by circulatory collapse). Today sodium benzoate and metabisulfite are the most used preservatives, and are prominent in the FAO/WHO List (Table 5.1). Benzoic acid which is a constituent of berry fruits has a long record of innocuousness. Unfortunately, a small but significant proportion of the population is sensitive to either benzoic acid or sulfur dioxide, which is why these preservatives have to be declared on the label in most countries.

The *p*-hydroxybenzoic esters have been found to be safe and efficient preventers of the growth of moulds in many kinds of food. Calcium propionate is much used in breadmaking to protect against growth of moulds. In Britain, the addition of antimicrobials to food is closely controlled by the Preservatives in Food Regulations Act of 1979 (SI 1979, No. 752) as amended (SI 1980, No. 931, and SI 1982, No. 15). In the USA, the corresponding statutory control is exerted by the Food and Drugs Authority which acts on advice from SCOGS (the Select Committee on GRAS substances (p. 82) of the Federation of American Societies for Experimental Biology).

Quite the most controversial preservative in use at the present time is sodium nitrate, which is much employed in the curing of meats, fish and poultry for sale in delicatessens small goods shops, and charcuteries. An important feature of its use is the trace of sodium nitrite produced by the reducing action of the meat. The nitrite is valued for two reasons, (a) it inhibits *Clostridium botulinum*, an anaerobic bacterium which greatly favours such flesh and whose toxin has often killed whole communities who feasted on infected food, and (b) the meat assumes a customer-pleasing pink appearance instead of turning the usual dark grey. A few processors choose to add the nitrite directly; in either case the FAO/WHO schedule limits the proportion present (Table 5.1).

We have already discussed the concentration, by some vegetables, of nitrate from soils rich in this anion, the risk of its easy reduction to nitrite by infants under 4 months, and its general harmlessness to the average adult (p. 60). The likely human intake from cured meats has been put at 1–2 mg a day, although this must vary from community to community (White, 1976). The first steps to reduce the nitrite content of food were prompted by the occasional appearance of a nitrosamine in cooked bacon, and the suspicion that this nitrosamine, or nitrite itself could be carcinogenic.

We noted (p. 60) that the normal adult does not convert nitrate to nitrite in his stomach, because the low pH prevents the growth of nitrate-reducing bacteria. However these bacteria tend to grow freely in the upper gastrointestinal tract of those individuals who suffer from *achlorhydria*. This numerous segment of the population is made up of three strands, (a) the elderly who have lost their oxyntic cells, (b) those who have undergone gastrectomy, and (c) those with chronic atrophic gastritis, a condition often caused by excess intake of ethanol.

Swallowed nitrate is recycled through the salivary glands, more so in some subjects than in others. This oral nitrate is, in many individuals, partly reduced to nitrite by organisms living in the mouth. In such people, salivary nitrite concentration can reach several hundred milligrams per litre after nitrate-rich foods are eaten (Walters, *et al.*, 1979).

Only 4 nitrosamines have been found in food: nitrosopyrrolidine, nitrosopiperidine, diethylnitrosamine and (principally) dimethylnitrosamine (Crosby, *et al.*, 1972). Analyses carried out by the International Agency for Research on Cancer (Lyon, France) found up to 80 ppb of dimethylnitrosamine in nitrate-preserved meat and up to 180 ppb in nitrate-preserved fish (IARC, 1978). Nitrosamines commonly occur in the faeces of healthy human beings (Wang, *et al.*, 1978).

Many types of nitrosamine have been tested in a wide range of laboratory animals and found, after initially producing liver damage, to give rise to malignant tumors (Druckrey, *et al.*, 1967; Magee, 1971). This high incidence of cancer, induced at low doses of nitrosamines, suggests that a hazard may exist for man, not only from the nitrosamines that he consumes in processed foods, but also from any that he may synthesize in the stomach.

When nitrous acid produces a nitrosamine by reaction with a secondary amine, the nitrosating agent is nitrous anhydride (N_2O_3) at any pH from 0 upwards. The amine being nitrosated reacts faster in the molecular (non-ionized) condition than when ionized (Sander, Schweinsberg and Menz, 1968). Thus weak bases are much more susceptible to nitrosation than strong ones. Examples of such weak bases would be diphenylamine (pK_a 0.79) and N-methylaniline (pK_a 4.85). Fortunately, such weak amines are seldom present in the human stomach which receives stronger ones (pK_a 8–10) in food by the deamination of amino acids, and as medicinal substances.

Laboratory results, such as those abstracted above, have suggested links, for man, between cancer on the one hand and nitrate, nitrite and/or nitrosamines on the other. However, only epidemiological studies (p. 288) can test the significance of each hypothesis for the human situation. As a start, it has been shown that populations (as in China) that experience a high incidence of gastric cancer do not have unusually high exposure to nitrates; alternatively, populations exposed to excess of nitrate (as in fertilizer works) do not have an increased tendency to gastric cancer (Forman, Al-Dabbagh and Doll, 1985). Neither conclusion implies that nitrate-intake plays no role in the generation of cancer, but only that it is not the limiting factor. It should be kept in mind that both gastric and primary (i.e. non-metastatic) liver cancers are relatively uncommon in Europe and the USA, and rapidly disappearing in Japan. Further epidemiological surveys are under way to test alternative hypotheses. Meanwhile the significance of nitrate, nitrite and nitrosamines for the causation of human cancer remains unclear, and affords no basis for immediate, drastic legislation. To sum up: three sectors of the community may be most at risk (a) those consuming high concentrations of nitrate in food or drinking water, (b) those who have ceased secreting HCl in the stomach, and (c) those who produce high concentrations of nitrate in their saliva. For the others, that is to say: for the great majority of people, the risk is generally assessed as small. For further reading, see Rowland and Walker 1983, pp. 242–46; Forman, Al-Dabbagh and Doll, (1985); Tannenbaum and Correa (1985); Gibson and Ioannides (1981).

Emulsifiers and suspension-stabilizers

These useful substances enable one phase (such as oil) to remain finely dispersed in another (such as water). They are controlled in Britain by the Emulsifiers and Stabilizers in Food Regulations of 1980 (as amended in 1982), and are similarly supervised in other industrialized countries.

Is irradiated food wholesome?

The use of ionizing radiation offers an alternative method of preservation in food storage and processing. The usual sources, ^{60}Co and ^{137}Cs, have been found to cause no induced radioactivity. A low dosage (up to 1 kGy*) inhibits sprouting of grains, kills insects and delays over-ripening; a medium dosage (1–10 kGy) reduces the microbial count; and higher dosages are not authorized. It was concluded that, 'Irradiation of any food commodity up to an overall average of 10 kGy presents no toxicological hazard' (FAO, 1981). In 1985, the US FDA allowed pork to be treated with gamma radiation to control the tapeworm, *Trichinella spiralis*; it is expected that more uses will soon be sanctioned.

Some quantitative aspects of additives

Of all the additives used in the USA, 93% (by weight) consist of four traditional ingredients: sucrose, glucose, corn syrup and salt. Together these provide 127 lb (56 kg) of total additives, annually (Larkin, 1976). Another 3 lb each year is made up of the following eight ingredients: carbon dioxide, sodium bicarbonate, caramel, citric acid, mustard, pepper, starches and yeast. Only 7 lb is contributed by the other 2800 (approx.) permitted additives, which are mainly spices, flavours, emulsifiers and extenders (Roberts, 1981, pp. 242–46).

Further reading

Food Safety (Roberts, 1981)
Xenobiotics in Foods and Feeds (Finley and Schwass, 1983)
Martindale, the Extra Pharmacopoeia (Reynolds, 1982) pp. 370–79 for emulsifiers, 423–33 for colouring, flavouring and sweetening agents; 1281–93 for pre-servatives and antioxidants
Handbook of Food Additives (Furia, 1979–80).

Follow-up

Make a small survey of ten people. Choose them from widely different walks in life, and ask them what they understand by the words 'food additives'. Then ask how they regard the presence of these substances in what they eat, and where they find information on additives.

5.3 Enhancement of mood at table

Meals seem to go more pleasantly when consumed in good company. This elevation of mood is relished particularly when economic or geographical conditions furnish only monotonous, or even quite unpalatable, food. If this observation seems close to a psychological interpretation, let us keep on solid ground by discussing three quite material euphoriants that often accompany eating: carbohydrates, ethanol and caffeine.

---

*1 Gy (Gray) equals 100 rads (old nomenclature) and is a measure of radiation.

Carbohydrates

It has been well said that 'Food is without doubt the oldest and most widely used tranquillizer' (Brobeck, 1960). Yet this relationship depends on the nature of the food. When 184 normal adult subjects were tested for mood and performance, greater relaxation, even sleepiness, was reported after a high carbohydrate, than after a high protein, meal (Spring, *et al.*, 1983). This effect was attributed to the carbohydrate-induced release of insulin and the linked increase of tryptophan level in the serum. In rats, it has been found that this amino acid penetrates into the brain where it is acted on by tryptophan-5-hydroxylase; the product is then decarboxylated to 5-hydroxytryptamine (serotonin). Protein meals are also accompanied by tryptophan release, but they furnish other neutral amino acids that compete with tryptophan for uptake into the brain, which consequently receives little serotonin (Fernstrom and Wurtman, 1972).

The calming and euphoric effects of serotonin in the brain are well established, and a whole series of antidepressant drugs acts by inhibiting the re-uptake of serotonin when this neurotransmitter is released from synaptic terminals in the brain (Iversen, 1985). The turnover time of serotonin in the brain is quite short – about one hour.

The following observations seemingly linked to the above may repay closer study. Depressed people tend to elevate their mood by excessive recourse to carbohydrates (Wurtman, *et al.*, 1985). The effect appears sooner when the ingested carbohydrate is a soluble one. The Koran, sacred book of the Muslim faith, forbids the taking of ethanol; in its place a sherbet (highly sweetened fruit drink) is offered in hospitality. The children of most countries, once they have tasted sucrose, tend to crave it and are noticeably pacified after some has been consumed!

Ethanol

We have discussed ethanol as a food (Section 3.1) and shall later note how it functions as a medicine (p. 63) and as an habituating poison (p. 307). Here we note a low-dose use of this substance, namely to add to the jollity of the repast. Early tribal groups in many parts of the world (although not in Australia, North America or Oceania) learnt how to produce ethanolic drinks and formulated rules limiting their use. Early civilizations insisted on strict moderation in drinking (e.g. in ancient Greece, Egypt, Mesopotamia).

Ethanol, most unusually for a substance taken orally, is rapidly absorbed through the lining membranes of the mouth, oesophagus and stomach. At blood alcohol levels of 30 mg/dl (0.03%) a mild euphoria is usually experienced, but at 50 mg/dl some uncoordination tends to set in; at 100 mg/dl ataxia is noticeable and the diner often upsets his chair on rising; at 200 mg/dl the subject is drowsy and confused (Miles, 1922). The blood alcohol level seen after ingesting a certain amount of an ethanolic beverage is approximately twice as high if it is taken before rather than during the meal. A chronic alcoholic subject often requires higher blood levels of ethanol to display these characteristics.

In general it cannot be denied that the partaking of ethanol with meals has been appreciated by many civilized men as a valued social agent that promotes good fellowship. Both men and women 'come out of themselves' and act more sociably. Moreover in moderation ethanol promotes appetite. However even the moderate use of ethanol impairs judgment and the attendant euphoria usually prevents the subject from appreciating his loss. Because the consumption of ethanol can be specially dangerous for motorists the driver's blood level is, in a great many countries, subject to legal control (p. 310).

Caffeine

Although they are often taken with sugar, and sometimes with milk or cream as well, caffeinaceous drinks have of themselves no food value and are consumed exclusively for the stimulating effect of the caffeine that they contain. It is revealing that these outright medicines have now found a place at the meal table. Prehistorians report that paleolithic man, in many regions of the world, made use of caffeinaceous plants. Of these tea and coffee are the most used today, although 20 million South Americans are said still to drink maté. Tea, from *Camellia sinensis*, has been drunk in China for over 2000 years but it came to be used in Europe (at first only as a luxury) in the seventeenth century. Coffee, from *Coffea arabica* (a native of Ethiopia), developed more slowly for it required the discovery of first a fermentation process to liberate the beans from their tight, scarlet capsule, and second, the roasting process to impart aroma. Used by Arabic people for perhaps only the last 500 years, it was later taken up by Europeans, at first hesitatingly.

Today, an average cup of coffee contains about 90 mg of caffeine (*5.17*), whereas a cup of tea is likely to have about 50 mg of caffeine and 1 mg of theophylline. A 360 ml bottle of cola drink has about 50 mg of caffeine of which about half may come from cola seeds (*Cola nitida*, a native of West Africa now thriving in Jamaica) and the rest is derived from the manufacture of decaffeinated coffee. Not more than 5 mg of caffeine is likely to be present in a cup of cocoa whose principal methylxanthine, theobromine, has little pharmacological action.

After consuming a caffeinaceous drink, people usually experience less drowsiness, less fatigue, and a rapider and clearer flow of thought. There is an increased capacity for intellectual effort but some mental and physical skills are decreased. The stimulating effect of caffeine is bought at the expense of subsequent tiredness usually relieved by taking another cup. Apart from this food-like use of caffeine, it also exhibits medicinal (p. 165) and poisonous (p. 305) properties, thus illustrating all three aspects of the Paracelsian doctrine.

At the molecular level the stimulating effects of caffeine seem to arise from its blockade of adenosine receptors (Daly, Brons and Snyder, 1981). Caffeine also inhibits the action of phosphodiesterase but at concentrations not usually achieved by the coffee drinker. For more on the caffeine-containing drinks and the pharmacology of methylxanthines see Rall (1985).

Investigations into possible deleterious effects of caffeine have recently been concentrated on whether or not it causes birth defects, a teratological project. Retrospective study of 14 000 human mothers found no association, between intake of caffeine and abnormalities in offspring (Federation of American Societies for Experimental Biology, 1978a). These investigators found also no teratogenic effects from caffeine in laboratory animals in doses of 50 mg/kg body weight, the equivalent of 130 cups of coffee daily for a woman of average weight. Other retrospective studies showed that coffee even in a large daily dose is not a factor in developing coronary thrombosis, as had been speculated.

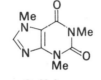

Caffeine
(1, 3, 7-Trimethylxanthine)
(5.17)

What gives the different commercial types of coffee their characteristic aromas? The roasting process causes extensive pyrolysis that forms some 500 new substances most of them of unknown toxicity. They have been isolated in small amounts by gas chromatography and identified by mass spectra. They include several thiophenes, thiazoles, oxazoles, furans, pyrroles, pyridines, quinolines, quinoxalines and indoles. More recently investigators have isolated a family of seventeen odoriferous cyclopentano- and cyclohexano- pyrazines (Walter and Weidemann, 1969; Vitzthum and Werkhoff (1974, 1975). A list of about 450 of these pyrolytic products can be seen in Furia and Bellanca (1975).

Drugs

'I have called this principle, by which each slight variation, if useful, is preserved, by the term of Natural Selection'. (Charles Darwin, in Chapter 3 of *The Origin of Species*)

6

Introduction to Part Two: Drugs as foreign substances

In this book, the word 'drugs' is used interchangeably with 'medicines', 'medicaments' and 'remedies'. A certain overlap exists between what is popularly considered to be a drug and what a food. For example caffeine (as in tea or coffee), although indisputably a drug (Section 5.3), tends to be regarded as a food because it is commonly consumed with food. Conversely, all sorts of medicinal properties are popularly attributed to particular foods. In the medicine of tradition and folklore, foods and drugs tend to merge, as exemplified by the saying: 'An apple a day keeps the doctor away'.

Clinical medicine makes much use of what are called 'diets of omission' in conjunction with specific drugs. An example is the low carbohydrate diet prescribed in diabetes. Special diets are adding to the life-span of millions of sufferers from coronary disease. In Sections 4.1 and 5.1 will be found indications for dietary plans for several other constitutional disorders.

In passing we may note the short-lived 'fashion diets', of popular origin. Such a one was the 'weight-watchers grapefruit diet' of the early 1980s. An earlier one, 'the glucose supplement' began in the 1920s with a claim that it was healthier to eat glucose than sucrose, and that the former provided quicker and greater energy. (Glucose was also more expensive). Research soon showed that these claims were untrue. Sucrose gives more energy per gram than glucose, and the slower absorption of the fructose half of the molecule (liberated by almost instantaneous digestion) puts far less strain on the eater's metabolism (p. 24); the other half of the molecule is of course glucose!

In spite of a limited area of overlap, foods and drugs constitute two distinct classes of xenobiotic, for the following reasons:

1. Foods have to be taken daily to furnish energy and to supply the building blocks for growth and repair whereas medicines are used to treat an illness, are needed only so long as that illness persists and contribute nothing to energy, growth or repair.
2. The metabolism of foods and that of drugs proceed by two very different biochemical pathways. Chapter 7 explains what happens to a drug, from the moment of its ingestion to the final act of its excretion.

How drugs are named in this book

Generic names are used and of these preference is given to INN names, that is the International Non-Proprietary Names issued by the World Health Organization after consultations with member Nations. In Appendix II help is provided for searching the literature to locate more drugs than are mentioned in this book, together with their formulae, names and physical and chemical properties.

Further reading

Foods and Drugs, Interactions, Toxicology and Safety (Basu and Stiles, 1985).

6.1 The three classes of drugs currently used in therapy: some useful definitions

So that living cells can perform efficiently a set of small molecules has evolved during the several thousand million years of evolution. These are naturally-occurring agonists, a word derived from the Ancient Greek for participants in games. In conjunction with much larger molecules (their complementary biopolymers), these agonists control the cell's nutrition, growth, repair and reproduction. The principal types are the vitamins (often seen working as coenzymes), the hormones and neurotransmitters, the inorganic ions, the photosynthetic and respiratory pigments, the metabolic fragments derived from food (e.g. acetyl residues), the purine and pyrimidine bases of nucleic acid and that most remarkable storer of the cell's energy adenosine triphosphate.

There are three kinds of drugs currently used by man: (a) the naturally-occurring agonists, (b) some man-made agonists, and (c) a great many man-made antagonists. The naturally-occurring agonists are used only in replacement therapy, to restore supplies of vitamins, minerals or hormones lost by depletion. Examples are the use of folic acid and calcium in pregnancy and of thyroxine in hypothyroidism. Man-made agonists are those based on the natural agonists but with molecules subtly altered to obtain a more prolonged action, e.g. by slowing elimination or destruction. They are usually based on hormones or neurotransmitters. An example is provided by methacholine (*6.1*) whose extra methyl group makes it a poorer substrate for acetylcholinesterase. Hence its action persists in the human body much longer than that of the neurotransmitter,

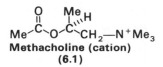

Methacholine (cation)
(6.1)

Acetylcholine (cation)
(6.2)

acetylcholine (*6.2*). However, the majority of man-made drugs are antagonists which are essentially inhibitors of natural agonists.

Antagonists are designed (a) to eliminate invading organisms, or (b) to suppress pain, or (c) to restore normality in one of those biochemically-unbalanced states typical of the sick body. All antagonists are by their nature toxic (poisonous). However, provided that their toxicity is selective, this is their most valuable property. In short, antagonists can enlist toxicity in the service of man. Naturally toxicity in a drug is valuable only when it is selective. Chapter 9 describes how selectivity is introduced into the design of a new drug molecule.

What is *selectivity*? A drug is selective if it can influence one kind of living cell without affecting others even when these cells are close neighbours. Selectively toxic effects can be either reversible or permanent, just as desired. It is convenient, when discussing selective toxicity, to distinguish between economic and uneconomic cells. The economic cells are those that should remain completely unaffected by the drug, whereas the uneconomic cells are those on which the drug has to exert its effect, whether only temporarily (as in producing anaesthesia) or permanently (as in killing bacteria).

Pharmacology, that branch of science which studies the action of drugs, is divided into chemotherapy and pharmacodynamics. In chemotherapy, the aim is to kill all the uneconomic cells, which are usually parasites invading their host, man. The term is extended to include the drug-treatment of cancer. Pharmacodynamics deals with the opposite situation where the uneconomic and economic cells are part of the same organism (man) but the drug-affected uneconomic cells must eventually be restored to normal.

Many 'stimulants' which were once thought to be agonists have been found on scientific examination to be antagonists. Thus ethanol damps down inhibitory nerves in the central nervous system so that the related excitatory nerves escape from normal balance. Strychnine, strongest of the known convulsants, is similarly a blocker of inhibitory nerves and hence, like ethanol, an antagonist.

The selective use of toxicity is excellently illustrated by general anaesthetics which suppress all feelings of pain by exerting a toxic action on the central nervous system. The more toxic an anaesthetic is the more it is valued, provided that it is (a) selective for the central nervous system only and (b) completely reversible in a short time. Morton's introduction of ether as a general anaesthetic in 1846 was an early and convincing demonstration of the power and possibilities of selective toxicity. When almost a century later muscle relaxants were introduced to enable surgeons to operate with lighter anaesthetics both types of drug underwent further refinement to reach the highest degree of selectivity.

Most of man's currently used drugs are synthetic and of low molecular weight (usually under 500). However a few (principally antibiotics)* are of natural origin. Also several vaccines are used as prophylactics against certain bacterial and viral infections: the active principle is usually a protein of molecular weight well over 100 000. New immunological agents of this kind are becoming harder to discover but their specificity is remarkable.

How much medication is being practised? The following figures relate to the pure drugs (synthetic and antibiotic, but not herbal) consumed by the whole world in 1982. The total was estimated as 214 million kg. Of this the USA consumed 34%, Western Europe 32%, Japan 4% and the rest of the world 30% (the respective populations were 228, 336, 117 and 4120 million) (Anon., 1985a).

In industrialized countries, about half of this usage took place in hospitals (by both in- and out- patients) and in the home as the result of physicians' prescribing. The other half was consumed as over-the-counter (OTC) remedies for minor ailments, which were purchased on the initiative of the patient or of his advising pharmacist.

How do people react when they realize they have developed a medical problem? A survey of such responses was made by the US Proprietary Association and reported by their President at the 21st Meeting of the European Proprietary Association in Munich, May 1985. Replies from 1500 people over the age of 12 disclosed an average of nine health problems a month. Only for 9% of the problems was a physician consulted and slightly more than a third were tolerated without recourse to medication. However about one third were treated with OTC remedies quite satisfactorily but the remainder unsatisfactorily. Delegates from other lands thought that these figures might roughly represent the situation in their countries, too (Cope, 1985).

For a major newly-discovered drug to traverse the uncertain path from discovery in the laboratory to being regularly prescribed takes something like ten to twelve years. The cost of finding, developing, and marketing a new drug, taking into account all the unsuccessful early approaches, has been estimated at about £90 million, of which about £26 million would probably have been used before clinical trials can be started (Dench, 1981). More recently it has been internationally agreed that the cost of bringing a new drug from its discovery to the market lies between £50 and £100 million (Wells, 1985). Such expenditure requires financial sources on a historically unprecedented scale, as well as confidence in the long-term investment.

The following eight nations (alphabetically listed) seem to be the principal developers of new drugs: Britain, France, Italy, Japan, Sweden, Switzerland, the United States and West Germany.

Such high costs used to deflect drug research away from such relatively rare conditions as multiple sclerosis, narcolepsy, Huntington's chorea and *Pneumocystis* pneumonia. However thanks to lobbying by the US National Organization for Rare Diseases the 'Orphan-Drug Act' became law in January, 1983. It

---

* Bleomycin–A$_2$, seemingly the most complex of all antibiotics has a molecular weight of only 1356.

provides finance for industrial firms to develop and market drugs to treat the rarer diseases. The Food and Drug Administration, which supervises this act, defines such diseases as those with fewer than 200 000 sufferers (Asbury, 1985).

6.2 A brief history of drug discovery, from early man to the present time

Early man, confronted with illness, must have tried desperately to find remedies in the plants and animals that surrounded him. For the most part, the results could only have been disappointing because of the limited terrain surveyable, the lack of means to estimate concentrations of active agent (either in plant or patient), and sheer ignorance of the cause of any disease. Nevertheless any information on lethal or curative properties acquired by chance would be passed on to following generations by oral tradition.

Some time after the agricultural revolution of about 10 000 years ago (Section 2.2), current medical practices began to be written down. For example the Ebers Papyrus, a roll inscribed in Egypt about 3500 years ago, commences with the words: 'Here begins the treatise on the preparation of medicine for all parts of the human body'. It describes more than 50 medications based on faeces and urine (of both human and non-human origins) for both external and internal use. Blindness was treated with a paste of pigs' eyes poured into the patient's ear. All of this is a far cry from present-day practices most of which have been devised remarkably recently.

Of all the potent drugs in use today the ancient Greek and Roman civilizations knew of only three: opium (the analgesic latex of *Papaver somniferum*), belladonna (leaves of *Atropa belladonna*) which was more used as a poison than a medicine, and ergot (the fungus, *Claviceps purpurea*, a contaminant of rye) regarded purely as a poison. Prescribing practice changed little through the centuries that followed. What was in use after the Renaissance may be gleaned from the London Pharmacopoeia of 1618, one of the first books of drug standards to be printed. Alongside a few remedies that have stayed in use, such as magnesia and senna, most others seem quaint and futile, such as the fat of dogs, storks, eels and hedgehogs, the excrement of several animals, also stones from a patient's bladder.

Soon, penetration of Europeans into the Americas was to yield some new remedies, notably cinchona bark (from Peru) used against malaria in the seventeenth century; and the botanically-related ipecacuanha rhizome from Brazil, which was used to treat amoebic dysentery.

It began to be postualted by some (but denied by many) that every crude drug relied for its effect on an active principle contained in it. This thesis triumphed when Sertürner extracted morphine from opium in 1804, Pelletier and Magendie isolated emetine from ipecacuanha in 1817, Pelletier and Caventou obtained quinine from cinchona bark in 1820 and Mein isolated atropine from belladonna in 1831. It was soon shown that these alkaloids were indeed the active principles, and analysts devised processes for determining them quantitatively so that dried plants, or crude extracts, of known alkaloidal strength could be purchased and prescribed. The next advance was administering the active principle free from the many contaminants present in crude plant material.

European folk medicine continued to be explored, but yielded only one prize, namely digitalis (foxglove leaves) which Withering showed in 1785 to alleviate dropsy. Its value in boosting cardiac insufficiency was soon realized but it proved treacherous in use because the toxic dose lay so close to the effective dose. The active principle, a lactone glycoside named digitoxin, at first proved too chemically unstable to isolate, but this was accomplished about 1925.

Recalling the Chinese origin of tea (Section 5.3) has often prompted the hope that the medical practices of China, some of them more than 2000 years old, could provide useful new drugs for the Western world. Chen, who was based in the USA, reviewed this situation and in 1924 successfully introduced ephedrine (from the herb *ma huang*) for treating asthma. However, nothing else of consequence came to light from this Eastern repository until artemisinin, a sesquiterpene peroxide from the herb qinghaosu (*Artemesia annua*), was re-examined in the late 1960s and found to have promising antimalarial properties (Klayman, 1985).

South America yielded another useful drug, tubocurarine. This was extracted from curare, a blowpipe poison, used to immobilize prey by muscular relaxation. Curare was brought to Europe as a curiosity in the late sixteenth century, but its active principle was not used in medicine until 1940, and the exact chemical constitution discovered only later (Everett, Lowe and Wilkinson, 1970).

Whereas one of the most sought-after qualities in food is palatability it was considered until well into the 1920s, that medicines acted more effectively if they tasted unpleasant. This doctrine gave plenty of scope for the vegetable bitters (gentian, quassia and calumba) and the utterly disgusting herbs, valerian and asafoetida.

Slowly without any fanfare a quite new source of drugs was found in the mid 1800s, namely *organic chemical synthesis*. This departure from tradition began with the general anaesthetics, whose benefits became quickly appreciated. Next simple chemical substances quite different from anything isolated from plants were found to relieve insomnia, notably chloral hydrate (1869), paraldehyde (1882) and the first of the barbiturates (1903). They were accompanied by a whole series of synthetic analgesics such as phenacetin (1888) and Dreser's aspirin (1899) which is not only analgesic but also an efficient anti-rheumatic.

The first local anaesthetic, cocaine, extracted from an Andean plant, was introduced by Koller in 1884. When its sinister addictive properties were recognized chemists volunteered to remove the offending part of the molecule, a startlingly new concept. This goal was achieved in 1905 when Einhorn synthesized procaine (issued at first, under the trade name 'Novocain'). This successful outcome spurred many improvements on such natural products as atropine, morphine, quinine and emetine. This logical and highly productive quest continues (for a summary see Albert, 1985, pp. 271–81).

As the present century started to unfurl interest in seeking new drugs from plants noticeably slackened because so few potent but selective medicaments had come to light from this source in spite of two millenia of exploration in countries near and far. However in the early 1920s new discoveries in biochemistry started to change the prescriber's habits. Hormones and vitamins began to be prescribed. The superstitious not to say unhealthy use of strychnine and arsenic as 'tonics', and of mercury for internal medication of trivial disorders began to be replaced by what biochemists indicated was essential in the cell's economy. Isolation of epinephrine (Adrenaline') from the adrenal medulla by the Japanese biochemist Takamine and its synthesis by Stolz in 1904 led eventually to a rich field of hormone extraction followed by synthesis and then by molecular improvement. Later the discovery of penicillin by Fleming in 1929, its isolation by Chain in 1940 and introduction into the clinic by Florey in 1941, led to rewarding exploration of other micro-organisms for other antibiotics.

Pharmacodynamics and chemotherapy

These two disciplines could at first be studied only with the very few drugs available. However, as they found their scientific basis, such studies began to indicate what substances should be synthesized as an aid to discovering new structure-action relationships, and from this work new candidate-drugs soon began to appear. While evolving independently, chemotherapy and pharmaco-dynamics have from time to time exerted much influence on one another.

Pharmacodynamics, the older of the two studies, was itself influenced by the teachings of astute physicians from Paracelsus to Magendie. However its establishment as an independent branch of science began with Rudolf Buchheim (1820–1879) (Fig. 6.1), who was born in Saxony, the son of a physician. At the Baltic University of Dorpat, he established the world's first pharmacological laboratory and attracted many brilliant young men to work in it. In 1867 he transferred to a comparable position at Giessen, in Germany where he remained until his death.

Before Buchheim the study of drugs had been termed Materia Medica and had been kept very much in the background but Buchheim consistently worked for a more rational approach to the study of drug action and therapy, and strove to translate the accumulated, random observations of cures and poisonings into contemporary physiological language. To him too must be assigned praise for a startlingly modern thought: 'Scientific recognition of the action of a given drug would imply our ability to deduce each of its actions from its chemical formula'. He was the first to emphasize the need to experiment with the simplest possible model, and advocated parallel studies of metabolism and statistics. No outstanding discovery is coupled with his name, but Buchheim is revered as a teacher, for his students moved on to win recognition for pharmacology as an exact discipline. For a biography see Habermann (1974).

The term *chemotherapy* was coined by Paul Ehrlich (1854–1915) (Fig. 6.2), who defined it as '*The use of drugs to injure an invading organism without injury to the host*'. It

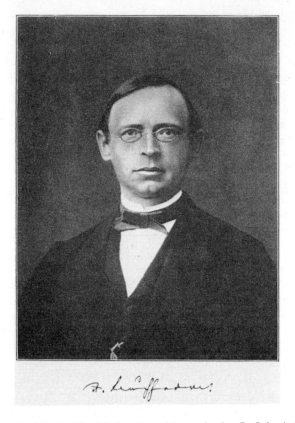

Fig. 6.1 Portrait of Rudolf Buchheim (from biography by O. Schmiedeberg, 1912).

implied a contrast between the small, simple molecules which he visualized as suitable chemotherapeutic agents, and the much larger antibodies (MW about 150 000) which the host's cells produce in reaction against the infecting organism (Browning, 1929). Although in a human infection much of the struggle has to be borne by the host's leucocytes and other of his immunological defence forces, Ehrlich aimed for drugs that could tip the balance in the host's favour by attacking the invader directly. The study of chemotherapy was to be greatly helped by the separate existence of the economic and the uneconomic species (p. 101), which enabled them to be studied independently. Consequently the governing principles of chemotherapy were brought to light much sooner than those of pharmacodynamics.

Before starting his work on chemotherapy Ehrlich had already achieved fame through outstanding discoveries in immunochemistry. He was the first to show that the neutralization of an antigen by an antibody could be effected in a test-tube and did not require the presence of a living mammal as had been thought.

He also devised a chemical interpretation for the immune process, and went on to discover an accurate method for standardizing vaccines. His ability to master so difficult a field led to his appointment as Director of the new Royal Institute for Experimental Therapy in Frankfurt (Germany) in 1899.

However Ehrlich's active mind was not prepared to continue along lines that he thought he had sufficiently explored. Visiting the Hoechst chemical works near Frankfurt, he found a chemical industry which, typical of Germany in that period, was turning out a profusion of synthetic antipyretics, analgesics, hypnotics, antirheumatics and local anaesthetics. Because these simple molecules could obviously differentiate between the various tissues of the human body, Ehrlich postulated that other simple molecules could be found to differentiate between man and his invading parasites. At that time this was a new and startling thought, although the success of quinine in malaria did provide one solitary example.

From 1904 onwards Ehrlich devoted his time mainly to chemotherapy, working first with the protozoal disease, trypanosomiasis, and later with the bacterial disease, syphilis. These two taxonomically remote organisms have one thing in common. Unlike other protozoa and bacteria they are highly motile and burn up vast reserves of energy in the process. In 1906, a benefactress built Ehrlich a new institute especially for these chemotherapeutic studies. This 'Georg Speyer Haus' (named in honour of her late husband) adjoined his other institute, so that Ehrlich was able conveniently to direct them both. In 1908, he received a Nobel Prize in Medicine 'in recognition of his work on Immunity'. It was not until 1910 that his chemotherapeutic project produced a useful drug. This was one that provided the first cure for syphilis, a disease that raged as an epidemic in those days more than now. This success owes much to Hata who, in Tokyo, had managed to produce this disease in the rabbit, thus providing the first basis for drug trials. This is but one example of many where progress in chemotherapy had to await discovery of a suitable laboratory model. Ehrlich brought Hata to Frankfurt where they worked through a long series of organic arsenicals which a team, directed by Bertheim, was producing. It turned out that selectivity depended on presence of a benzene ring with *meta*-amino and *para*-hydroxy substituents. The most selective candidate was arsphenamine (No. 606, or 'Salvarsan') (*6.3*). The Hoechst works lost little time in marketing this remedy, now seen as the opening event in a chemotherapeutic revolution that was to transform the treatment of infectious diseases.

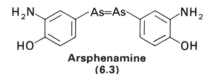

Arsphenamine
(6.3)

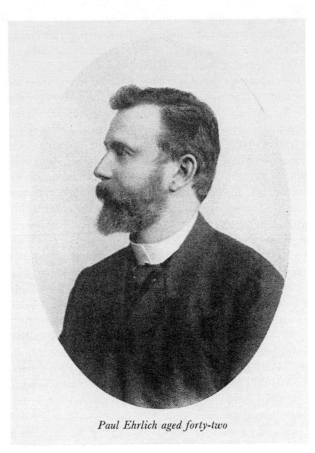

Paul Ehrlich aged forty-two

Fig. 6.2 Portrait of Paul Ehrlich (from biography by M. Marquart, 1949).

This happy result owed much to Ehrlich's introduction of a quantitative measure of selectivity, namely his 'chemotherapeutic index' defined as the ratio:

$$\frac{\text{minimal curative dose}}{\text{maximal tolerated dose}}$$

Thus a substance which cured trypanosomiasis in mice at 2 mg/kg, but did not kill the mice below 50 mg/kg, had an Index of 1/25 (Ehrlich, 1911). He quickly recognized that a drug acted on the invading organism by combining with a receptor (p. 124), which he defined as a small chemical group on a biopolymer normally engaged in the cell's metabolism. He established too that such unions were in general readily reversible. The discovery of *drug resistance* (Section 7.3) in Ehrlich's laboratories gave support to this hypothesis. Thus Ehrlich observed that those trypanosomes which had, through graded exposure to one of his trypanocidal agents, become resistant to it, did not absorb this substance, whereas susceptible trypanosomes still did. Thus he reasoned the resistant protozoa by selective breeding had lost the chemical group that normally took up the drug.

For a biography of Ehrlich see Muir (1921) or Himmelweit (1956).

After Ehrlich's death in 1915, the next twenty years produced effective drugs against almost every kind of protozoal disease thanks to the principles that Ehrlich had established which were applied to the various problems by the brilliant scientists whom he had gathered around him. Regrettably the organic arsenicals, although useful in treating trypanosomiasis and amoebiasis, provided no remedy against bacteria other than the spirochaete that caused syphilis. Although aminoacridines such as proflavine (*8.41*) were found by Ehrlich's Scottish associate, Browning, to deal selectively with bacteria in deep wounds, no antibacterial was discovered that was active in the bloodstream and deep tissues.

This situation was remedied in 1935 when Domagk, in Germany, discovered a yellow substance, sulfachrysoidine (Prontosil) (*6.4*), the first systemic broad-spectrum antibacterial (Domagk, 1935, 1936).

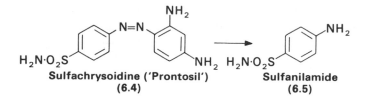

Sulfachrysoidine ('Prontosil')   **Sulfanilamide**
(6.4)   **(6.5)**

As this discovery was almost ignored in Germany, the first large clinical application of sulfachrysoidine took place in London where Colebrook and Kenny (1936) demonstrated its unprecedented ability to save moribund mothers from death by puerperal sepsis. Sulfachrysoidine surprisingly had no effect against bacteria in the test tube. A group of scientists in the Pasteur Institute (Paris) recalled that Ehrlich had shown that pentavalent arsenicals did not act on spirochaetes until reduced, in the body, to oxophenarsine (*6.6*). Therefore they reduced sulfachrysoidine to sulfanilamide (*6.5*) which proved to be the vital part of the molecule, active both *in vitro* and *in vivo* (Tréfouël, *et al.*, 1935). This drug was the forerunner of a whole series of sulfonamides each bearing a *N*-heterocyclic ring (e.g. the pyrimidine ring in sulfadiazine). These new derivatives of sulfanilamide were much more powerfully antibacterial but retained the selectivity.

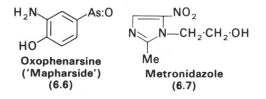

Oxophenarsine   **Metronidazole**
('Mapharside')   **(6.7)**
(6.6)

Seven years after the sulfonamide antibacterials appeared on the scene, penicillin (the first antibiotic) began to be used in the clinic. Antibiotics are toxic substances secreted mainly by the bacterial species *Streptomyces* but also by a few fungi (moulds). It was in 1929 that Fleming noted that a mould *Penicillium notatum*, that had blown into his London laboratory through an open window, gave a watery extract which was toxic to bacteria but not to mammals. However he found the active principle too unstable to isolate so he did not pursue it. Several years later Florey, Chain and their colleagues in Oxford University succeeded in obtaining pure penicillin and introduced it into clinical medicine in 1942. This, and related, work is summarized in a book (Florey, *et al.*, 1949). For their respective parts in the discovery, Florey, Fleming and Chain were awarded the Nobel Prize in Medicine for 1945. Penicillin, both as original benzylpenicillin (*9.31*) or as one of its more recently introduced derivatives, remains the most often prescribed of all antibiotics.

The high selectivity of penicillin and its outstanding success in curing systemic bacterial infections led to a worldwide search for other antibiotics which were discovered mainly in *Streptomyces*. Very many of these isolates turned out to be too unselective for clinical use. Of those that proved acceptable most are active against bacteria, a few against fungi and a very few are used in treating cancer. Of the antibacterial examples the tetracyclines are valued for their broad spectrum of activity and have become (after the penicillins) the most widely prescribed antibiotics. Tetracycline also attacks the malarial parasite but in general, antibiotics have not proved useful against either protozoa or viruses.

The great success of antibiotics did not inhibit progress with synthetic drugs which are usually less expensive and whose simpler molecules facilitate endless small alterations ('tuning'). Among such triumphs was the simple substance, isoniazid (*7.7*), which played the leading part in reducing human tuberculosis from a dread scourge to an easily treated complaint (Offe, Siefken and Domagk, 1952). Exploration of the nitro-heterocycles, a hitherto neglected territory, produced nitrofurantoin which is an excellent urinary antiseptic, and metronidazole (*6.7*) which besides combatting anaerobic bacteria in the bowel rapidly cures amoebic dysentery. Nalidixic acid and trimethoprim (9.14) represent further but quite distinct lines of effective synthetic oral antibacterials. Success is at last being obtained with drugs for the systemic treatment of *viral* diseases, such as acyclovir (*7.44*) in herpes infections. Many excellent synthetic drugs have been introduced for worm infections (anthelmintics), including the highly pathogenic schistosomiasis (p. 114).

(*a*) *Pharmacodynamics and chemotherapy contrasted.* We noted that the well-established manufacture of pharmacodynamic drugs provided Ehrlich with the confidence to launch a new branch of pharmacology, to wit chemotherapy (p.107). Yet once the latter was established as a useful source of drugs against infections its progress outran that of pharmacodynamics. How did this reversal of positions come about? It happened because the problems of chemotherapeutic research turned out to be less than those of pharmacodynamic research.

Pharmacodynamics has to deal with three difficulties that have no counterpart in chemotherapy. In the first place its results are usually required to be reversible, for example an anaesthetized patient must not be permanently deprived of feeling. On the other hand the action of a chemotherapeutic drug is most esteemed when the toxic action is irreversible. In the second place pharmacodynamic drugs are required to act with a *graded* response (i.e. the effect should be proportional to the dose) whereas chemotherapeutic drugs need an all-or-nothing response. In the third place it is unusual in pharmacodynamic research to be able to isolate the test object as a uniform population of single cells, whereas in chemotherapeutic research this is standard practice.

This relatively slow progress of pharmacological research became greatly accelerated about 1945 by adoption of chemotherapy's quantitative measure of selectivity which had in the meantime undergone refinement. The following equation was adopted by the whole of pharmacology:

$$\text{therapeutic index} = \frac{\text{average tolerated dose}}{\text{minimal effective dose}}$$

It should be noted that this equation differs in two ways from Ehrlich's original equation (p. 108). (a) It is expressed reciprocally, so that the larger the index the safer the drug, and (b) the *maximal* lethal dose (which in practice differed from animal to animal) has been replaced by the *mean* tolerated (or lethal) dose (LD_{50}) which is the dose that affects (or kills) 50% of the test animals.

Compared to what is easily obtainable in physics and chemistry, the reproducibility of biological tests may seem to be poor. The main factor that makes values spread within a single experiment is the genetically-based variation in the rate of metabolic transformations (p. 126) between individuals, even in inbred strains of laboratory animals. When one is comparing the results of different experiments one finds diversification arising from variations in feed, lighting, bedding, crowding and handling by the investigator. Variation is minimized by using as many animals, organs or cells as possible, and analysing the results statistically.

The LD_{50} concept was introduced by the English mathematician, Trevan (1927), who showed that members of a set of cells, organs or intact animals respond to a fixed dose of a drug according to a log normal distribution curve as in Fig. 6.3. When such responses were summed for a series of logarithmically increased doses a sigmoid curve was obtained (Fig. 6.4) which represents a cumulative log normal distribution. Some more recent workers prefer to denote the safety of a drug by that dose which elicits recognizable toxicity but permits more than 90% survival. For more on the widely-used LD_{50} test, see Section 10.3.

The response plotted in Fig. 6.4 may be the percentage cured, or killed or it may be a physiological response, such as muscular contraction. Because of the logarithmic plotting, the portion of the sigmoid correlation curve that lies

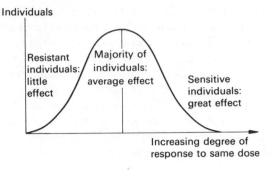

Fig. 6.3 A log normal distribution curve.

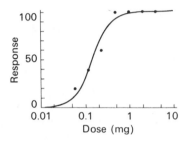

Fig. 6.4 A cumulative normal distribution curve (sigmoid). The response is plotted against the logarithm of the dose.

between 20 and 80% response is likely to be a straight line which makes a convenient starting point for comparisons.

For further reading on quantitative aspects of pharmacology see Barlow (1980).

We noted in Part One how people benefit today from eating the wholesome, nutritious and satisfying foods that our ancestors, at no little risk to themselves, long ago introduced into our diets (e.g. wheat has been cultivated for about 10 000 years). Yet, when we consider medication, we find that most of the safe, powerful and effective drugs that are in use today were discovered only in the last 50 years.

That so many excellent drugs are now available owes much to the comparatively recent discovery of the relations that link structure to biological activity as discussed in Chapter 8. That the newer drugs constantly tend to higher standards of safety is due to the even more recent understanding of what properties make for selectivity (discussed in Chapter 9), and to the excellent methods for measuring selectivity as described above.

6.3 The current state of world health, and how drugs are helping

As was noted in Section 4.1, the people in industrialized countries are steadily increasing their life span in spite of all that the news media say about poisoned food, polluted air and uncontrollable epidemics. The facts are that in the 1850s, one quarter of all children born in Britain were dead by the age of 5, and another quarter by 40. Today, however, only 1% of all Britons die in childhood and only 2% before 40; indeed 70% are still alive in their seventies. Other industrialized countries have parallel statistics.

In this remarkable prolongation of human life, vaccination, refrigeration, and hygeine have all played a part, to which improved medication has added a powerful contribution in the present century. As a result fewer than 1% of these inhabitants die of an infectious disease. Instead most of them are lost much later in life, through the degenerative diseases: stroke, coronary occlusion and cancer, diseases whose dietetic links were discussed in Section 4.1.

Yet as recently as the early 1930s, before the advent of the sulfonamides and antibiotics, bacterial diseases still reaped a grim harvest in industrialized countries. In their central hospitals, the medical wards always had many patients untreatably ill, even dying, with pneumonia and on the outskirts of cities there were other hospitals for highly contagious diseases such as diphtheria and scarlet fever while far removed from the cities were hospices for the many patients dying of tuberculosis. In the surgical wards of the central hospitals one saw many chronic, often unresolving, infections of the arms and legs and much chronic bladder infection. Peritonitis was a dreaded, and often fatal, complication of abdominal surgery. In obstetric hospitals mothers acquired septicaemia from which they and their children often died. In children's hospitals, intractable osteomyelitis and middle ear infections abounded.

Today children are no longer immunized against scarlet fever (a once dreaded streptococcal infection) because penicillin can so rapidly cure it. In this example we penetrate to the very heart of the changes from which the more advanced countries reaped great benefit.

In complete contrast, the developing countries which constitute about three quarters of the world's population are overrun by infectious diseases of which they are exposed to a truly enormous variety. Their people who in many cases suffer from malnutrition and an infected water supply have a relatively short span of life.

A useful summary of the present state of the world's health can be found in the Biennial Report of the Director General to the World Health Assembly and to the United Nations. Issued in the May of even-numbered years, this Report is available as a separate publication and also as part of an annual *The Work of WHO*. The following brief account of the world's health is based on these reports, published in Geneva (Switzerland).

Diseases caused by protozoa

Diseases caused by protozoa (single-celled animals) are common in developing countries. Of these diseases, malaria (which is caused by several species of the genus *Plasmodium*) is the one which leads to more debility, illness and deaths than any other disease in the world. It has been eliminated from Europe and the USA only within living memory, and it is not beyond the bounds of probability that it will return, propagated by the ever-increasing air-traffic with tropical regions. At the present time about 200 million people are infected with malaria, some of them in countries which at first had the disease under control but have since lost ground. This retrogression has in some countries occurred through diminished vigilance in the essential four-prong attack: prophylactic medication, curative medication, spraying against the mosquito (whose every bite starts a new infection) and draining the swamps where it breeds. In other cases, retrogression has occurred through the increased resistance of the *Plasmodia* to medication and of the mosquitos to insecticides. This resistance phenomenon has led to vigorous research for more effective drugs and sprays.

In 1966 the world's annual death rate from malaria was estimated as about one million. It has not fallen appreciably since then for the stated reasons.

Whereas malaria is prevalent in the majority of tropical countries, another group of dreaded protozoal diseases, the trypanosomiases, is confined to Africa (in a wide belt between the latitudes 10°N and 25°S) and to Latin America. Powerful drugs exist for treating these insect-carried diseases but more selective examples are needed. About 45 million people annually suffer from trypanosomiasis in Africa and about 12 million in Central and South America, from Mexico to Argentina.

Leishmaniasis and amoebiasis are other grave protozoal diseases, which fortunately respond well to existing drugs. In general, the human body makes only a feeble immune response to invasion by protozoa. Discovery of a vaccine against malaria, though vigorously pursued, still seems far away (Bruce-Chwatt, 1985).

Diseases caused by worms

Of these the most devastating is schistosomiasis which stands second only to malaria in producing debility, economic loss and death. All species of the worm follow a similar life-cycle, passing through snails in the water supply. Of the 600 million people at risk in Egypt, Arabia, West Africa, China and neighbouring countries, about 180 million are severely infected. Other sufferers are located in Brazil, Venezuela, and the Caribbean. Excellent drugs are now available for treatment, but where problems of hygiene still contaminate the water supply, reinfection is common. The use of molluscicides against the snails is providing a second line of attack.

Filariasis is caused by a worm (*Wuchereria*) which in miniaturized form is carried by a mosquito and injected into the human victim in whose lymphatics it grows to about 10 cm. This causes obstruction and eventually the gross enlargement of limbs known as elephantiasis. There are about 200 million sufferers in tropical Africa, Asia, Indonesia, the Americas and the West Indies. Diethylcarbamazine is a selectively toxic drug that is efficient as a prophylactic and useful in treatment. Recently, the antibiotic, avermectin, has been used for a related disease, onchocerciasis which is transmitted by biting flies in tropical Africa, Arabia, South Mexico and Guatemala. It is estimated that 20 million people are infected, many of them blinded. Spraying with insecticide helps to break the cycle.

Hookworms, which affect about 600 million people throughout the tropics and subtropics, develop in warm, moist soil, penetrate the skin of field labourers and are carried to the lungs and bronchi from where some are coughed out, but many are swallowed to mature in the wall of the small intestine from where they are finally voided in the faeces to begin another cycle. Many effective and selective drugs are known but very many of those who need them cannot afford even the least expensive.

Of the pathogenic intestinal worms the human race is estimated to have at any one time about 1000 million cases of *Ascaris* (roundworm), *Enterobius* (pin and thread worms), and *Trichuris* (whipworm). These are common in every country in the world, and are easily abolished by selectively toxic anthelmintics in all communities that can afford them.

Diseases caused by viruses

It is heartening to know that smallpox, one of the most contagious and devastating diseases ever experienced by man, has been completely wiped out thanks to WHO's strategy of worldwide vaccination. Although similar immuno-prophylaxis is used to give children lifelong protection against some other virus diseases such as poliomyelitis, there are many viral diseases that cannot be prevented in this way and *none* of them can be cured with an immunological treatment (e.g. a serum) once infection has occurred. Fortunately, it seems that the present period is leading to discovery of several effective antiviral drugs, just as Ehrlich's work led eventually to the great array of antibacterial drugs (p. 109). The excellent anti-herpetic effect of acyclovir (*7.44*) seems to point the way. However selectively toxic agents active against the following virus diseases are needed: hepatitis, yellow fever, rabies, dengue, influenza, AIDS, mumps and the common cold. Some progress has been made with influenza. For a review of the chemotherapy of virus infections see Came and Caliguiri (1982).

Diseases caused by bacteria

It might be supposed that tropical countries, because of their burden of protozoal and worm-caused diseases, would be spared the additional thrust of bacterial illnesses. Unfortunately that is not so and cholera, leprosy, tuberculosis and trachoma (which often leads to blindness) are quite common. Even the industrialized countries have yet to eliminate brucellosis (contracted from farm animals) and urethritis (both gonococcal and chlamydial), nor has syphilis been completely eradicated. Excellent drugs exist for treating all these bacterial diseases.

Diseases caused by fungi

Systemic fungal diseases, although they can be life-threatening, are rare. Localized fungal infections such as tinea are common in all countries. Several selective drugs are available for their treatment, although the cure is often slow.

Diseases caused by man

This (possibly unexpected) heading covers the self-inflicted injuries such as cigarette smoking, overeating, excesses of ethanol and use of illicit drugs. From there we move on to the nosocomial* infections that patients pick up in a hospital to which they had been admitted on account of some other illness (*Staphylococcus aureus* provides a common example). Finally there are the iatrogenic[†] diseases which are those inadvertently introduced by a physician in the course of his treating a more serious malady. For more on this subject *see Iatrogenic Diseases* by D'Arcy and Griffin (1985). In all these diseases prevention is simpler than cure.

---

* Greek *nosos* disease, hence *nosokomeion* hospital.
[†] Greek *iatros* physician and *genos* birth.

7

The distribution and metabolism of drugs

The concentration attained by a drug at the site of action usually determines the degree of its effect there. This concentration at the receptor depends in the first place on the size of the dose and then on the rate of the drug's passage through intervening cell membranes. The amount of drug that arrives at the receptor is much less than the original dose because of early losses through (a) simple excretion (b) localization in non-target areas and (c) metabolic inactivation. Quantification by pharmacokinetics of these various effects can lead to specification of the size of the ideal dose and of the ideal dosing interval. All of these factors will be discussed in turn in this Chapter which will conclude with a brief account of the steps by which a promising candidate drug can be introduced into medical practice.

The competing effects that influence a drug on its journey from the site of administration to the site of action are shown diagramatically in Figure 7.1. Each arrow in this figure represents an equilibrium or (more often) a steady state. Many steps are reversible.

7.1 The uptake of medicaments from the bloodstream and gastrointestinal tract: permeability of natural membranes

When a drug is given orally it usually traverses the cytoplasmic membrane of those cells that form a single layer lining the gastrointestinal tract. From these

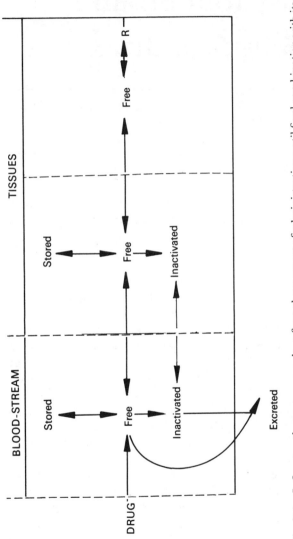

Fig. 7.1 Influences that act upon a drug from the moment of administration until final combination with its specific receptor (R). The broken vertical lines represent selectively-permeable membranes.

cells the drug passes by the portal vein to the hepatocytes of the liver (p. 16) where it is exposed to the full battery of metabolizing enzymes to be described in Section 7.3. Any drug that is, from its chemical constitution, particularly susceptible to such biotransformations may be so diminished in concentration (before it can escape into the general circulation) that very little is likely to reach the target receptor. Such a fate is described as 'almost total loss during first-pass'. Such a drug would better be administered by injection into the patient's arm, from which it can diffuse into the bloodstream and circulate around the body for a brief time before being destroyed by the liver. It is a skill required of the drug designer to devise drugs that are not too susceptible to first-pass losses. Yet drugs should not be completely resistant to the liver enzymes because the patient needs to become quickly free of medication when a particular substance is no longer needed in his treatment.

Each time a drug crosses a selectively-permeable membrane it is said to enter a new compartment some of which are quite large. Examples (in litres) are the circulating plasma of blood (3), the erythrocytes (3), extracellular water other than blood (11) and all the intracellular water (24). This adds up to 41 litres or 58% of total body weight (average values for a 70 kg man) (Goldstein, Aronow and Kalman, 1974). Three such compartments are represented in Fig. 7.1. Equilibration is usually rapid between all of these compartments. The macroporous nature of capillaries ensures that any drug in the bloodstream, unless bound to protein there, can instantly enter the extravascular area. From that vantage point most commonly-used drugs are sufficiently lipophilic to penetrate the plasma membranes of cells in tissues and they do so rapidly.

Equilibration between these various compartments allows the drug molecules to return to compartments which they have left if the concentration decreases there. A different kind of compartment houses each secretory fluid: urine, tears, saliva, milk, bile and sweat, which provide little opportunity for equilibration.

A useful value that helps us picture *where* the drug is distributed is the apparent volume of distribution (V_D). This represents the volume of water in which a measured amount of drug is dissolved. It is obtained by dividing the weight of administered drug by the plasma concentration of the free drug, experimentally determined after equilibrium has been established. A value of V_D that is compatible with the known volume of a body compartment indicates that the drug could be confined to that compartment. On the other hand, a value of V_D that is greater than the total body fluid-volume indicates that the drug is also deposited in a tissue (Goldstein, *et al.*, 1974). Most often the distribution lies between these extremes.

Four types of selectively permeable membranes are known in the human body. The commonest type is conveniently referred to as Type 1 membrane. It is so constituted as to ensure simple diffusion, which means that the transport velocity is proportional to the concentration difference across the membrane. Thus, when equilibrium is reached, the internal and the external concentrations of drug are the same. Temperature has little effect on the equilibrium, nor on the transport velocity which is increased by liposolubility of the drug but decreased if it is ionized; this property also falls off with increase in molecular weight of the drug. In short this type of membrane hinders the passage of ions, permits that of neutral molecules and favours those with a high oil/water partition coefficient. However if the partition coefficient is too high the substance enters the membrane freely but cannot escape from it (Hansch, 1971). For more information on liposolubility and partition coefficients *see* Appendix I.

Type 1 membranes are about 5 nm thick and consist mainly of lipid molecules. A few protein strands dip into them whereas other proteins, often arranged as ion pores, run right through. The best representation of a Type 1 membrane so far seems to be that of Singer and Nicolson (1972), shown in Fig. 7.2. The commonest lipid constituents of membranes are triglycerides (fats) and phospholipids such as lecithin (phosphatidylcholine) (*7.1*). Variations on this ground-pattern provide the membranes of particular tissues with their selectivity. For example the central nervous system's membranes contain much cholesterol (Chacko, *et al.*, 1976). The plate-like rings of this steroid become intercalated between the long chains of the phospholipid molecules, restricting their motion. In this way, cholesterol increases the rigidity of a membrane and

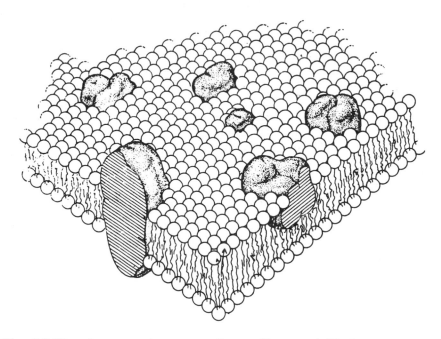

Fig. 7.2 The plasma membrane according to Singer and Nicolson (1972). The triglycerides and phospholipids are represented as a continuous bilayer; some of their polar head-groups are in contact with extracellular water and the others with intracellular water. The randomly distributed stippled bodies represent the protein components.

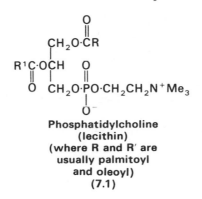

Phosphatidylcholine
(lecithin)
(where R and R' are
usually palmitoyl
and oleoyl)
(7.1)

raises the temperature at which it becomes fluid. The high cholesterol content of the brain's membranes causes hypnotics and general anaesthetics to accumulate in that organ preferentially over other tissues.

Many substances that are important for the body's economy are made of molecules that are well endowed with oxygen or nitrogen atoms. As a result they are too poorly liposoluble to penetrate a Type 1 membrane. For these essential metabolites, Type 2 membranes are present, often as patches in Type 1 membranes. In Type 2, specific carrier molecules occur for each of the following classes of hydrophilic metabolites: sugars, amino acids and the purine and pyrimidine bases. Thanks to the operation of these carriers, the metabolites can enter the cell against a concentration gradient. That is to say, when the concentration is higher on the inside than the outside, entry is not halted. However carriers are saturable and one can easily see from the kinetics when they are fully occupied.

Such carriers are glycoproteins of MW about 100 000, which operate by conformational change (Kyte, 1981). They exercise considerable, but not absolute, selectivity. Thus the carrier for D-glucose can also transport D-mannose, D-ribose and D-xylose but not fructose nor inositol. Although drugs intended to operate inside cells are usually designed to be slightly lipophilic, use is also now being made of Type 2 membranes. For example the successful anti-cancer drugs 6-mercaptopurine, 5-fluorouracil and cytarabine enter cells with the help of the three carriers provided for the normal metabolites, hypoxanthine, uracil and deoxycytidine respectively.

Type 3 membranes closely resemble Type 2 except that they consume energy, derived usually from glucose, for transporting the inorganic ions that are their usual cargo. Type 4 membranes differ sharply by being riddled with little pores which retain a molecule of 70 000 daltons (such as albumin) but let one of 50 000 pass. These carriers are found in three situations: in the capillaries of the blood supply, in the glomerulus of the kidney (Fig. 7.3), and in the parenchyma cells of the liver (hepatocytes).

Let us now review how drugs penetrate various human organs and tissues. Simpler rules govern the passage of a foreign substance than those which exist to guide the products of digestion and metabolism of food. Thus Type 1 membranes regulate the passage of most foreign molecules through the following structures: the gastrointestinal lining-membranes, the membrane lining the renal tubules, the epidermis and the blood-brain barrier (Schanker, 1961). Some examples follow.

The human stomach which, during a meal, may have a pH as low as 1, permits absorption into the bloodstream of drugs that are acids, and hence not ionized at that pH*. Examples are aspirin, the barbiturates and the coumarin anticoagulants. Naturally neutral substances such as ethanol and the benzodiazepine sedatives (e.g. diazepam) are also absorbed from the stomach. On the other hand drugs that are bases are not absorbed because they are totally ionized at this low pH. Examples are the alkaloids such as atropine and the sympathomimetic amines such as ephedrine. Fortunately these basic drugs are readily absorbed from the duodenum and jejunum where near-neutrality reigns whereas any acidic drug that escaped absorption from the stomach cannot be absorbed to any extent from the small intestine because the pH obtaining there will keep it ionized. To sum up, a drug can be absorbed readily from the stomach or intestine if (a) the drug is sufficiently lipophilic to be acceptable to a Type 1 membrane (say P lies between 0.1 and 10)[†], and (b) the difference between the pK_a of the drug and the pH of the organ is such that the drug is not substantially ionized (see Albert, 1985, pp. 384–89). These rules also help the designing of drugs intended *not* to be absorbed but to act on the walls or contents of the gastrointestinal tract.

The transfer of drugs from blood plasma to *tissues* follows a pattern similar to the above. Only the fraction *not* strongly bound by plasma albumin is free to diffuse in this way (p. 125).

The skin offers a major barrier to absorption because the outer layer (called stratum corneum) consists of tightly-packed dead cells. The selective barrier of the skin, the epidermis, lies below this and has a mainly Type 1 character.

Human erythrocytes have mainly Type 1 permeability but possess a special carrier for glucose. Inorganic anions have a most unusual ease of entry because they exchange with bicarbonate ions which are then lost as carbon dioxide.

The lungs are highly effective absorbing areas for liposoluble material such as the general anaesthetics. Absorption occurs through the 200 m^2 of alveoli (air spaces) which are richly provided with capillaries.

The kidney has a fundamental unit known as the nephron of which each human being carries about one million. If uncoiled and placed end-to-end, our nephrons would stretch about 80 km (50 miles). Each nephron consists of a porous tube within a non-porous tube, and has a U-shape (Fig. 7.3). Near the

---

*For the effect of ionization on the action of drugs see Albert (1985, Chapter 10); for the determination of ionization constants and tables of pK values see Albert and Serjeant (1984).
† For more on partition coefficients see Appendix I.

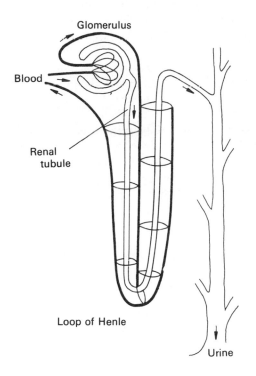

Fig. 7.3 Unit structure of the human kidney.

upper end of each nephron there hangs a little tuft of blood capillaries known as the glomerulus. Blood flows into this tuft which has a Type 4 (highly porous) membrane that retains all the corpuscles and proteins but feeds the rest into the nephron. The latter directs useful constituents back into the bloodstream and then sends the rest (urine) down the ureters into the bladder. The kidney handles about 185 litres in this way, every day; but the tubules resorb all but about 1.5 litres. These tubules have a normal Type 1 membrane, so that liposoluble substances can pass through in either direction depending on the concentration gradient. They also have special patches of Types 2 and 3 for secreting many kinds of organic ions even against a gradient and these are not resorbed. Other patches resorb water and also inorganic ions such as bicarbonate and chloride.

The capillaries of the blood supply have porous Type 4 membranes, similar to those of hepatocytes and the kidney glomerulus. Diffusion of drugs from the blood to the brain is more restricted than elsewhere in the body thanks to the existence of the blood-brain barrier which consists of a Type 1 membrane that lines the supplying capillaries which overlap more closely than in other parts of the body (Rapoport, 1976).

The *liver* excretes in the bile those drugs whose molecular weight is too high for excretion by the kidneys. The pathway followed is: blood → liver interstitial fluid → hepatic parenchyma cells → bile → small intestine. In this way molecules of MW 250–5000 pass readily from blood to bile. Unfortunately many such substances are resorbed from the bowel and recycled as before; in this way a dangerously high blood level of a drug can be built up if dosing is continued and the drug is not appreciably metabolized in the liver. Such points have to be considered by any drug designer who ventures into this molecular weight area. For more on diffusion and transport across cell membranes see Stein (1986).

7.2 The eventual union of a drug with its receptor

The origin of the idea of receptors and their chemical nature are outlined in Section 8.2. Most drugs combine very loosely with their receptors. Thus when a test organ in the laboratory is washed briefly, the physiological effect of the drug usually disappears at once. This ready reversibility was noted by Ehrlich as early as 1900. A few drugs, notably penicillin and the organic phosphates, form covalent (and hence relatively irreversible) bonds with their receptors.

It is widely accepted that many agonists (but few antagonists) act by bringing about conformational change in their receptors and that it is this change that triggers any positive pharmacological result (Karlin, 1967; Levitzki, 1973).

7.3 Hazards encountered between uptake and reception

Simple elimination

As was indicated in Section 7.1 many hydrophilic drugs are excreted by the kidney unchanged. However much excretion takes place after metabolic alteration particularly for drugs that are at least slightly lipophilic. Isotope labelling helps to locate and measure drugs after administration. Usually metabolic products are isolated by high-performance liquid chromatography, identified by mass spectrometry and confirmed (where necessary) by comparison of infrared spectra. The electrophoresis of urine furnishes another useful technique. After isolation radioisotope-labelled products can be measured by scintillation counting, by scanning or by autoradiography. The most-used radiolabel is carbon-14, or the less expensive (but more mobile) tritium; labelling with *both* of these isotopes is practised in difficult cases. Alternatively the convenient and inexpensive technique of measuring carbon-13 (natural abundance, not radioactive) by using several relevant peaks of nuclear magnetic resonance spectra is often practised.

Storage

Many drugs enter into equilibrium with a storage site while they are still circulating in the bloodstream. This diversion of resources lowers the initial blood concentration and diminishes the amount free to proceed immediately to the receptor. There are three principal types of storage substances. Let us now consider each of these potential sites of loss in turn.

Drugs that are highly liposoluble (such as thiopental and dibenamine) are stored in body fat (see Table 3.1 for the composition of this fat). Such storage arises through simple partition between lipid and water (Brodie and Hogben, 1957). Anaesthetists have to deliver above-average volumes of anaesthetic gases to an *obese* patient and they alert the patient's nurse to the likelihood of his relapsing into unconsciousness after apparently complete recovery.

Those drugs that are cationic are stored on anionic biopolymers such as α-acid glycoprotein and chondroitin. Cationic drugs whose molecules are flat become stored to some extent between the purine and pyrimidine bases of RNA in the nuclei of capillaries. The antimalarial, mepacrine (quinacrin, 'Atebrin') is stored in this way where it does no harm but helps to replenish the blood level when this begins to fall (Hecht, 1936).

Those drugs that are anionic, provided that they are at least slightly lipophilic, become stored in serum albumin – a protein that constitutes 4% of human blood and has a MW of 69 000. The binding occurs through an ionic bond to an arginine residue that is situated in a lipophilic cleft; flat molecules supplement this by van der Waals binding to a tryptophan residue. The strength of binding of anionic drugs to serum albumin increases with (a) increase in lipophilic property of the drug as measured by the usual octanol/water partition coefficient (see Appendix I) and (b) increase in flat area of the drug. Typical anionic drugs bound in this way are: aspirin, the coumarin anticoagulants (e.g. warfarin, dicoumarol), the penicillins, the antibacterial sulfonamides, the thiazide diuretics and the pyrazolone analgesics (e.g. phenylbutazone). Binding follows the law of mass action – it is saturable and readily reversible. Just how the binding of a series of penicillins increases with increasing partition coefficient was demonstrated by Bird and Marshall (1967).

The dissociation constant (K_D) (of the drug with respect to the protein) is obtainable from the equation:

$$K_D = C(n-r)/r$$

where C is the concentration of the drug, n is the number of binding sites on the protein and r is the ratio of molecules of bound drug to molecules of albumin. Values of K_D vary from 900 for sulfadiazine, which is rather poorly bound, to 11 for sulfadimethoxine which is almost too well bound to be a useful drug. However unless more than 90% of a drug is bound by albumin the renal clearance is not slowed and the serum protein acts as a depot and not a site of loss. K_D can be obtained experimentally by enclosing a buffered solution of albumin in a dialysis bag which is left to equilibrate with a solution of the drug in the same buffer. A control experiment is run in which the protein is omitted. The value of r is calculated from the difference between the two final concentrations. A plot of r/C against r (i.e. bound/free against bound) should be a straight line with a slope of $-(1/K_D)$. From this plot values of K_D and n can be read (n equals r when $r/C=0$). For more on calculations of such equilibria see Barlow (1980).

A potent drug adsorbed on the patient's albumin can be displaced by a less potent one if the latter has more affinity or (as often happens with less potent drugs) is taken in larger doses. A common example is that of a patient who is under medication with an anticoagulant drug such as dicoumarol, warfarin or phenindione. Should this patient innocently take some aspirin tablets for a headache, the anticoagulant, by becoming displaced, lowers the level of prothrombin in the bloodstream and a crisis of bleeding may ensue. Similarly with young patients undergoing methotrexate treatment for leukaemia, self-administration of aspirin has often released a toxic concentration of the anticancer agent into the circulation. The anti-arthritic drug, phenylbutazone, acts similarly to aspirin in such circumstances. For a comprehensive listing of the percentage of all common drugs bound by plasma protein see Table A-II-1 in Gilman, *et al.* (1985).

Drugs that chelate with calcium, such as the tetracycline antibiotics (also some heavy metals such as lead), become stored in bone particularly in infants. Such substances are at first adsorbed to the bone-crystal surface but later become incorporated into the crystal lattice. Liberation of lead from these stores into the bloodstream continues long after exposure to the metal has ceased. For more on the toxicity of lead see Chapter 12.

Metabolic deactivation

During the long evolution of the various animal species, probability of survival was enhanced by the development of deactivating mechanisms. These were required for two purposes: (a) to terminate the action of hormones once their immediate task was accomplished and (b) to detoxify poisonous substances present in foods derived from plants. Much later when man introduced his medications (p. 103) he came to prefer those drugs whose life in the body was reasonably short. Hence existing pathways of metabolic deactivation were unconsciously utilized (Brodie, 1956).

As an example of (a) we may note that the male hormone, testosterone, although steadily synthesized in the human testis, has an average half-life in the bloodstream of only 15 minutes (determined by radioimmunoassay). It is inactivated in the liver by oxidation of the 17-OH group to give androstene-dione. The human male also manufactures the principal female sex hormone, estradiol, to which he accords an even shorter half-life, excreting it as a mixture of its sulfate and glucuronate – two changes for which the liver again is responsible. In the human female much testosterone has to be biosynthesized in the ovary as raw material for bio-oxidation to estradiol. Metabolic inactivation of both hormones follows the same pathways as in the male but at quite different rates (Murad and Haynes, 1985).

Here our principal concern is not with hormones but with substances foreign to the human body. Many chemical reactions take place (most of them in the liver) which result in a drug becoming more hydrophilic*, and hence more readily eliminated by the kidney. Many drugs are at least slightly lipophilic and these, after passing through the renal glomerulus, become resorbed into the bloodstream through the renal tubules (p. 123). Without any biotransformation their probable fate would be to remain in the body for several weeks, an embarrassment to prescriber and patient alike. Not only does biotransformation help to eliminate a drug but it usually inactivates it as well. Yet in some cases the transformed drug does retain some pharmacological action, often different from that of the parent drug, and a few drugs (e.g. phenacetin) have been discarded because they were found to be transformed into distinctly toxic substances.

A few transformations are effected in the human bloodstream, notably the rapid hydrolysis of an ester group to the corresponding acid. This change is accomplished by the non-specific esterases that are abundant there. The free acids are usually biologically inert and are in any case rapidly excreted by the kidneys (p. 123). Familiar examples of this detoxication mechanism are provided by aspirin, by the local anaesthetic, procaine and by the insecticide, malathion.

Mostly however the transformation of drugs is accomplished in the liver. There some types of reaction take place in the *cytosol* of the hepatocytes whereas others take place in those cells' endoplasmic reticulum (abbreviated here to ER but often referred to as 'microsomes' Fig. 3.1). Because the drug will first encounter the cytosol we shall begin with the former series of transformations.

Of the most frequently encountered conjugations those proceeding by sulfation or acetylation take place in the cytosol, whereas those leading to glucuronides occur in the ER. The term conjugation refers to the condensation of a drug with a hydrophilic substance to improve the hydrophilicity of the drug. Hydrophilic alcohols and phenols (and a few amines) become sulfated by a sulfokinase that transfers an active sulfate group from 3'-phosphoadenosine 5'-phosphosulfate. Thus phenol (*7.2*) is converted to phenyl sulfate (*7.3*) but it is also sufficiently lipophilic to enter the ER, where a comparable amount is converted to the glucuronide (*7.4*). *p*-Acetamidophenol (paracetamol, acetaminophen), a popular headache remedy, is similarly converted to both sulfate and glucuronide as happens also with the female sex hormone, estradiol.

---

* Some drug workers say 'polar' when they mean 'hydrophilic'. In chemistry 'polar' means having a definite dipole moment. For example methyl chloride is highly polar ($\mu = 1.86$ D), whereas carbon tetrachloride is not ($\mu = 0.0$ D). Yet neither substance is hydrophilic, in contrast with methanol ($\mu = 1.70$ D) which is both polar and hydrophilic.

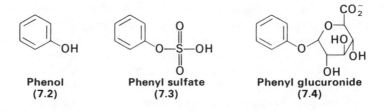

| Phenol (7.2) | Phenyl sulfate (7.3) | Phenyl glucuronide (7.4) |

Aromatic primary amines and hydrazines are acetylated in the cytosol by two or more acetyl transferases which utilize acetyl coenzyme A (p. 23). These transferases are specified by different genes; consequently the human race is divisible into fast acetylators and slow acetylators. Because acetylation usually deprives a drug of all its therapeutic activity it follows that different people may require different doses of acetylatable drugs to achieve the same blood level. Examples of susceptible drugs are the antibacterial sulfonamides, of which sulfanilamide (7.5) is converted to the acetyl derivative (7.6); the tuberculosis remedy, isoniazid (7.7), and the anti-hypertensive drug, hydralazine (7.8).

Patients who acetylate isoniazid rapidly produce acetylhydrazine (after further metabolism) which can cause liver damage (Mitchell, Thorgeirssen and Black, 1975). Whereas about 90% of Japanese and Chinese people are rapid N-acetylators, only about 40% of the white and black citizens of the United States show this trait (Kalow, 1962). Studies of this kind are classed as pharmacogenetics (Kalow, 1962; Albert, 1985, p. 377). Sulfathiazole, one of the early antibacterial sulfonamides, produced an acetyl derivative that was poorly soluble and hence blocked the kidney tubules leading to many deaths. It was replaced by sulfadiazine, a newly introduced drug that lacked this property. Slow acetylators convert a high proportion of primary amines to glucuronide in the ER.

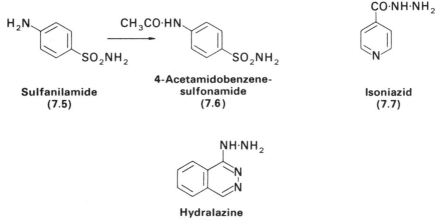

| Sulfanilamide (7.5) | 4-Acetamidobenzene-sulfonamide (7.6) | Isoniazid (7.7) |

Hydralazine (7.8)

Organic acids become conjugated with glycine in the mitochondria of hepatocytes. Thus benzoic acid (often consumed as a food preservative, or by eating berry fruits or by taking a drug that is a benzoyl ester or amide) is converted to N-benzoylglycine (7.9). This reaction occurs in competition with some glucuronide formation inside the ER, from which benzoic acid emerges as the glucuronide (7.10).

Glutathione (which is the tripeptide L-glutamyl-L-cysteinylglycine) forms conjugates in the cytosol, in the mitochondria and in the ER of hepatocytes. It converts aliphatic and aromatic halogenated hydrocarbons into easily excreted mercapturic acids. Thus, bromobenzene is changed to S-phenylcysteine (7.11) which is then acetylated to phenylmercapturic acid (7.12) and excreted by the kidneys (Hirom and Millburn, 1981). Epoxides are similarly converted to mercapturic acids.

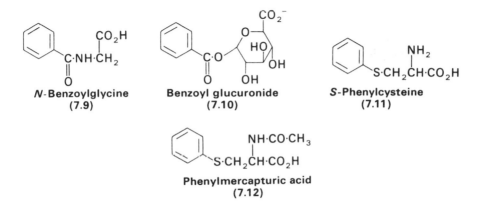

N-Benzoylglycine
(7.9)

Benzoyl glucuronide
(7.10)

S-Phenylcysteine
(7.11)

Phenylmercapturic acid
(7.12)

Alcohols and aldehydes are oxidized in both cytosol and mitochondria to the corresponding acids. Thus toluene, of which house-painters inhale a great deal without apparent harm, is converted in the ER to benzyl alcohol which is then oxidized in the cytosol to benzoic acid; this acid is disposed of as indicated above. Reduction of nitro groups and the cleavage and reduction of azo groups can take place in both cytosol and ER. However these reductions are more often accomplished by bacteria in the small intestine (Scheline, 1973). It was in this way that the first antibacterial sulfonamide, a prodrug named sulfachrysoidine ('Prontosil') (6.4), became activated to the true drug sulfanilamide (6.5). Hydrolysis of amides occurs mainly in the cytosol of hepatocytes.

One of the most important reactions for the designers of anticancer drugs is the formation of ribonucleosides of those purine and pyrimidine analogues which they submit for biological testing, confident that this biosynthesis will occur. This takes place in the hepatocyte cytosol alongside any O-, S- or N-methylations of phenols, mercaptans and aromatic amines respectively.

Multifarious as these various reactions may seem to be, the most diverse and important of the metabolic changes effected by the liver are generally considered to be those that take place in the endoplasmic reticulum (ER). To enter these organelles the drug must possess at least a small degree of lipophilicity whereas this property is not required for entry into the hepatocyte which is contained by a highly porous Type 4 membrane (p. 121).

As mentioned above a characteristic reaction of the ER is the conversion of alcohols, phenols and carboxylic acids into their glucuronides. This reaction is carried out by glucuronyl transferases which receive the carbohydrate fragment from uridine diphosphate glucuronate (made from glucose in the cytosol). These glucuronides are usually biologically inactive and are rapidly eliminated in the urine.

Still more characteristic of the ER are its oxidases which are a set of proteins each linked to the haem known as cytochrome P-450. This distinguishing number (450) is derived from the strong absorption at 450 nm of the carbon monoxide adduct. It is a spectral characteristic much used in the recognition and estimation of the cytochromes P-450. They are all monooxygenases, that is to say they use only one of the two oxygen atoms present in the molecules of atmospheric oxygen for oxidizing the drug (the other atom is removed with the help of NADPH). Because these enzymes are concerned simultaneously with two substrates they have been called mixed function oxidases. The cytochromes P-450 constitute a set of about 8 isoenzymes, separable electrophoretically. Each is specific for a particular type of substrate (Boobis, *et al.*, 1985; Ruckpaul and Rein 1985).

Typical reactions of these oxidases are (a) aliphatic *C*-hydroxylation, as in the conversion of the barbiturate, pentobarbital (*7.13*) to the hydroxy-derivative (*7.14*); (b) aromatic *C*-hydroxylation, as in the oxidation of acetanilide (*7.15*) to paracetamol (*7.16*); (c) *N*-oxidation, as in the transformation of trimethylamine (*7.18*) to its oxide (*7.19*); and (d) *S*-oxidation, as in the conversion of chlorpromazine (*7.20*) into its sulfoxide (*7.21*). In each case, reaction with the enzyme has made the substrate more hydrophilic; moreover the creation of a hydroxy group has provided a new substrate for glucuronide formation; all these circumstances favour elimination. A mechanism exists for conveying these hydrophilic products into the cytosol through breachable pits in the membrane that surrounds the ER.

Further reactions accomplished by these 'microsomal oxidases' include (e) the *N*-hydroxylation of primary and secondary amines, as in the conversion of the $-NH_2$ of 2-naphthylamine into a $-NHOH$ group; (f) *O*-dealkylations, as in

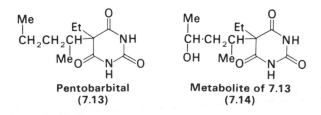

Pentobarbital
(7.13)

Metabolite of 7.13
(7.14)

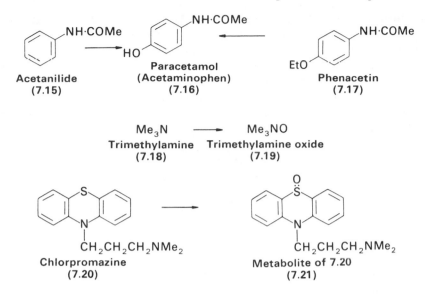

Acetanilide
(7.15)

Paracetamol
(Acetaminophen)
(7.16)

Phenacetin
(7.17)

Me₃N ⟶ Me₃NO
Trimethylamine   Trimethylamine oxide
(7.18)   (7.19)

Chlorpromazine
(7.20)

Metabolite of 7.20
(7.21)

changing phenacetin (*7.17*) to paracetamol (*7.16*) (also similar *S*-dealkylations); (g) *N*-dealkylations as in the transformation of ephedrine to norephedrine (*7.22→7.23*) (in (f) and (g) each alkyl group is oxidized to the corresponding aldehyde); and (h) the deamination of primary amines to aldehydes or ketones, as in degrading the side-chain of amphetamine (*7.24*) to the corresponding ketone phenylacetone (*7.25*) and ammonia. The responsible enzyme, mono-amine oxidase (MAO), is also active in kidneys, nerves and intestinal walls.

Compared to mammals fish manage with very little cytochrome P-450, presumably because they excrete foreign substances directly through their gills into the surrounding water. Lacking this facility, human beings have come to depend on a large and complex P-450 system as a main line of defence against

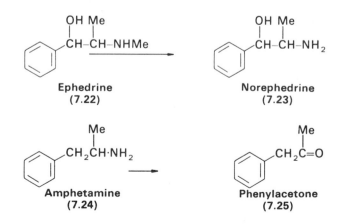

Ephedrine
(7.22)

Norephedrine
(7.23)

Amphetamine
(7.24)

Phenylacetone
(7.25)

foreign chemicals. In fact, biologists think that the development of a metabolizing enzyme system in the liver was one of the main evolutionary advances that enabled animals to transfer from sea to land. How severely tested this protective system has been since the industrial revolution began surrounding us with increasing quantities of man-made chemicals! The spectacular success of our metabolizing system in dealing with this onslaught has depended on the relatively non-specific nature of the enzymes that have evolved. This latitude has provided the potential for degrading many poisons long in advance of their discovery. Long may this happy state of affairs continue!

A parallel has been pointed out between the cytochrome P-450 system and the body's immune response to bacteria in that increased quantities of an appropriate enzyme can often be induced fairly rapidly after a foreign chemical enters the human body. For example phenobarbital (7.26) gradually stimulates production of increased amounts of several P-450 enzymes. One result is that this drug becomes increasingly destroyed. In addition other drugs that are metabolizable by these enzymes are increasingly destroyed too. Thus when the anticoagulant, warfarin (7.27), and phenobarbital are administered together (as often happens for a patient who has just experienced a stroke), the plasma concentration soon falls below the level that exists when warfarin is administered alone. The latter drug is not a vigorous enzyme inducer, so that if its blood concentration is restored by increasing the dose of this drug, the desired therapeutic effect reappears. Should the phenobarbital medication then be stopped the blood level of warfarin will rise to a dangerous height at which severe bleeding is liable to occur (Cucinell, *et al.*, 1965). The following substances similarly catalyse their own destruction and that of many other drugs given at the same time: aminopyrine, chlorcyclizine, chloridiazepoxide, chlorpromazine, glutethimide, meprobamate, phenylbutazone, probenecid, tolbutamide, the general anaesthetic methoxyflurane and the insecticide DDT.

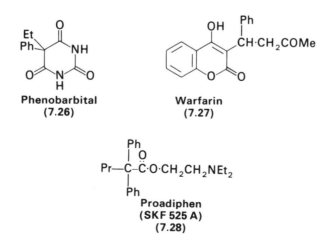

Phenobarbital
(7.26)

Warfarin
(7.27)

Proadiphen
(SKF 525 A)
(7.28)

Phenobarbital also accelerates destruction of the following (non-inducing) drugs: diphenylhydantoin, griseofulvin, aminopyrine and digitoxin.

Knowledge of this inducing effect provides insight into some kinds of drug dependence. It is well known that a given dose of a hypnotic barbiturate such as pentobarbital (7.13) when taken nightly for chronic insomnia can result in shorter and shorter periods of sleep. Should the patient then increase his dose, the accustomed degree of sedation will return, but only for a few nights, by which time the induction of barbiturate-destroying enzyme in the ER will have escalated. If the patient continues to increase the dose, dependence characterized by withdrawal symptoms is to be expected. On the other hand the patient may decide to discontinue the drug as soon as he feels the first loss of action. After about a week the enzyme level will have returned to normal and the original potency of the drug should return. It is now realized that chronic insomnia is not suitably treated with sedatives.

The potentially adverse effects of ER induction which have become clear during the last 20 years have placed two new obligations on the prescriber: (a) to suspend, from time to time, the use of any drug that is on the list of those that engineer their own destruction, and (b) to avoid prescribing together two drugs if one of them is enzyme-inducing and the other is enzyme-susceptible. The practising physician will most likely consult *Drug Interactions* (Hansten, 1985) for such information.

Another type of adverse reaction can arise through saturation of the customary metabolizing enzymes with the result that any excess of the drug is shunted to a normally less favoured enzyme. This occurs for example in overdosage with the mild analgesic paracetamol (7.16). Normally this drug is excreted as a mixture of two conjugates: the sulfate ester and the glucuronide. However a dose higher than that recommended on the label can saturate the conjugating enzymes leaving the drug to become a substrate for a N-hydroxylase that converts it to N-acetyl-benzoquinonimine (7.29). This highly reactive intermediate is at first detoxified by combination with hepatic glutathione. However when supplies of the latter are exhausted the liver proteins become attacked and hepatic necrosis results (Hinson, et al., 1981).

(a) *Synergism.* The above examples of drug antagonism prompt thoughts about the opposite effect, synergism, where one drug potentiates the effect of another most often by blocking the site of loss (Veldstra, 1956). Proadiphen (7.28) has been found a useful laboratory tool for the study of synergism although it has no use in medicine. It prevents the destruction of many drugs when they are exposed to isolated microsomes (p. 127). Metabolism of the drug by cytochrome P-450 enzymes is prevented by competitive inhibition of the hydrolytic enzymes and non-competitive inhibition of the oxidizing enzymes (Gillette, 1966). Many drugs cause toxic responses in the patient by inhibiting metabolic activation of another simultaneously administered drug. Thus the anticoagulant drug dicoumarol, by inhibiting the destruction of the anti-epileptic drug, phenytoin, converts a safe dose of the latter into an overdose which is manifested as drowsiness and ataxia.

Similarly many patients suffer crises of raised blood pressure from simultaneous administration of a monoamine oxidase inhibitor and an amine drug that is not toxic on its own. Thus the MAO inhibitor phenelzine (phenylethylhydrazine, which is used to treat mental depression) has caused death after a usually safe dose of amphetamine, pethidine, or amitriptyline *or* after the patient has consumed such amine-rich foods as cheese, red wine or yeast extract.

These are examples of unfortunate synergism but many favourable examples are known. Thus the action of the penicillins can be increased when the presence of a highly resistant bacterium necessitates it by simultaneously administering the enhancer probenecid (7.30). The latter, which is a moderately lipophilic carboxylic acid like the penicillins, blocks facilitated transport of the latter through the patient's kidney tubules thus raising the level of the penicillin in his blood. An effect similar to this use of a synergist can be achieved by inserting a sterically-hindering group such as methyl into a drug to slow its metabolic degradation. This device is much used by designers of steroid drugs (Ringold, 1961).

The endoplasmic reticulum with its cytochrome-450 enzymes is not confined to the liver although that is its principal site of action. It is also active in the lungs and to a smaller extent in the kidney and gastrointestinal lining.

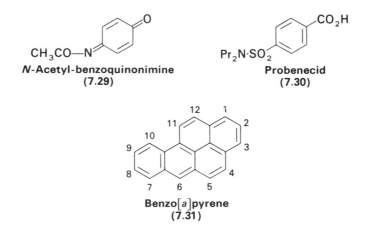

N-Acetyl-benzoquinonimine
(7.29)

Probenecid
(7.30)

Benzo[a]pyrene
(7.31)

(*b*)   *The cytochrome P-448 enzymes.* Less well-known than their P-450 analogues, the P-448 cytochromes of the hepatic ER system exhibit a more sinister aspect in that they are induced by flat, polycyclic molecules (such as dibenz[a, h]anthracene, 3-methylcholanthrene, and tetrachlorodibenzo-*p*-dioxin), which they oxidize to carcinogens. These oxidations take place in positions that are so conformationally hindered as to make the substrates inaccessible to the cytochrome P-450 enzymes. Thus benzo[a]pyrene (*7.31*) which occurs in tar and soot is converted by the P-448 system to the proximate (i.e. true) carcinogen, benzo[a]pyrene-7,8-diol-9,10-epoxide, which damages nuclear DNA (Parke and Ioannides, 1984; Ioannides, Lum and Parke, 1984). The normal functions of P-448 cytochromes are not yet well understood.

(c) *The contribution of gut flora.* Quite apart from changes that the human metabolic system can inflict on drugs a whole battery of chemical attacks can be launched on them by the bacteria normally resident in the patient's gastrointestinal tract. The stomach makes little contribution to this assault, but from that point onwards many species of bacteria exhibit activity. The principal changes effected are hydrolysis, reduction and degradation (Rowland and Walker, 1983). Among the materials hydrolysed are esters, glycosides and amides. Because the host is a large contributor of hydrolysing enzymes the hydrolytic function of resident bacteria gives little concern to the drug designer. The helpful effect of intestinal bacteria in reducing sulfachrysoidine (*6.4*) to sulfanilamide (*6.5*) was mentioned (p. 109); and nitro groups, in such drugs as chloramphenicol and metronidazole, are also reduced. Bacterial degradations deserve attention. They include N- and O- dealkylations and the decarboxylation of the amino acids that arise from digestion (some of the ensuing amines are elevators of blood-pressure but most people are able to deaminate them by monoamine oxidase in the intestinal wall). The reduction of nitrate (to nitrite) in food has been mentioned in two connections (pp. 60 and 89).

(d) *Gene deficiencies limit deactivation.* Because of genetic differences, individuals (and even whole races) may show a very different response to a fixed dose of several commonly prescribed drugs. One example, the slow and the fast acetylators of isoniazid was discussed on p. 128. Another type of genetic inadequacy is affecting about 100 million people throughout the World, notably in the Mediterranean Basin and Western Asia. These individuals inherit a deficiency of the enzyme glucose-6-phosphate dehydrogenase in their erythrocytes. Such people suffer incapacitating haemolysis if medicated with phenacetin, or the antimalarial drug, primaquine (their similar reaction to eating broadbeans was described on p. 74). Another genetic variation, affecting about one person in 2000, is lack of the enzyme that hydrolyses suxamethonium (succinylcholine) after its use as a muscle-relaxant during surgery.

It is common knowledge among travellers that the enzyme alcohol dehydrogenase is inherited in fast and slow types. The former is commoner among East Asians who can show embarrassment from the prickling and flushing caused by sudden release of acetaldehyde (Propping, 1978).

For further reading on this topic which is known as pharmacogenetics see Kalow (1962, 1980); World Health Organization (1973).

(e) *Biotransformation: detoxification or intoxication?* The early investigators of drug metabolism encountered mainly detoxifying effects from the many metabolic processes that they investigated (Brodie and Axelrod, 1949; Williams, 1959).

From the wider viewpoint of today we note that although most biotransformations are detoxifying (and their evolutionary selection and persistence depended on this), enough aberrant examples exist to alert us to a possibility of
intoxication arising when detoxification was expected. With all their defects,
biotransformations have continued through the millennia to safeguard our
species since we first reached out into the unknown, consuming what fruits and
berries came to hand and inhaling the smoke of our first fires. Today we
understand enough of the wide specificity of the concerned enzymes to feel
confident that they will continue to protect the human race, even from chemicals
yet to be discovered. Those who feel this hope is over-bold should cheerfully note
the ever-increasing span of human life in the more industrialized nations (p. 40).

Table 7.1 exemplifies how biologically-active substances range from those
which receive strong metabolic detoxification to those where mammalian
metabolism actually increases the toxicity. Fortunately the latter type is
relatively uncommon.

In human medicine, it has sometimes proved advantageous to devise pro-
drugs, biologically-inert substances which are converted to the active drug by the
body's metabolism. See Section 7.4 for examples of this artifice.

Further reading

On the metabolic alteration of drugs: LaDu, Mandel and Way, 1971; Brodie,
Gillette and Ackerman, 1971; Gillette and Mitchell, 1975; Mitchell and
Horning, 1984; Caldwell and Paulson, 1984; Gibson and Skett, 1986.

See also the following periodicals: *Progress in Drug Metabolism* (1976 onwards),
Bridges, J. W. and Chasseaud, L. F. (eds.), Taylor and Francis, London. *Drug
Metabolism Reviews* (1972 onwards), Di Carlo, F. J. (ed.), Marcel Dekker,
New York. *Drug Metabolism and Disposition* (1973 onwards), Zannoni, V. G. (ed.),
Williams and Wilkins, Baltimore for the American Society of Pharmacology.

Table 7.1 The metabolism of a drug may not detoxify it. (Average
lethal doses, g/kg mouse, of drugs and of their principal metabolites)

Substance	LD_{50}	Metabolite	LD_{50}
Cyanide	0.002	Thiocyanate	0.4
Benzoate	2	Benzoylglycine	4
p-Aminobenzoate	3	p-Aminobenzoylglycine	3
Sulfadiazine	1.5	N^4-Acetylsulfadiazine	0.5
Pyridine	1.2	N-Methylpyridinium cation	0.2

(After Reeves, 1981)

Drug resistance

Colonies of microorganisms have evolved several ways of surviving otherwise lethal drugs. This phenomenon called drug resistance was discovered in 1905 in Ehrlich's Frankfurt Institute as follows. Mice suffering from trypanosomiasis were treated with an inadequate dose of a normally curative drug such as trypaflavine. Surprisingly, renewal of treatment with a normally effective dose of the same drug failed to cure the mice. This resistance in the trypanosomes proved to be hereditary and irreversible. Thus a genetic change had occurred. Similar phenomena came to light in many other organisms, notably bacteria, cancer cells and insects.

Today we distinguish two mechanisms of resistance, mutation and gene transfer. The first mechanism takes place through natural selection in which the drug plays no part. Such a mutation must have occurred by a random event long before the organism encountered the drug. Although a culture of one million bacteria may contain only one organism resistant to a certain drug, the killing of all the susceptible organisms presents this solitary resistant cell with the opportunity to multiply without any competition.

Two techniques have demonstrated that resistance to a drug antedates the organism's first encounter with the drug. One is the examination of freeze-dried bacteria in culture banks that were laid down before the drug came into use. The other is the Lederberg technique of replica-plating, as follows. First some bacteria (*E. coli*) were grown on an agar plate. Then replicas of the colonies were transferred to several other plates by printing with a velvet pad. One of these nutrient plates contained streptomycin. When, after incubation, the position of a colony resistant to streptomycin was found in the antibiotic-containing plate, colonies were harvested from the identical position in the streptomycin-free plates. These proved to be streptomycin-resistant although they had never encountered this antibiotic (Lederberg and Lederberg, 1952). That bacteria can be resistant to a drug in advance of meeting it need cause no surprise, for these organisms are resisting only the biochemical change that the drug brings about and such changes are relatively limited in number.

Resistance by gene-transfer takes place either through transduction or conjugation. A third mechanism, transformation, seems to be largely confined to the laboratory. In transduction a bacteriophage (a bacterium-infecting virus) carries a gene which confers drug-resistance from one bacterium to another. *Staphylococcus aureus*, more than any other bacterium, takes in plasmids (extra-chromosomal DNA) of this kind, coding for penicillinase. Other plasmids similarly confer resistance, in the same organism, to erythromycin and tetracycline. In conjugation genes pass from one bacterium to another through the bridge of conjoined sex-pili. Conjugation occurs primarily among Gram-negative rod-shaped bacteria in the colon. Resistance to several drugs can be transferred simultaneously in this way, and usually operates by chemical elaboration (not by degradation). Thus streptomycin is inactivated by esterification with adenylic acid, chloramphenicol by acetylation and kanamycin by phosphorylation. Such resistant bacteria can be isolated in quantity from rivers. The practice of feeding extracted antibiotic mats to farmyard animals to increase their weight by suppressing what used to be thought of as 'natural dysentery' seems to be the main source of this genetic pollution, so easily transferred from beast to man.

Resistance is a widespread but far from universal phenomenon. In all the years that syphilis was treated with arsenicals or (since 1943) with penicillin, no discernible resistance arose. Again very little resistance has been encountered with *Streptococcus pyogenes*. Yet resistance of *Staph. aureus* was noted soon after penicillin began to be used against that organism. Today, about 80% of strains of *Staph. aureus* resist penicillin G (the original penicillin). Selection of the resistant mutants occurs quite naturally in clinics where the susceptible strains are suppressed by under-dosing, or dosing for too short a period; these deficiencies encourage the resistant strains to proliferate. Resistance is also encouraged by prescribing an antibacterial for a disease that it could not possibly benefit (a viral disease for instance).

In many hospitals more than 80% of the nursing staff are harbouring strains of *Staph. aureus* that resist penicillin by containing an enzyme (penicillinase, which is a β-lactamase) that inactivates the drug by hydrolysing it. This state of affairs has arisen from continual inhalation of traces of penicillin dust, which destroys the sensitive strains thus liberating the nostrils to be an ideal culture-medium for growing the resistant strains (Gould, 1957).

Troublesome resistance has also emerged, although much more slowly, in *Neisseria gonorrhoeae* and *Streptococcus pneumoniae*, the bacteria which cause gonorrhoeae and pneumonia respectively. Conversely highly resistant mutants occasionally emerge rapidly for particular bacterium-drug combinations, e.g. *E. coli* and rifampicin. Some resistant strains are much less pathogenic than their susceptible counterparts whereas others seem to be just as virulent.

To describe more fully the biochemical manoeuvres by which resistance is accomplished it is convenient to distinguish four main types:

In Type 1 resistance the drug is excluded from the site of action often quite simply by changing the composition of the cytoplasmic membrane. This was the first type of resistance discovered. Ehrlich found that the arsenic-containing medium that surrounded his resistant trypanosomes, without their suffering any harm, was rapidly lethal to susceptible strains of trypanosomes. Similarly *Staph. aureus* can become resistant to tetracycline by modifying the plasma membrane which normally facilitates uptake of this drug. In this way the organism is protected from the drug's action, even though the drug's target (the ribosomes) remains as susceptible as ever.

The physical basis for Type 1 resistance is indicated by the work of Haest, *et al.* (1972) who showed that the plasma membrane of *Staph. aureus* can adjust its net charge by varying the proportion of phosphatidylglycerol (anionic) to lysylphosphatidylglycerol (cationic). In this way either anionic or cationic drugs can be excluded by the operation of Coulomb's law. This change can be brought about either by the proliferation of a favourable mutant or by gene-transfer.

In Type 2 resistance the amount of drug-destroying enzyme is increased. In this way *Staph. aureus* becomes resistant to penicillin in the clinic, sometimes by clone-emergence, sometimes by capture of a helpful plasmid. Similarly the treatment of acute leukaemia with cytosine arabinoside fails in proportion as malignant cells with a higher concentration of cytosine deaminase appear. Again treatment of this disease with 6-mercaptopurine lapses when the cells manufacture enough alkaline phosphatase to degrade all the tumour-inhibiting nucleotide to which the cell normally converts this pro-drug.

In Type 3 resistance the amount of a target enzyme is increased. This type is exemplified by those situations in which an enzyme is the receptor for a drug which has been designed to inhibit it. The now widespread resistance of malarial parasites (protozoa) to drugs acting on dihydrofolate reductase has this origin. For example the Uganda strain of pyrimethamine-resistant *Plasmodium falciparum* was found to contain 30–80 times as much of this enzyme as the susceptible strain. In human leukaemia the malignant white blood cells can develop resistance to methotrexate by manufacturing a great excess of dihydrofolate reductase, the enzyme that this drug is employed to block.

Type 4 resistance is exemplified by the synthesis of an excess of the metabolite to which the drug is a planned antagonist. Thus staphylococci, pneumococci and gonococci can become resistant to the usual concentration of sulfonamide antibacterials by secreting extra amounts of p-aminobenzoic acid.

No general way is known for overcoming drug resistance but it can often be prevented by medication with two or more drugs at the one time, each drug being chosen to act on a different receptor. Ehrlich was already recommending such multiple therapy in 1909.

In pharmacodynamics, a phenomenon arises that is parallel to the resistance encountered in chemotherapy and is known as tolerance (closely-related terms include down-regulation, desensitization and tachyphylaxis). This is shown when a standard dose of a drug starts to lose its full effect. It occurs either through the liver enzymes undergoing induction (p. 132) or through loss of sensitivity in the receptor through phosphorylation (Levitzki, 1986).

Further reading

On drug resistance: Albert, 1985, pp. 256–65;
Mitsuhashi, 1982 and Bryan, 1982 for bacteria;
Fox and Fox, 1984 for cancer cells.

Follow-up

Write a short essay comparing and contrasting the fate of (a) food and (b) orally-administered drugs, in the human body.

7.4 Metabolic activation of a pro-drug

From time to time it has proved useful to alter the molecule of a drug in such a way that it no longer has any effect at the site of administration but is converted to the true drug at the site where it is required to act. The name pro-drug was devised for masked substances of this kind (Albert, 1958).

The first example methenamine (hexamine) (*7.32*) was introduced in Germany as long ago as 1899. This cage-shaped molecule, easily synthesized by mixing formaldehyde and ammonia, has no biological action of its own but liberates the true drug, formaldehyde, as soon as it is acidified. If taken before meals, it meets no acid environment until it enters the urine, the low pH of which (often 4.5) liberates formaldehyde which functions as a urinary antiseptic. Methenamine continues to be used for this purpose.

In spite of this promising start very little designing of pro-drugs was pursued until the 1960s. Some of these more recent examples will now be presented. Parkinsonism, a disease characterized by deficiency of dopamine (*7.33a*) in the brain, cannot be treated with dopamine directly because this neurotransmitter does not penetrate the blood-brain barrier. However excellent results are obtained by oral administration of levodopa (*7.33b*). This pro-drug enters the brain thanks to an amino acid carrier and it is decarboxylated there to dopamine (Costzias, Van Woert and Schiffer, 1967).

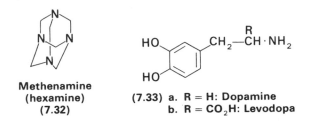

Methenamine
(hexamine)
(7.32)

(7.33) a. R = H: Dopamine
        b. R = CO$_2$H: Levodopa

When attempting to use 6-mercaptopurine (*7.34*) to protect donor grafts by suppressing the human body's immune reactions, the drug was eliminated too fast to yield a sustained effect. Of less easily eliminated derivatives the best was azathioprine (6-(1-methyl-4-nitroimidazol-5-yl)thiopurine) (*7.35*). This pro-drug is slowly cleaved (non-enzymatically) in the body to 6-mercaptopurine, for which it serves as a depot. The electron-attracting properties of the nitro-group give the desired lability to the C–S bond (Elion, 1967). Many successful kidney transplants have been carried out under its influence.

Metrifonate (*7.36*), an organic phosphate that is highly effective in curing the incapacitating worm disease schistosomiasis, is a pro-drug from which the active drug, dichlorvos (*7.37*), is liberated in the patient.

Another pro-drug, pargylene (*7.38*), is used in the aversion therapy of alcoholism to inhibit aldehyde dehydrogenase. This action causes an almost

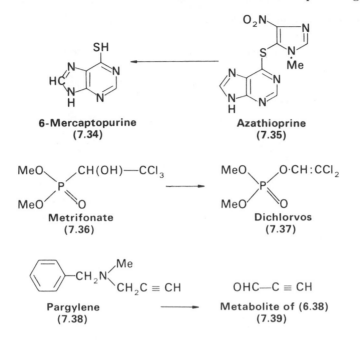

6-Mercaptopurine
(7.34)

Azathioprine
(7.35)

Metrifonate
(7.36)

Dichlorvos
(7.37)

Pargylene
(7.38)

Metabolite of (6.38)
(7.39)

unbearable concentration of acetaldehyde to build up. Pargylene acts in this way only after conversion, by the *e.r.* of the liver, into propiolaldehyde (*7.39*), a substance far too irritant to administer directly (Shirota, DeMaster and Nagasawa, 1979).

Several of the most used benzodiazepine (sedative) drugs are thought to act only after being metabolized to nordazepam (*7.40*) which has the same sedative action as the original substances but acts much faster. In degradation to nordazepam, diazepam ('Valium') (*7.41*) loses the 1-methyl group whereas chlordiazepoxide ('Librium') loses oxygen from position 4 while undergoing hydrolysis of the 2-methylamino group to an oxygen atom. While nordazepam has been made available for prescribing, diazepam is more highly valued for its sustained action.

Ampicillin, a semisynthetic penicillin, is often administered as an ester, such as pivampicillin. The more lipophilic properties of these esters ensure better absorption from the digestive system than occurs when ampicillin (a carboxylic acid) is taken orally. These esters of course are pro-drugs, inactive until converted back to ampicillin by the non-specific esterases in the bloodstream. Esters of erythromycin survive the stomach's hydrolysing acidity which the free antibiotic does not. These pro-drugs lack antibacterial properties but some are hydrolysed to the active drug in the duodenum whereas other, more lipophilic, examples are hydrolysed to erythromycin in the bloodstream.

Cyclophosphamide (*7.42*), the most selective anticancer drug in the nitrogen-mustard class, and much used clinically, remains inert until it is converted (in several steps, at first in the ER of the liver, but finally in the tumour itself) into phosphoramide-mustard (*7.43*). Many attempts are currently being made to couple anticancer drugs to an antiserum raised against cancer cells. The goal is that the drug should be ferried quite specifically to the tumour where, it is hoped, it will be liberated.

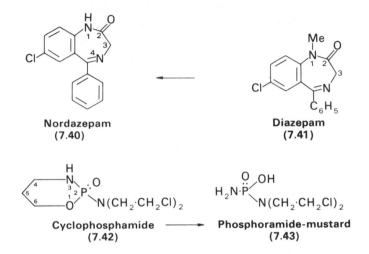

Nordazepam
(7.40)

Diazepam
(7.41)

Cyclophosphamide ⟶ Phosphoramide-mustard
(7.42)   (7.43)

A new era in the treatment of viral disease began in 1981 with the introduction of acyclovir (*7.44*) to treat all forms of herpes. This pro-drug, 9-[(2-hydroxyethoxy)methyl]guanine is converted to the true drug by phosphorylation in the affected cells. The triphosphorylated product is highly toxic to the virus-infected cells but has no effect on healthy cells (Elion, *et al.*, 1977). What is quite remarkable about this form of medication is that transformation of pro-drug to drug is delayed until the pro-drug has reached the infected cell. An even greater refinement of action is achieved in chemotherapy when the pro-drug makes use of the normal mechanism of an enzyme to become changed to a permanent inhibitor of that enzyme (Abeles and Maycock, 1976). Such a drug is called an irreversible mechanism-based inhibitor or IMBI (or somewhat facetiously and quite inaccurately, a 'suicide inhibitor'). Such drugs are designed to have a group that sufficiently resembles part of the normal substrate to become concentrated on the enzyme's active site. This group in the pro-drug must be designed to have a further property, namely it must allow the enzyme to convert it to an active group of such a nature that it can quickly form a covalent bond with the active site on the enzyme thus permanently deactivating it. Now we see why such drugs are classed as mechanism-based inhibitors. One of the best studied IMBIs to date is 2-(difluoromethyl)ornithine (*7.45*) ('Eflornithine'), which irreversibly inhibits ornithine decarboxylase, the enzyme that converts ornithine to putrescine in protozoa. The enzyme removes one fluorine atom to

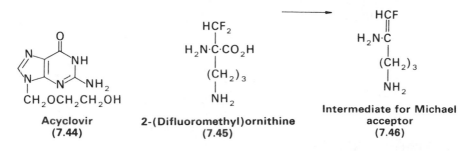

Acyclovir
(7.44)

2-(Difluoromethyl)ornithine
(7.45)

Intermediate for Michael
acceptor
(7.46)

form the double bond shown in (7.46) and a Michael reaction covalently attaches this metabolite to the enzyme (Prakash, *et al.*, 1980).

In Sections 6.2 and 7.3, we noted some medicinal substances that were thought at the time of their discovery to be drugs, but which turned out to be only pro-drugs. Thus the mild analgesic acetanilide (7.15), which acts only after metabolic conversion to paracetamol (7.16), has been replaced by the latter. Likewise, sulfachrysoidine (6.4), which became antibacterial only after reduction, in the gut, to sulfanilamide (6.5), was replaced by the latter. As a general rule drug designers and investigators try to avoid pro-drugs unless they offer a large advantage. This policy is followed because the pharmacokinetics (Section 7.5) are greatly complicated when the distribution and elimination of *two* substances has to be optimized to ensure the ideal dose and the least toxicity to the patient.

Organic arsenicals are available at three levels of oxidation, as exemplified by the formulae (7.47–7.49). Paul Ehrlich (1909) showed that phenylarsonic acids, e.g. (7.47), were inactive until reduced in the body to phenylarsenoxides, e.g. (7.48). The special therapeutic value of phenylarsonic acids lies in their property of passing through the blood-brain barrier (p. 124) on a phosphate carrier, with the happy result that the change from pro-drug to active drug occurs in the target area. In this way cerebral trypanosomiasis is selectively treated without exposing the rest of the body to toxic amounts of active arsenicals. Curiously Ehrlich did not realize that his history-making drug, arsphenamine (6.3), whose discovery was outlined on p. 108, had to be oxidized from the arsenobenzene level (7.49) to the arsenoxide level (7.48) before it became biologically active. When this was eventually established by Carl Voegtlin (1925) in the USA, the arsenoxide form (oxophenarsine) (6.6) began to replace arsenobenzene in the treatment of syphilis, because the patient could be cured with much smaller doses, thus increasing the margin of safety (Tatum and Cooper, 1934). However in 1943 penicillin began to replace arsenical drugs for treating this disease.

For further reading on metabolic activation and pro-drugs see Albert, 1985, pp 97–109; Higuchi and Stella (1975); Bundgaard (1985); Mitchell and Horning (1984). For examples of the biotransformation of harmless into harmful substances see p. 136.

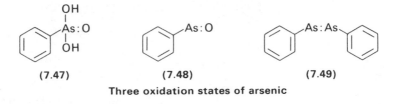

(7.47)   (7.48)   (7.49)

Three oxidation states of arsenic

7.5 Pharmacokinetics

So far this chapter has been only qualitatively describing the processes that regulate access of a drug to its receptor, as indicated in Fig. 7.1. To obtain full, practical value from this information, it needs to be expressed quantitatively by performing experiments to establish the constants governing every process depicted in Fig. 7.1. Two kinds of constant are relevant, (a) rate constants, which indicate the speed of the process and (b) equilibrium constants which refer to the composition of the mixture after attainment of equilibrium. These are the kinetic and the thermodynamic treatments respectively. However in the living cell equilibria are constantly changing; hence rate constants are preferred, especially as they are easier to determine and can provide a basis for calculating effective dose schedules.

The first goal of these rate studies is to affix constants to each arrow in Fig. 7.1. Ideally one could determine two constants for each double-headed arrow, one for the forward and one for the backward movements. In practice a single overall constant often suffices, in fact (as we shall see) it is sometimes possible to neglect one arrow, or even take two or more arrows into consideration in a single constant. On the other hand any overall constant can later be split into its two 'microscopic constants' by further experimental work if the nature of the investigation points to an advantage.

Pharmacokinetics is a study of the time course of drug absorption, distribution, metabolism and excretion. Its principal aims are to discover the ideal dose and the ideal interval between doses so that the patient can experience the most beneficial, and the fewest adverse, effects. Such studies were little pursued until E. K. Marshall in Baltimore showed that the curative effect of an antibacterial sulfonamide was proportional to its blood concentration. He also pointed out that for a given dose the optimal blood level varied from patient to patient (Marshall, 1937). Brodie, working in the National Institutes of Health, Bethesda, showed that Marshall's results applied to many (though not all) drugs.

Pharmacokinetics made rapid progress in the 1960s through the introduction of new techniques for measuring very small amounts of drugs, and of appropriate calculations for dealing with the results. These results, in turn, were often used to refine the experimental methods. Outstanding pioneers in these activities were Krüger-Thiemer (1960) in Germany, and Nelson (1961) in the United States. Brodie also showed that the blood level of a drug represents the pharmacological status of the body far better than the dose does. Apparently the large differences in effective dosage that exist between man and laboratory animals depend more on differences in the rate of metabolic destruction that on any difference in sensitivity of the target organs or their receptors (Brodie, 1964).

Before procceding to a mathematical treatment of pharmacokinetics the reader may care to re-read, in the first pages of this Chapter, about the speed of transfer of drugs between compartments and the volume of distribution (V_D). For most drugs given intravenously elimination* occurs so much more slowly than distribution that we can treat the human body as one single compartment thus simplifying our calculations. In these circumstances the plot of log concentration (log C) versus time becomes a straight line and can be described by first-order kinetics.

In other cases (and this happens more frequently after oral dosage) a significant fraction of the drug is eliminated before distribution has reached equilibrium. Such behaviour produces a plot characteristic of a two or three compartment system. To describe this plot would require two or three exponential terms, because the curve is seen to consist of two or three distinct zones. This is because the initial concentration of the drug in the plasma declines rapidly until eventually a linear relationship is established between log C and time. This somewhat complicated situation is seen also with intravenously administered drugs if the physician prefers a continuous infusion, spread over one hour or more, to the traditional bolus injection where all the drug is given at once. The behaviour of theophylline in Fig. 7.4 illustrates how differently a drug

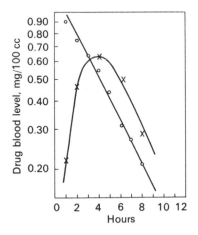

Fig. 7.4 Different distribution patterns of a drug (theophylline) depending on whether the dose is given intravenously (circles) or orally (crosses). (From Swintowsky, 1956).

* The term *elimination* refers to the whole of metabolism and excretion considered together. In more subtle analyses, these components can be separated.

may become distributed and eliminated depending on the mode of dosage (an intramuscular injection usually yields a curve intermediate between the oral and intravenous curves).

Any mathematical treatment of pharmacokinetics conveniently begins with the simplest case where a rapidly-distributing, slowly-eliminating drug is administered as an intravenous bolus.

The relationship between the amount (A) of a drug in the human body to the concentration (C) of that drug in the blood plasma is normally given by the equation:

$$A = C V_{\mathrm{D}}$$

where V_{D} is the volume of distribution. The rate of elimination of the drug from the body may be described by differentiation as follows:

$$-\mathrm{d}A/\mathrm{d}t = kA$$

where $-\mathrm{d}A/\mathrm{d}t$ refers to the loss of a minute amount of drug in a very short period of time and represents the rate of change of the amount of drug in the body. If, instead of A, we write E for the amount of drug eliminated from the body the above equation becomes:

$$\mathrm{d}E/\mathrm{d}t = kA$$

Here k is the first-order rate constant whose dimensions are reciprocal time (e.g., per hour). Instead of starting with A we can use the concentration (C) as follows:

$$-\mathrm{d}C/\mathrm{d}t = kC$$

The linear plot of log C versus t has the slope $-k/2.303$. The intercept on the y axis at $t = 0$ corresponds to the concentration at the moment of injection (C_0) which is almost impossible to determine experimentally. Also available from this plot is the *half-life* of the drug ($t_{0.5}$), which can be read directly from the plot. The half-life is the time needed to reduce the concentration to half its former value. It is independent of the initial plasma concentration. The elimination rate-constant is equal to $0.693/t_{0.5}$. The half-life and the elimination rate-constant tell us how long a drug is persisting in the body. These values are used to calculate the ideal dose and the ideal frequency of dosing. Some $t_{0.5}$ values are presented in Table 7.2.

When the drug is given by intravenous infusion instead of a bolus (as above), the plasma concentration increases slowly to a maximum and, when infusion ceases, declines linearly. The rate of change of the amount of drug in the body can be represented as:

$$\mathrm{d}A/\mathrm{d}t = k_0 - kA$$

where k_0 is a constant rate imposed by the mechanics of the delivery apparatus and expressed as amount per unit time.

When the drug is given orally (or intramuscularly) the drug concentration

Table 7.2 Half-lives of representative drugs in the human body.

Drug	Half life (hours)	Drug	Half life (hours)
Amitriptyline	16	Indomethacin	2.4
Amoxycillin	1	Isoniazid	
Aspirin	0.3	slow acetylators	3.1
		fast acetylators	1.1
Bleomycin	3.1	Methadone	35
Bromide (ion)	7 days	Methotrexate	7.2
Chlorpromazine	30	Methyldopa	1.8
Chlorthiazide	1.5	Metronidazole	8.5
Cimetidine	1.9	Morphine	3
Cisplatin	0.6	Phenobarbital	99
Clonidine	9	Prednisolone	2.2
Cyclosporin	16	Propranolol	3.9
Dapsone	28	Rifampicin	
Diazepam	2 days*	(rifampin)	3.5
Digoxin	39	Sulfadiazine	7
Doxorubicin		Tetracycline	10.6
(adriamycin)	36	Theophylline	9
Erythromycin	1.6	Thiopental	9
Gentamicin	2.5	Trimethoprim	11
Haloperidol	18	Tubacurarine	2
Hydralazine	1	Warfarin	37
Imiprimine	18		

(Compiled from Table A-II-1 of Gilman, *et al.*, (1985) where very many other half lives are listed)
*The sedative action often continues due to a metabolite (demethyldiazepam) that has a half-life of 2–10 days.

profile is more complex because absorption does not occur at a constant rate but usually displays first-order kinetics. The plot for orally-administered theophylline shown in Fig. 7.4 is representative of this type of profile. The shape of the curve reveals that the rate of change of the amount of drug in the body $(\mathrm{d}A/\mathrm{d}t)$ depends on both the absorption rate $(\mathrm{d}A_A/\mathrm{d}t)$ and the elimination rate $(\mathrm{d}A_E/\mathrm{d}t)$ thus:

$$\mathrm{d}A/\mathrm{d}t = \frac{\mathrm{d}A_A}{\mathrm{d}t} - \frac{\mathrm{d}A_E}{\mathrm{d}t}$$

where A_A is the dose and A_E is the amount of drug eliminated. The peak concentration in the plasma occurs at the moment when the absorption rate and the elimination rate become equal*. Usually the absorption rate is much faster

* The area under the curve (AUC) represents the amount of absorbed drug less what the liver may have destroyed.

than the elimination rate. As soon as all of the drug is absorbed, the rate of change of the amount of drug in the body depends solely on the elimination rate which is the first-order expression already derived for intravenous bolus injections:

$$-\mathrm{d}C/\mathrm{d}t = \mathrm{k}C$$

This relationship determines the linear character of the final portion of the (oral) curve in Fig. 7.4. (Note that when the drug is only feebly soluble or is given in a sustained-release form this type of plot may fail to yield values for k or $t_{0.5}$).

(a) *The ideal dose.* For most diseases a blood concentration is known below which no therapeutic effect is obtainable. The prescriber aims to calculate such a dose as will maintain this concentration (or 10% above it) as a steady state. In this way, the patient can obtain the drug's typical benefit without being exposed to side-effects arising from overdosage. Because the plot of dose versus beneficial effect is usually a hyperbola there is often little to be gained by increasing the dose above one that will establish the minimal therapeutic concentration, although this is a matter for careful experiment early in the history of use of any new drug.

A steady state is most easily achieved by a continuous intravenous infusion at a constant rate. However this technique is labour-intensive and most inconvenient for staff and patient alike. Recourse is usually had to oral therapy which gives rise to a 'saw-tooth' pattern of plasma concentrations; in short the drug concentration rises after each dose but soon declines through distribution and elimination. The equations that express these changes are too complex to be useful. A useful approximation can be made by concentrating on the minimal concentrations $(C_{\min})$ shown during the fluctuations. In this way the following useful expression has been derived for the amount accumulated (A_Z):

$$A_Z = (C_{\min})_{ss}/C_{\min} = 1/[1 - \exp(\mathrm{k}\tau)]$$

where $(C_{\min})_{ss}$ is the minimal drug concentration at steady state, $C_{\min}$ is the minimal concentration achieved after the first does, k is the elimination rate-constant and τ is the dosing interval. By giving the drug once every half life, τ becomes $t_{0.5}$ and the accumulation obtained when steady-state has been achieved will be twice that found after the first dose.

Alternatively use can cautiously be made of a simpler expression:

$$\bar{C}_{ss} = F r_{av}/V_D \mathrm{k}$$

where F is the fraction of the dose that reaches the bloodstream, r_{av} is the average dosing rate, and V_D is the volume of distribution. $\bar{C}_{ss}$, the average drug concentration, is analogous to the steady-state concentration so easily attained by continuous infusion.

No matter how a drug is administered it usually takes a time equal to four half lives to reach the desired steady-state concentration ($\pm 10\%$). For any drug that has a long half life, achieving the steady-state by simply waiting for it leaves the patient untreated for too long. To overcome this defect the initial dose is increased to give a 'loading dose' (also called 'priming dose'). If the drug is being administered every half life, a loading dose of twice the maintenance dose is given. Such dosage at half life intervals is typical of antibiotic (particularly of penicillin) therapy in order to enable persisting bacteria to re-enter the growing phase when they are more susceptible to the drug. In general though it is undesirable to allow the blood concentration to drop so far and the ideal loading dose is obtained by dividing the maintenance dose by $1 - \exp(-k\tau)$. For example digitoxin, whose half life is 6 days, requires a loading dose of about 1.6 mg followed by a daily dose of about 0.2 mg. In the clinic such a loading dose is often divided into three well-spaced portions to avoid a possible untoward reaction in the patient.

(b) *Ideal dosing interval* (τ). This is available from the expression:

$$\tau = 3.32 t_{0.5} \log(1 + C_0/C_{av})$$

where C_0 is the *initial* blood concentration and C_{av} is the average *required* blood concentration. Should the dosing interval furnished by this equation be too difficult for the nursing staff (or the patient) to observe (e.g. every 19 hours), a more convenient interval can be substituted, as τ, into the following equation (Wagner, 1967):

$$D = \tau V_D C_{av}/1.44 t_{0.5} F$$

where all terms retain their previous meaning. The ideal dosage interval can also be read from plots of blood levels against time such as Fig. 7.4. This is done by drawing a line parallel to the baseline at a height corresponding to C_{av}, and noting the time it takes for the plot to plunge below this line.

Treatments are most securely based when an *ideal dosage schedule* has been determined for each patient based on the results of blood and urine analyses performed at the beginning of treatment. This approach links the dosage pattern to the patient's own, genetically-determined handling of absorption, distribution and elimination. When this individual approach is not possible, for reasons of urgency or economics, recourse must be made to the averaged data found in published Tables. Recommended dose ranges are available from pharmaco-poeias and (for newly introduced drugs) reports of clinical trials. Tables are also available for recommended dose intervals such as those in Table 7.3.

Reliance on a recommended average dose-range is slowly being replaced by recommended plasma concentrations such as: 10–20 μg/ml for the use of theophylline in asthma or 0.5–2.0 ng/ml for treating congestive heart failure with digoxin. Wider use of such concentrations would represent a great advance over reliance on recommended doses. Without such guidance the physician is at risk of presiding over a treatment that has been made ineffective by under-dosage or of harming the patient by over-dosage.

Because information of this kind is indicated only in the most general way by preliminary animal experiments the help of healthy human volunteers is greatly valued. A historical study of this kind was conducted by Nelson and O'Reilly

Table 7.3 Recommended dose intervals of some antibacterial sulfonamides. Recommended ratios of loading dose (D^*) to maintenance dose (D) for obtaining a steady blood level.

Drug	Average half life (hours)	Dose interval (hours)	D^*/D
Sulfisoxazole	6.1	6	2.0
Sulfanilamide	8.8	8	2.1
Sulfadiazine	23.5	24	3.0
Sulfamerazine	23.5	24	3.0
Sulfadimethoxine	41.0	24	3.0

(From Krüger-Thiemer and Bünger, 1961, 1965)

(1960) with the assistance of their pharmacy students. Various sulfonamide antibacterials similar to those in Table 7.3 were given orally and specimens of blood and urine were taken at intervals and analysed. Four types of rate constants were obtained for each drug: (a) for reversible binding to serum albumin, (b) for metabolism of the drug by N-acetylation, (c) for excretion of the drug and (d) for excretion of the acetylated drug. By fine timing of the sampling procedures constant (c) was split into two microscopic constants: (e) for secretion of the drug by the kidney glomerulus, and (f) for resorption from the kidney tubules into the bloodstream.

More than ever before, medicines are being taken orally as solids. Some of these, such as aspirin and paracetamol, need extra time to dissolve before their absorption can occur. The absorption of dissolved drugs from the gastrointestinal tract usually follows first-order kinetics. The kinetics of dissolving drugs are more complex; they are reviewed by Wagner (1961). Poorly soluble drugs often differ in bioavailability. This happens when different batches of the drug have different particle size or crystal type; both these factors affect the rate of solution very much. Trouble of this kind has been encountered with (for example) digoxin, phenytoin, dicoumarol, paracetamol, nitrofurantoin and the tetracyclines. In most cases the remedy has been to reduce the particle size by ultrasonic treatment; in some other cases (notably nitrofurantoin) crystals of an intermediate size have provided the desired absorption rate.

(c) *Prolonged release (sustained release)*. It often happens that a single dose is required to act over a long period, particularly from bedtime until daybreak. The ideal solution to this problem lies in the zero-order kinetics of constant-rate medication. Soon after the introduction of penicillin in the 1940s it was found advantageous to give it as a depot. This took the form of a deep, intramuscular injection of its insoluble procaine salt in aqueous suspension, from which the drug was slowly released during the next 12 hours or so. A still slower release, covering several days, was provided by replacing the procaine with another base, benzathine (*NN'*-dibenzyl ethylenediamine). Another fairly early example of sustained release is provided by testosterone propionate injected intramuscularly in peanut oil. Prolonged action can also be provided by a pro-drug, as in the use of the sedative, diazepam (*7.41*), which has a half life of 43 hours in the body whereas its active metabolite, the true drug nordazepam (*7.40*) is rapidly eliminated.

However for oral therapy it is more usual to surround the dosage form, whether tablet, pill or capsule, by a physical barrier in order to limit the drug's rate of diffusion. Originally the desired restraint was sought by coating each tablet with a well-adhering polymeric carboxylic acid such as shellac or a half-ester of cellulose. In this way an acid-sensitive drug such as erythromycin was protected from the gastric juice but became liberated in the mild alkalinity of the duodenum. This technique led to the use of concentric coatings designed to provide a small initial dose followed by delayed doses.

A considerable improvement in performance took place when tiny pellets of the drug, some timed for instant release others for release at 3, 6 and 9 hours, were placed in an untreated capsule, which instantly dissolved in the stomach (Ballard 1980). One well-regarded brand of products engineered in this way has become known as 'Spansules'. Such devices work well in the majority of patients but individual variability has produced a sprinkling of failures. Slow-release tablets of potassium chloride merely have this salt embedded in wax. The kinetics of the weeks-long dissolution of steroid drugs when implanted as pellets under the skin has been reviewed by Ballard and Nelson (1962).

Another sustained-release system widely used in Europe consists of a compressed tablet made from the drug mixed with a resinous plastic powder. In the digestive tract the drug is slowly leached out of the plastic matrix which retains its shape and is eventually voided with the faeces. Physicians find that theophylline, presented in this way, is particularly effective in controlling bronchial symptoms in children.

Non-oral medication can often be advantageously effected with drugs embedded in silicone rubber, polymerized in the presence of the drug (Zaffaroni, 1974). The medication reliably diffuses out of the polymer at a slow, steady rate in a moist situation. These devices can be moulded to any desired shape and are used mainly in the body's cavities. One such device (the 'Ocusert'), charged with pilocarpine, is inserted by a glaucoma patient under the lower eyelid where it steadily delivers the drug for a whole week. (This improves upon the usual practice of instilling drops of a 2% aqueous solution of pilocarpine 3–4 times daily, a time-consuming procedure that yields little overnight protection.) Unfortunately a significant proportion of patients cannot retain this device.

Long-term contraception, sometimes attempted with intramuscular injections or implants of steroids, has also been achieved with a T-shaped device made from silicone rubber designed to release about 65 μg of progesterone daily in the uterus. Other contraceptive devices, in the form of steroid-impregnated silicone rubber capsules, are being implanted under the skin experimentally.

Liposomes which are hollow oil drops of radius about 20 nm can be filled with drugs and then injected into the bloodstream (Gregoriadis, 1977). They usually discharge their contents in the liver or spleen and are used for selectively delivering antimonial drugs to those suffering from visceral leishmaniasis (Alving, *et al.*, 1978).

A new device, named the 'elementary osmotic pump' or EOP, is essentially a tablet intended to release its contents at a steady rate during about 12 hours in the gastrointestinal tract. It consists of a core of solid drug, coated with a rigid membrane made from a water-permeable polymer and containing an orifice about 0.2 mm in diameter (Theeuwes, 1975). As soon as this device has been swallowed water slowly enters through the membrane and begins to dissolve the drug. The internal pressure produced by the entry of the water forces this solution out of the orifice. It has been used to deliver the β-adrenergic-blocking drug, metoprolol, at substantially zero-order rate (Kendall, 1982).

Research continues into *micro-pumps* to be attached to the human body for release, on biochemical demand, of the medication with which they have been charged. Campbell (1982) reviews the use of insulin pumps for treating diabetes.

(*d*) *Transdermal medication*. Transdermal medication consists of applying a drug to the skin in order to obtain a systemic effect. It is effective only for highly potent drugs which must be lipophilic as well. Better performance can sometimes be obtained in this way for drugs which are readily degraded in gut or liver. Two well established uses are for nitroglycerin in treating angina, and scopolamine (hyoscine) to prevent motion sickness. The nitroglycerin plasters are rate-limited only by the skin whereas the hyoscine plasters are more intricately constructed in order to control the rate internally. Less expensively, nitroglycerin is often applied to the skin as a simple ointment and works reasonably effectively.

(*e*) *The pharmacokinetics of two or more compartments*. This is a complication that we have so far avoided because of the more difficult mathematical treatment. However many drugs such as the benzodiazepine sedatives and cardiac glycosides undergo this type of distribution. For barbiturates the second compartment is lipid not water. Kinetics for two-compartment distribution were first worked out by Loo and Riegelman (1968), and received a fuller treatment from Gibaldi (1984).

Even on intravenous bolus injection such drugs do not give the usual straight line when log dose is plotted against time. This occurs because a significant fraction of the dose is eliminated before distribution has reached equilibrium. Although this is the normal behaviour for orally-administered drugs (Fig. 7.4) it is unusual for an intravenous bolus-administered drug to depart from a first-order controlled linear plot. In these bicameral (two compartment) drugs the apparent volume of distribution (V_D) slowly increases with time whereas the rate constant of decline in plasma (drug concentration) itself declines. Eventually when equilibrium is reached drug concentrations in the plasma decline by first-order kinetics and continue to do so. That portion of the curve presents neither novelty nor difficulty in the calculations.

For bicameral drugs given orally, the situation is more complex, but workable approximations are available. The zero moment method which is based on the theory of statistical moments can be used to calculate availability and clearance of a drug. This approach begins with calculation of the area under the curve (AUC) in the looped plots of dose (not log dose) against time. This calculation may be done by systematically running a planimeter over the area, or by cutting out the AUC and weighing it, or (most accurately) by (a) ruling the AUC with lines, one running through each experimental point, parallel to the dose axis, then (b) calculating the areas of the several trapezoids produced in this way (area = width times averaged height), and summing them.

This area can be used in calculating mean residence time (MRT) which may be regarded as the statistical equivalent of a drug's half life. This MRT provides a measure of the persistence of a drug in the body and is a function of both distribution and elimination. Obtaining the MRT, which is the ratio of AUMC to AUC, requires calculation of the former (Area Under First Moment Curve) from the plot of the product of concentration and time against time (area is measured as detailed above).

AUC is also used in the calculation of $\bar{C}_{ss}$ which is the average drug concentration at steady state. It is obtained from the small AUC available after a single dose of the drug has been administered; this mini-AUC is then divided by the dosage interval that it is proposed to be used. Several other values useful in clinical pharmacology can be established by similar applications of zero moment methods.

Between two drugs that differ from one another by as little as a methyl group, large kinetic differences can operate at one or more of the stages of distribution shown in Fig. 7.1. Such differences are availed of by drug designers to improve selectivity. Among the antibacterial sulfonamides, most of those kinetics that are helpful to the host are favoured by a moderate increase in the lipophilicity of the drug. This property particularly favours the volume of distribution and the rate of absorption after oral dosage. The elimination of these drugs depends equally on ionization (with a maximum near pK_a 6) and lipophilicity. Binding to serum albumin is another property that increases with lipophilicity and is useful for designing prolonged action into the molecule. When short-acting examples are required however use is made of the fact that *ortho* substitution in the heterocyclic ring, even though it increases lipophilicity, decreases protein binding because of the steric effect. Increased lipophilicity also inhibits wasteful N-acetylation of the drug (Seydel, 1981). For discussion of the often profound changes in biological properties engineered by a single methyl group see Section 8.4.

Studies such as these have shown that members of a family of look-alike drugs can have individual *independently variable* physical properties. Hence the pattern of drug distribution (also the therapeutic index) can be varied at will by making a series of planned changes (quite small ones usually suffice) in the molecular structure.

(*f*) *Conclusion*. Today pharmacokinetics is seen as one of the most significant branches of drug studies. Pharmacokinetics can determine the best dose for the patient and the right timing intervals between doses. By monitoring the drug and its metabolites at every phase of distribution it can expose areas where selectivity needs to be improved and can indicate how this may be accomplished.

Further reading

For modification of a drug's structure to improve its pharmacokinetics see Notari, 1973.

For the theory and calculations underlying kinetic studies of drugs see Krüger-Thiemer, 1966, *Biopharmaceutics and Clinical Pharmacokinetics*, (Gibaldi, 1984).

For controlled drug delivery and release see Bruck, 1983.

Table A-II-1 in Gilman, *et al.*, 1985 provides, for very many commonly-prescribed drugs, the following data: volume of distribution; percent availability after oral administration; percent urinary excretion; percent bound in plasma; half life in plasma; effective plasma concentration; lowest plasma level for display of toxic effects and clearance in $ml \, min^{-1} \, kg^{-1}$.

7.6 Stages in the introduction of a new drug into medical practice

The placebo effect

'Placebo' means I shall please. Until the threshold of the present century, when very few effective drugs were known, a physician's treatment depended very much on placebos, always administered with the strong suggestion 'This will do you good'. Such treatment was a form of faith healing and has two dis-advantages. Only a fraction of the population is susceptible to it and even that minority cannot be helped by placebos if the illness is really serious. Within these limitations much contemporary faith healing is conducted, by religious sugges-tion, homeopathy, herbal treatments, and many other types of alternative medicine. See further Section 10.2.

Clinical trials

The scientific basis of all drug therapy rests on clinical trials. When different mammalian species are compared little connection can be seen between dosage and a standard degree of activity. However activity is usually well correlated with blood level. As soon as a potential remedy (candidate drug) has shown that it is both effective and harmless in laboratory animals, nothing short of administering it to man can give useful new information. The first task is to see what dose in healthy human beings can produce the blood level found to be effective in laboratory animals. From kinetic data obtained by analysis of blood and urine specimens after a single dose, suitable continuing doses for patients can be calculated (Section 7.5).

Provided that the drug is unquestionably more promising than existing remedies the next step is to introduce it into a selected group of volunteer patients who have given their informed consent. The ensuing studies have to be conducted with all the usual precautions such as the use of placebos (as unmedicated doses for the control patients) and cross-over tests (where the control volunteers become the medicated ones, and vice versa). It is also best to use the *double blind technique* where the observing physicians are kept as much in the dark (concerning which patient gets the medication and which the placebo) as the patients are.

The patients are randomly divided into two groups of which one receives the drug the other the placebo. Ideally a cross-over procedure is initiated after the first trial is complete.

Clinical trials proceed in three stages: they begin as soon as toxicity tests on experimental animals, and then on healthy volunteers (whether laboratory staff or medical students) have established that giving potentially therapeutic doses to patients is unlikely to cause untoward effects. In Britain these trials cannot start until the Government Committee on Safety of Drugs has given written consent. Similarly in the USA the FDA (Food and Drug Administration) must approve an IND (application for Investigation of a New Drug) which shows that adequate pharmacological and toxicological research has been carried out (this IND is based on the Harris-Kefauver Amendment of 1962).

(*a*) *Phase 1*. With healthy human volunteers observed by professional clinical pharmacologists the dose is ascertained that gives the same blood level as was found optimal in experimental animals. It is then learnt how the drug is distributed and metabolized, and side-effects such as diarrhoea, constipation, digestive disturbance, palpitation of the heart or blood-pressure change are noted.

(*b*) *Phase 2*. This may last for three or four years. In it, a small number of patients, selected and observed by professional clinical pharmacologists are watched to see if, in the first place, the drug effectively relieves the symptoms or (if the disease is a curable one) initiates and sustains the cure. Depending on the results, the dose is refined and any new side-effects noted. Care is taken to see whether distribution and metabolism differ from that observed in healthy subjects. If all has gone according to plan up to this point (which could be at the end of the first year) this investigation is repeated with a larger number of patients and for a longer period.

(*c*) *Phase 3*. This is known as the broad clinical trial. Before it begins, results will be scrutinized from studies in animals of chronic toxicity, reproduction and fertility. In Phase 3 supervision is not by pharmacologists as in the earlier phases but by experienced clinical physicians. A larger number of patients, from 500 to 3000 in the USA, is treated with the drug for 3–6 months. The intention of this initial period is to establish the efficacy and safety of the new drug in the eyes of the physicians. This broad clinical trial is then continued for up to two years.

(*d*) *Surveillance and ethics.* In the USA once Phase 3 is complete a New Drug Application (NDA) is required by Law. Evidence submitted with the NDA is considered by the Food and Drug Administration who may ask for extra evidence. Alternatively they may give approval but one or other of these decisions has to be made within six months of the NDA being received. The approval given by FDA may limit the drug to selected medical centres only or it can release it for use by all physicians who are willing to submit organized reports (postmarketing surveillance).

In Britain, Government postmarketing surveillance is supervised by the Committee on Safety of Medicines (CSM) of the Department of Health and Social Security. This Committee has the power to withdraw the product licence to manufacture and supply. Adverse reactions at the 1 in 1000 patient level are taken into account with the severity of the treated disease and the availability of safer alternatives. Notable withdrawals in recent years included benoxaprofen (1982), zomepirac (1983), osmosin (1983), zimeldine (1983), fenclofenac (1984), feprazone (1984) and oxyphenbutazone (1984) in which year also the licence for phenylbutazone was restricted to fewer diseases.

All human trials have to be conducted within the ethical framework of the Declaration of Helsinki, as laid down by the World Medical Association in 1964. The informed consent of the patient, after all aspects of the trial have been explained to him by several responsible officials, is imperative.

About 5000 drugs are in regular use at the present time in the industrialized countries. However there may seem to be many more because of the plethora of trade names and synonyms. Medical scientists use only the generic names, preferably INN names (International Nonproprietary Names) which are agreed on by an international committee of the World Health Organization in Geneva. This body issued a major compilation of INN names in 1982. Supplements to this book are distributed to all who write and ask to be put on the free mailing list for INN names.

Follow-up

Compare and contrast how the human body handles (absorbs, distributes, metabolizes and excretes) (a) drugs, (b) the calorigenic constituents of food and (c) the flavourings and other minor constituents of food.

Further reading

For side-effects in the clinic, see the annual *Side Effects of Drugs*, Elsevier, Amsterdam.

8

Activity: how the actions of drugs are related to their chemical structure

The common characteristic of drugs and poisons is that they both exhibit a powerful activity in man whereas food (in moderation) does not. Scientists have been labouring for more than a century to find how it is that even a small change in a molecule can trigger this difference. For instance why is olive oil (principally glyceryl trioleate) consumable in large amounts without noticeable activity whereas castor oil (glyceryl tri*ricin*oleate) precipitates violent defecation, even in small doses. Yet the only difference between these two molecules is a hydroxy group in the ricinoleic chain.

Another age-old question was 'How many kinds of biological activity can drugs provide?'. Outlines of the main types of known pharmacological effects, and medicinally useful drugs that make use of them, will be found in Section 8.1. Such a rich variety owes much to comparatively recently acquired knowledge of how biological activity springs from a substance's chemical nature. Useful correlations of this kind were established only slowly because clues were hard to find. The early attempts to assign each biological action to a particular substituent proved to be misleading. A better understanding was achieved in proportion as a central role was accorded to drug receptors (as told in Section 8.2). However structure–action relationships were not properly understood until about 1940 when the important role of physicochemical properties began to be established. After that, the function of chemical structure came to be seen as a provider of the requisite physical properties (properties that are available also from other structures). These aspects of the source of biological activity are outlined in Section 8.3.

How so small a molecular change as adding (or subtracting) a methyl group could create or abolish activity is discussed in Section 8.4.

8.1 Classification of drugs according to their site of action

The great majority of pharmacodynamic* drugs used in medicine act on one or other portion of the nervous system. To avoid losing sight of the minority that act elsewhere, many of which are drugs of importance, it seems prudent to describe these first. At once, a further specialization emerges, for most of those that do not act on nerves exert their effect on muscles or glands.

Apart from the activation of muscle by the two most-studied neurotransmitters acetylcholine (6.2) and norepinephrine (8.1a), the hormone epinephrine (adrenaline) (8.1b) which is constantly secreted by the suprarenal gland maintains the normal tone of involuntary muscles and also stimulates heart muscle. Histamine (5.2), a tissue hormone, contracts muscles of the uterus and intestines, dilates the muscular fibres of blood vessels and stimulates the secretion of acid by glands in the stomach wall. Anti-histaminic drugs are much used in medicine. Those, such as chlorphenamine (8.2), that inhibit the H_1 receptor are effective in treating coryza (hay fever) and several other allergic conditions whereas those that inhibit the H_2 receptor, such as cimetidine (8.3), have revolutionized the treatment of peptic ulcer.

Ergometrine, from a fungus that infests rye, stimulates the muscle of the womb and constricts the muscular fibres of the blood vessels. Many aliphatic amidines, guanidines and isothioureas, which are all strong bases, raise blood pressure and contract the intestines by direct action on muscle (Fastier, 1949).

The cardiac glycosides, extracted from digitalis and strophanthus, act directly and selectively on heart muscle, increasing the force of contraction. Quinidine and procainamide exert a direct depressant action on heart muscle and are used clinically to correct arrhythmias.

Several drugs that are used to reduce pathologically elevated blood pressure (hypertension) act by directly relaxing the muscles of the capillaries throughout the body; examples are hydralazine (7.8) prazosin, the organic nitrates and sodium nitrite (no longer used medicinally, but see p. 60). Drugs like verapamil (8.4) and nifedipine, that block the slow calcium channel in both smooth muscle and myocardium, are much used to reduce high blood pressure and also to prevent attacks of angina in those subject to them.

Drugs that relax skeletal muscle, whether through acting on spinal reflexes (as the benzodiazepines do) or directly on the muscle (as dantrolene does), find a useful place in treating acute spasm, although the patient may then complain of muscular weakness. Dicycloverine acts directly on the muscle of the bladder and effectively suppresses bed-wetting (Awad, Downie and Kirulata, 1979).

* Pharmacodynamics and chemotherapy are defined and contrasted on p. 101.

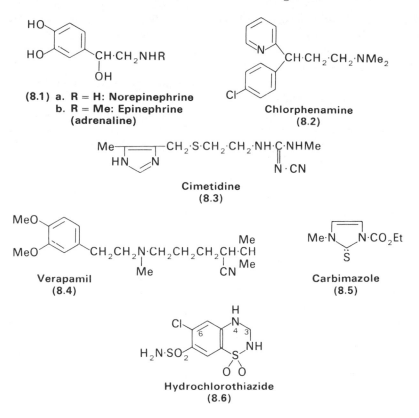

(8.1) a. R = H: Norepinephrine
      b. R = Me: Epinephrine
          (adrenaline)

Chlorphenamine
(8.2)

Cimetidine
(8.3)

Verapamil
(8.4)

Carbimazole
(8.5)

Hydrochlorothiazide
(8.6)

The thiocyanate ion which is often absorbed in sufficient amount from a generous helping of cabbage (p. 66), inhibits uptake of the essential iodide ion in the thyroid gland; but hyperthyroidism is more safely treated with thiourea-based drugs such as propylthiouracil and carbimazole (8.5). Many drugs such as hydrochlorothiazide (8.6) and furosemide are used for producing diuresis. They act by altering the permeability of the membrane that lines the kidney tubules to K^+ and particularly Na^+ (p. 122).

Anticoagulants such as warfarin (7.27) and antileukaemic agents such as methotrexate act on components of the bloodstream, whereas antiarthritic drugs such as salicylates and the corticosteroids, act by inhibiting prostaglandin synthesis.

Replacement therapy, e.g. with vitamins, minerals or hormones may be included here.

To this listing of therapeutic agents that act otherwise than on the nervous system can be added the majority of chemotherapeutic agents. These are designed not to act on the human body but to destroy invading organisms selectively by interfering with their metabolism, as outlined in Chapter 9.

Before reviewing the principal classes of drugs that act on the human nervous system it may prove useful to review the principal divisions of that system and to outline how the nervous impulse is conducted through it.

The first division is usually made into the central (brain and spinal cord) and the peripheral (all other nerves) portions. The peripheral system is divided into sensory (information collecting) and motor (providing action) portions. The motor system is divided into somatic (acting on voluntary muscles) and autonomic (acting on involuntary muscles and on glands). The autonomic nerves are divided into sympathetic and parasympathetic, traditional names into which much meaning should not be read. It is more important to note that the various organs are innervated by both sympathetic and parasympathetic nerves which act in opposition to one another thereby exerting a fine control. Which branch stimulates and which branch inhibits follows no rule but needs to be learnt for each organ. For example acetylcholine (the transmitter typical of a parasympathetic nerve ending) slows the heart whereas norepinephrine (the transmitter typical of a sympathetic nerve ending) stimulates this organ. The various divisions of the nervous system are conveniently set out in Fig. 8.1.

A typical nerve (neuron) consists of a single cell that has a central rather spherical portion whose periphery is drawn out into several fibres. Most fibres (dendrites) are short, but one of them, the axon, may be as long as 1 m (some axons however are only 20 mm long). At any junction with a muscle fibre, or with a second nerve, the axon is swollen into a presynaptic terminal which lies about 20–400 nm away from a corresponding postsynaptic area on the muscle or nerve with which the presynaptic terminal is to communicate. The nervous impulse is electrically propagated down the axon by a transient but progressive reversal of membrane potential at a rate that depends on the diameter of the fibre. The conduction velocity, which some may think rather slow, varies from 0.1 to 100 metres per second.

Across the gap between a pre- and a post- synaptic terminal, the nervous impulse is carried chemically. Whereas somatic nerves have only one such gap, namely at the surface of a muscle or gland, autonomic nerves require extra control because of their isolation from human willpower and they achieve this by having two such gaps. The earlier one is always a nerve–nerve junction, around which nerves of similar function tend to crowd, producing swellings known as

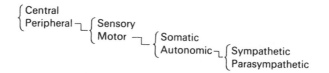

Fig. 8.1 Divisions of the nervous system.

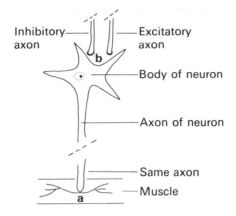

Fig. 8.2 Synapses (a) junction between a nerve and a muscle (b) junction between three nerves.

ganglia. Figure 8.2 shows (a) a nerve–muscle junction and (b) a nerve–nerve junction. The latter, situated in a ganglion, is controlled by two impulses, one excitatory and one inhibitory, because it is usually inefficient to stop an impulse merely by ceasing stimulation.

The following four chemical patterns apply to the relevant kinds of peripheral junctions. It may prove helpful, eventually if not now, to commit them to memory.

1. At the junction between a somatic nerve and a voluntary muscle, the neurotransmitter is always acetylcholine; its action can be mimicked by nicotine and reversed by tubocurarine.
2. At the junction between a parasympathetic (or a sympathetic) nerve and another nerve (i.e. at a ganglionic junction) the transmitter is always acetylcholine; its action can be mimicked by nicotine and reversed by hexamethonium.
3. At the junction between a parasympathetic nerve and a muscle or gland (this is one of the two kinds of postganglionic endings), the transmitter is always acetylcholine; its action can be mimicked by muscarine (*not* by nicotine!) and reversed by atropine.
4. At the junction between a sympathetic nerve and a muscle or gland (this is the other kind of postganglionic ending), the transmitter is always norepinephrine; its action can be mimicked by phenylephrine and reversed by propranolol.

A classification of drugs acting on the nervous system now follows.

Drugs that act on the central nervous system (CNS)

Clinicians divide such drugs into depressants and stimulants, according to the effect on their patients. It might be supposed that depressant effects are achieved with antagonists, and stimulant effects with agonists. This is not necessarily so, as the following samples of exceptions may indicate. Strychnine, which acts as an antagonist of inhibitory nerve fibres, is a violent convulsant. Likewise, the popularly styled 'stimulant' effects of ethanol arise from its inhibiting other inhibitory fibres. Similarly, morphine which acts as an agonist on an enkephalin receptor, is used clinically for its powerful depressant effects.

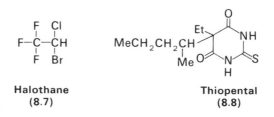

Halothane
(8.7)

Thiopental
(8.8)

(*a*) *The Central nervous system depressants*

General anaesthetics. These can either be inhaled (nitrous oxide, halothane (*8.7*)) or intravenously injected (thiopental (*8.8*)) and begin by depressing the higher centres in the brain; as the dose is increased centres in the medulla become blocked also. The introduction (about 1940) of muscle-relaxing drugs (of which tubocurarine was the first) abolished the need for *deep* anaesthesia during surgery.

Oxygen. This versatile substance could have been treated under 'replacement therapy' but is included here because it is the usual accompaniment of inhaled anaesthetics. For example anaesthesia is often maintained in an open system with a mixture of halothane (2%) and oxygen (98%). Oxygen also ranks as a poison because of the severe effects that an excess can cause on the central nervous system (p. 240).

In therapy, oxygen is generally used at a concentration of 50–100% under normal atmospheric pressure. Caution must be exercised because a strength of 80% or more begins to elicit toxic symptoms after about 12 hours of use. Indeed, oxygen admirably illustrates the Paracelsian doctrine (p. 1) of a substance being a food, a medicine or a poison, depending on the dose. Most oxygen is consumed as food (p. 8).

The principal therapeutic uses of oxygen are in lung and heart conditions. When a barrier exists to diffusion through the alveolar–capillary membrane oxygen provides effective treatment, e.g. in pulmonary fibrosis or pulmonary oedema. It also brings symptomatic improvement in pneumonia. Oxygen relieves the cyanosis of cardiac decompensation and it often alleviates acute symptoms in stroke and coronary occlusion. In poisoning by carbon monoxide

(Chapter 11) oxygen provides the logical and effective antidote. For more on the medicinal uses of oxygen see Smith, Gross and Wollman (1985).

Hypnotics. These are exemplified by the benzodiazepines (such as diazepam *(7.41)*) and by barbiturates milder than those injected for general anaesthesia (such as pentobarbital *(7.13)*). They are given orally to induce sleep but provide little analgesia. Because they tend to produce dependence they are unsuitable for treating chronic insomnia but they serve well on isolated occasions such as overnight air-travel. Benzodiazepines were introduced as anxiolytics and minor tranquillizers, but their hypnotic action is more characteristic. In lower doses benzodiazepines are used as *sedatives*.

Ethanol. The action of ethanol, while resembling that of the general anaesthetics and hypnotics, is more complex because its low molecular weight, low but definite lipophilicity and partial resemblance of the molecule to that of water, enables it to penetrate almost everywhere. Although much administered in those quick and crude forms of surgery that were practised before the discovery of ether (1846), no dose was found, orally or by inhalation, that did not risk respiratory arrest and death. Today ethanol is far less used in medical practice than as a household remedy where it is often valued as a hypnotic (often called a 'nightcap') and also as a stupefacient to make head-colds more bearable. However both medical and lay sources agree on its ability when taken before meals to improve appetite in debilitated patients.

Dehydrated ethanol is often injected near a nerve trunk or ganglion to relieve pain in inoperable cancer. Used outside the body ethanol forms a common vehicle for dermatological lotions. Also a wipe with 70% ethanol (stronger preparations are ineffective) is a standard antibacterial precaution before hypodermic injection.

Ethanol fits all three categories of the Paracelsian doctrine. We have explored its limited, but genuine, role as a food and its ability to elevate mood at table (pp. 25, 93). Here we treat it as a medicine and on p. 307 its role as an insidious poison will be discussed. For more on the various uses of ethanol see Ritchie (1985).

Anticonvulsants. The generalized convulsions of epilepsy are usually treated with phenytoin *(8.9)* (which has *no* sedative properties) or phenobarbital *(7.26)* (which is also a sedative). Epileptic absence-seizures (petit mal) are best treated with ethosuximide *(8.10)* or valproic acid.

Analgesics are classed as powerful, mild and intermediate. Powerful types such as morphine *(8.11a)*, methadone *(8.12)* and pethidine *(8.13)* act at the μ-

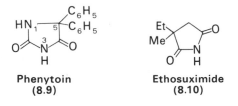

Phenytoin
(8.9)

Ethosuximide
(8.10)

enkephalin receptors which are unrelated to those occupied by the mild analgesics such as aspirin and paracetamol (*7.16*). Codeine (a methyl ether of morphine) and propoxyphene (*8.14*) are qualitatively similar in action to morphine but are classed as intermediate analgesics. Heroin (diacetylmorphine), a powerful analgesic no longer used in medicine, has found sinister recreational use (Section 13.2). Of all these analgesics only aspirin has an antirheumatic effect and this is exerted locally.

Drugs with an action confined to one action of morphine. Because morphine has several distinct actions on the human body, simpler molecules have been sought with a more limited range. Pentazocine represents a class of synthetic analgesics with a reduced proportion of the habit-forming euphoria of morphine. *Antitussive drugs*, such as dextromethorphan, retain only the cough-suppressing properties of morphine and codeine. Drugs used, as morphine and codeine traditionally have been, for the *reduction of intestinal mobility*, are exemplified by loperamide and diphenoxylate, chemically related to pethidine (meperidine) but lacking its habit-forming nature. The following *antagonists* of morphine and related opioids are used to reverse the effects of overdosage, also to diagnose dependence: nalorphine (*8.11b*), naloxone, and naltrexone.

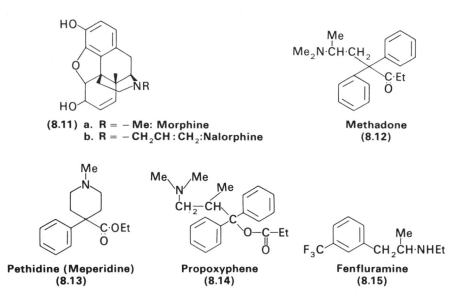

(8.11) a. R = − Me: Morphine
       b. R = − CH₂CH : CH₂:Nalorphine

Methadone
(8.12)

Pethidine (Meperidine)
(8.13)

Propoxyphene
(8.14)

Fenfluramine
(8.15)

Appetite suppressants. Appetite suppressants are sympathomimetic drugs (see below). Most of them have the additional property of stimulating the central nervous system and hence promoting insomnia. A typical example is the dextro-isomer of amphetamine (*7.24*). Fortunately one anorexic drug fenfluramine (*8.15*) lacks this side-effect.

Anti-Parkinsonism drugs. These fortify those regions of the brain that lack dopamine (*7.33a*) because of this degenerative disease; levodopa (*7.33b*) is the most used example.

Neuroleptic drugs. Also known as 'antipsychotics' or 'major tranquillizers' these are able to calm the disordered mind in schizophrenia by blocking dopamine receptors in the brain's corpus striatum. Much used examples are chlorpromazine (*7.20*) and haloperidol.

Hallucinogens. Lysergic acid diethylamide (LSD) and tetrahydrocannabinol (from *Cannabis* – marihuana – of which it is the active principle) have been discarded from medical practice but marihuana survives in the counter-culture (see Section 13.2).

(*b*) *Central nervous system stimulants.* These are less used in medicine than the depressants and are conveniently distinguished as follows:

Psychomotor stimulants. Caffeine (*5.17*) provides the mildest example of these drugs which produce euphoria, a sense of physical and mental well-being, an increased power of mental concentration and a lowering of the barrier against physical work. These gains are effected at the expense of the body's reserves of mental and physical energies and hence they lead to a tiredness that is usually eliminated by another dose of the stimulant, and so on. To drink tea or coffee in moderation is the mildest known form of this drug dependence. Yet dependence it certainly is because abstinence for about two days usually brings on typical withdrawal symptoms of which the commonest is severe, almost unbearable, headache. The stimulant action of caffeine depends on its blocking the adenosine receptor in the brain (Snyder, *et al.*, 1981). The use of caffeine to elevate mood at the meal table was discussed on p. 94 with notes on the caffeinaceous beverages. In domestic medication caffeine is often taken in compound tablets with aspirin or paracetamol. For abuse of caffeine see Section 13.2.

Theophylline which is at least as strong a CNS stimulant as caffeine, and chemically related to it, is used medicinally to relax bronchial smooth muscle in asthma and bronchitis.

The strongest psychomotor stimulants amphetamine (*7.24*) and cocaine (*8.16*) act powerfully on the cortex of the brain, wastefully releasing essential biogenic amines, of which norepinephrine comes away first. The abuse of these drugs, whose use in medicine has greatly declined, is dealt with in Section 13.2. Ephedrine (*7.22*) which is often prescribed in asthma is a less strong psychomotor stimulant and is not widely abused because the higher doses necessitated by down-regulation (desensitization; see p. 139) inhibit urination in many people.

Antidepressants used in treating psychoses. One type of these drugs inhibits monoamine oxidase and so allows norepinephrine and 5-hydroxytryptamine to build up in relevant parts of the brain; tranylcypromine (*8.17*) is an example. Another type, the tricyclic antidepressants such as imipramine (*8.18*), seem to control the same neurotransmitters but in a different way. Electroconvulsive therapy is thought to act by liberating dopamine and 5-hydroxytryptamine in the brain (Green, Heale and Grahame-Smith, 1977). Lithium carbonate,

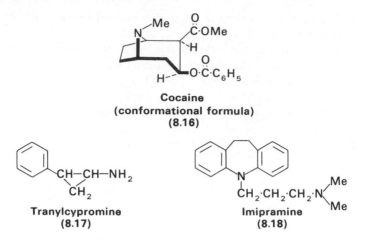

Cocaine
(conformational formula)
(8.16)

Tranylcypromine
(8.17)

Imipramine
(8.18)

historically the first of the modern psychotherapeutic agents, was introduced by Cade in Australia for the treatment of manic-depressive psychosis and rapidly spread throughout the world (Cade, 1949).

Antidotes against drug-induced CNS inhibition. Formerly used to resuscitate barbiturate-poisoned patients, these have largely been replaced by mechanical ventilation.

Centrally-acting drugs for lowering hyperpiesia. Pathologically high blood pressure can be treated at different physiological levels, from the capillaries to the brain, where clonidine and α-methyldopa *(8.29)* are used to stimulate catecholamine metabolism in a way that lowers hypertension.

The local anaesthetics

When applied to the exterior of any nerve, local anaesthetics promptly block all nerve conduction. Their use is followed by recovery without structural damage. As they are effective both centrally (as in spinal anaesthesia) and peripherally (as in dental work) this large family of drugs does not belong with the general anaesthetics but requires this special division. Local anaesthetics selectively block the smaller fibres so that sensory nerves are affected more than motor nerves. Fundamentally what local anaesthetics do is to elevate the threshold for excitation; in this way they block propagation of the nervous impulse without depolarizing (discharging) the fibre.

Local anaesthetics do not diffuse widely from the site of injection. They have none of the properties of hypnotics or sedatives and are unrelated to general anaesthetics both in chemical composition and in mode of action. Cocaine *(8.16)* the first of the local anaesthetics, was introduced in Vienna in 1884, but it soon aroused concern because its euphoriant side-effect often brought about dependence. Search for a simplified molecule, one that would exhibit the good action without the bad one, led to procaine (*8.19*) (Einhorn, 1905). This drug fulfilled most requirements for dental work up to the present time. Unfortunately for other classes of medical work, procaine does not penetrate mucous membranes. This difficulty was overcome by the later discovery of analogues that were more liposoluble and hence more penetrating. The most successful of these are tetracaine (*8.20*) and lidocaine (*8.21*), both of which are more powerful and long-lasting than procaine; both are much used as safe and effective spinal anaesthetics. No legitimate medical use now remains for cocaine, which has come under stringent legal control (see Section 13.2).

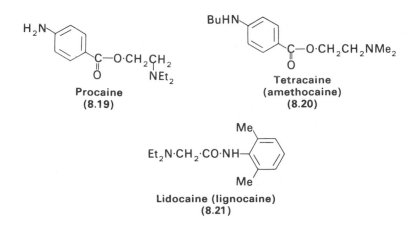

Procaine
(8.19)

Tetracaine
(amethocaine)
(8.20)

Lidocaine (lignocaine)
(8.21)

Drugs that act on peripheral nerve endings

Little is known of the chemical stimulation of sensory nerves and no therapeutic applications exist. On the other hand chemical stimulation of motor nerve endings plays a very important part in therapy. This subject will be discussed under two headings – cholinergic synapses and adrenergic synapses. These names were bestowed by Barger and Dale (1910) and remain convenient to use, although 'norepinephrinergic' could be more correct than 'adrenergic'!

(*a*) *Cholinergic synapses.* Because acetylcholine (ACh) (*6.2*) is hydrolysed by acetylcholinesterase (AChase) as soon as it is liberated from a nerve ending, cholinergic agonists had to be designed to give a longer action. This has been effected in two ways. The first way is to insert a group that will offer steric hindrance to hydrolysis, e.g. the methyl group in methacholine (*6.1*) or the replacement of acetyl by carbamoyl in carbachol. Methacholine acts only at those cholinergic receptors that are activated by muscarine (*8.22*) but these are the more useful ones in therapy. The second way is to inhibit AChase, as can be done with physostigmine (*8.23*), thus medicating the patient with his own ACh.

This stimulates the parasympathetic receptors that can be stimulated by nicotine
(*8.24*) as well as those activated by muscarine. (Muscarine and nicotine are
traditional pharmacologists' laboratory reagents; neither is used in medical
practice. For the recreational use of nicotine see Section 13.2.)

Therapy with cholinergic agonists is much used in correcting abnormal heart
rhythms and in overcoming postoperative retention of urine and faeces.
Organophosphates are AChase inhibitors used for treating the glaucoma of
elderly eyes. Neostigmine, a simplified structure derived from physostigmine, has
some direct action on voluntary muscle and hence is useful in overcoming the
neuromuscular block in myasthenia gravis, an autoimmune disease.

Although the stimulation of nicotinic receptors plays only a small part in
medication, nicotinic antagonists are widely used in surgery to provide the deep
muscular relaxation of voluntary muscle which permits much less of the general
anaesthetic to be used. The first such relaxant was tubocurarine (*8.25*) and was
introduced in 1942. Many other quaternary amines have since been introduced
for this purpose. Of these suxamethonium (succinylcholine) (*8.26*) is much
valued for the brevity of its action.

Atropine (*8.27*) which antagonizes the effect of ACh at parasympathetic nerve
endings (muscarinic ones) is a traditional drug with several different types of

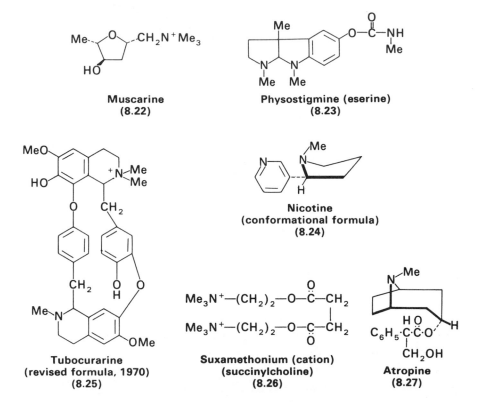

Muscarine
(8.22)

Physostigmine (eserine)
(8.23)

Nicotine
(conformational formula)
(8.24)

Tubocurarine
(revised formula, 1970)
(8.25)

Suxamethonium (cation)
(succinylcholine)
(8.26)

Atropine
(8.27)

action. Undesirable effects include dryness of the mouth, difficulty in urination, loss of visual accommodation and (in susceptible patients) stimulation of the central nervous system to the point of insomnia or even hallucinations or behavioural problems. One useful simplification of the atropine molecule produced homatropine which provided the ophthamologist with a means to paralyse the patient's pupil for a shorter, more practical duration. Other simplifications of the atropine molecule have given piperidolate, and dicycloverine (diclomine) which are used to relieve spasm and hypermotility of the colon. Propantheline, another simplified atropine, is used as a gastrointestinal sedative and is designed to act at a higher (ganglionic) level.

(b) *Adrenergic synapses.* Sympathomimetic drugs have achieved even more uses in medicine than parasympathomimetic* ones. The two starting points in their design are the suprarenal hormone epinephrine (adrenaline) (*8.1b*) and the neurotransmitter norepinephrine (*8.1a*). The receptors on which these act were found by Ahlquist (1948) to be of two kinds: The alpha receptors, stimulation of which constricts blood vessels, contracts the uterus and relaxes the intestine; and the beta receptors which, when stimulated, dilate blood vessels, relax the uterus, increase glycolysis in muscles and accelerate the heart. Norepinephrine stimulates the alpha receptors more than epinephrine does, whereas this order is reversed for the beta receptors. Synthetic analogues, in which the *N*-methyl group of epinephrine is replaced by a *tert*-butyl group, have a greatly enhanced betaagonist action.

Synthetic sympathomimetic drugs are designed to exhibit only a selection of the properties of the natural agonists so that each can find its special application in therapy. Clinically they are much used for treating hypertension, hypotension, shock, cardiac failure, anaphylaxis, allergy and asthma. They are also in frequent use to control bleeding, as nasal decongestants and to curb appetite.

The most used *alpha* adrenergic agonist is phenylephrine (*8.28*), which has the constitution of epinephrine minus one phenolic group. Unlike norepinephrine and epinephrine it is active by mouth. It is used in treating hypotension and shock and also as a nasal decongestant. It does not stimulate the central nervous system. Prazosin, an alpha adrenergic drug, is used to lower abnormally high blood pressure.

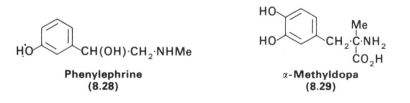

Phenylephrine
(8.28)

α-Methyldopa
(8.29)

---

* (Barger and Dale (1910) defined sympathomimetic and parasympathomimetic drugs as those which act on adrenergic and cholinergic synapses (or receptors) respectively.)

The beta receptors have been further divided into two types. Of these, the β_1-receptors, when stimulated, increase the force and rate of the heartbeat, dilate coronary blood vessels and relax the smooth muscle of the gastrointestinal tract. Stimulation of the β_2-receptors relaxes smooth muscle in the bronchi, uterus, and those arteries that supply skeletal muscle. Excellent β_2-agonists have been designed as bronchodilators and give great relief when inhaled during asthmatic attacks. Typical examples are salbutamol (albuterol) (*8.30*) and terbutaline. These drugs avoid the β_1-activated tachycardia that was the defect of earlier beta-agonists such as isoprenaline.

Sympathomimetic drugs are not confined to those that act, as the above do, directly on the postsynaptic receptor. Some of them use the presynaptic region of the adrenergic synapse (see Fig. 8.2) which normally exercises two functions: (a) it secretes norepinephrine and (b) it resorbs that substance after the impulse has acted. Metaraminol (*8.31*) prevents uptake of norepinephrine by the presynaptic terminal, and is used to raise abnormally lowered blood pressure and to combat shock. On the other hand, ephedrine (*7.22*) accumulates in the presynaptic terminal where it steadily pushes stores of norepinephrine out into the synaptic gap. Orally administered, ephedrine gives valuable relief in hay fever and other allergic states. It is best taken not too late in the day as its mild centrally-stimulating effect can invite insomnia. Amphetamine (*7.24*) has both of the actions of ephedrine but the central stimulation is much the stronger (p. 318).

The foregoing drugs act by giving the patient an overdose of his own norepinephrine; but guanethidine (*8.32*) acts differently. It accumulates in the presynaptic terminals but pushes out the stored norepinephrine at such an abnormally slow rate that this neurotransmitter is enzymatically destroyed as fast as it is liberated. Hence guanethidine, and the similarly acting bretylium, debrisoquine and bethanidine, are useful clinically for reducing moderately elevated blood pressure.

β-Adrenergic blocking agents are in daily clinical use for lowering hypertension and relieving angina pectoris and cardiac arrhythmias. The most used of these is propranolol (*8.33*) which acts as an antagonist at all β-receptors and is

Salbutamol (Albuterol)
(8.30)

Metaraminol
(8.31)

Guanethidine
(8.32)

Propranolol
(8.33)

without agonistic effect. Its molecular structure can be modified so that only a β_1 blocking action is exerted, as in metoprolol and atenolol; these are better tolerated by asthmatic patients than propranolol.

Many opportunities exist for designing drugs to act on less well-known parts of the nervous system than those activated by acetylcholine and norepinephrine. At least the roles of dopamine and 5-hydroxytryptamine (serotonin) in the central nervous system are partly understood and have led to new forms of therapy (p. 165). The part played by the purinergic adenosine receptor in the central effects of caffeine and theophylline were outlined on p. 165. The human gut, too, receives transmission from purinergic nerves, but ones whose activation stems from adenosine triphosphate. Pain centres in brain, spinal cord and intestines have receptors activated by the enkephalins and endorphins which were referred to during discussion of the action of opioids on p. 164. There is still much to investigate in seeking drugs to block or activate receptors for other natural agonists such as γ-aminobutyric acid, glycine, glutamic acid, bradykinin, substance P and bombesin. There are many other neurotransmitters and localized hormones to investigate, several of them common to both gut and brain.

8.2 The central role of receptors in the correlation of structure with biological action

Rapid progress made in the understanding of organic chemistry, during the second half of the nineteenth century kindled speculations about a possible connection between chemical structure and biological action. This was coupled to a related theme: How did medicines produce their various effects in the human body?

No correlation between structure and biological activity could be traced until 1869 in Scotland when Alexander Crum Brown and Thomas Frazer (1869) showed that a great many alkaloids, even convulsive ones, were converted to muscle relaxants when their tertiary nitrogen atom was quaternized by methylation. In fact, this simple chemical change had converted strychnine, bruceine, codeine, morphine, thebaine, nicotine, atropine and coniine into substances with the biological property of the alkaloid tubocurarine (curarine) (8.25), itself a quaternary amine.

Let us not underestimate the stimulating effect of this discovery on pharmacologists and medicinal chemists for at long last it seemed that a simple connection had been found between a constitution and a biological property. This correlation started the search for other chemical groups or nuclei (ring systems) to which a unique pharmacological action might be assigned. Hence for the next two generations a futile attempt was made to link every type of drug action to its own cluster of atoms. Futile because the true situation is fundamentally more complex and yet, as we shall see, possibilities for quantification have made it very much easier.

A more fundamental approach was begun by John Langley in 1878 when he put forward the concept of drug receptors in the human body. Langley was led to this idea by the results of his experiments, at the University of Cambridge, on the mutually antagonistic effects of pilocarpine and atropine on salivary flow. What he did was to give a little pilocarpine (*8.34*) to a cat then measure the excess saliva that it generated in a given time. Next he treated the cat with atropine (*8.27*) which promptly stopped the flow. He found that salivation could be started again with more pilocarpine and then halted with more atropine and so on.

Langley concluded: 'There is some substance or substances, in the nerve endings or gland cells, with which both atropine and pilocarpine are capable of forming compounds. On this assumption, then, the atropine or pilocarpine compounds are formed according to some law, of which their relative mass and chemical affinity for the substance are factors' (Langley, 1878). (Today we know that pilocarpine is an acetylcholine (ACh) agonist and atropine is an ACh antagonist, and that it is natural for these two alkaloids to exhibit opposed physiological effects in a constant ratio).

Langley's hypothesis was adopted and expanded by Paul Ehrlich in Germany at the turn of the century. It was he who coined the name receptor (Langley wrote 'receptive substance') and defined it as a chemical group, normally active in the cell's metabolism which, by combining with the drug, triggers the observed response. He showed that the receptors for arsenical drugs in trypanosomes were mercapto (–SH) groups and that the (reversible) formation of As–S bonds brought metabolic injury then death to the parasite (Ehrlich, 1909).

Several advances took place in the late 1920s. For some time Alfred Clark in London had been showing that the action of drugs on receptors quantitatively followed the Law of Mass Action, that is to say: the combinations were reversible and obeyed the law that Guldberg and Waage had worked out (for ordinary laboratory chemicals) in 1864. Because no receptor had ever been isolated, Clark was obliged to work with, at best, single cells; but the quantitative and repeatable nature of his results, which were derived from a great variety of drugs and many tissues, created a much wider acceptance of receptor theory (Clark, 1926, 1933).

Further evidence for the existence of drug receptors was provided by substances that form pairs of optically active isomers, as do atropine, morphine and epinephrine. The two forms of each of these bases, namely the dextro- and the laevo-rotatory isomers, differ strikingly in biological potency. Because the two members of such pairs have otherwise identical chemical and physical properties and differ only in that their molecules are built as mirror images of one another, it became evident that the shape of a drug molecule can be crucial for its action and that the bio-active part of the molecule must fit a structure complementary to it (Cushny, 1926). Another factor, seen at that time to favour the idea of receptors, was the low concentration at which many drugs act (several of them even at 10^{-9} M) which suggested that a complementary structure must exist in the cell to rescue the drug from so much solvent.

In 1926 the establishment of pharmacology was shaken when Otto Loewi, in

Vienna, discovered the constitution of the first neurotransmitter (Loewi and Navratil, 1926). It was acetylcholine (6.2), and the shock sprang from the following paradox: although a quaternary amine, acetylcholine was no muscle relaxant (like tubocurarine and all of Crum Brown's artefacts) but was actually nature's number one muscle activator! This discovery persuaded many people to renounce the dogma that one chemical group gives one type of biological action, others remained conservative.

That a given chemical group could produce either an agonist or an antagonist, depending on the remainder of the molecule, was explained by Raymond Ing, in London, as follows: acetylcholine and tubocurarine act on the same receptor but the smaller molecule exactly fits the site and activates it, whereas the larger molecule simply lies over the receptor and blocks access to it (Ing, 1936). We now know many series of drugs where the lower members are agonists whereas the homologues of higher molecular weight are antagonists.

In the late 1920s, drug scientists began to visualize an agonistic drug as relating to a receptor in much the same way that a coenzyme is related to an enzyme. Similarly an antagonistic drug and an enzyme antagonist were seen to have much in common.

In such a climate of opinion it was soon shown that at least one receptor was actually on an enzyme. In Scotland Edgar Stedman discovered that physostigmine (8.23) which acts like acetylcholine (ACh) does not act directly on the ACh receptor but blocks acetylcholinesterase (AChase), the enzyme that destroys ACh as soon as it has acted on the receptor. Blocking this enzyme by physostigmine allows natural ACh to accumulate so that the patient gets a continuing dose of his own neurotransmitter (Stedman, 1929).

Since that time many receptors have been found to be the active sites of enzymes. However the receptor for ACh is not on an enzyme but on a different kind of protein, one that regulates the passage of sodium and potassium ions in and out of the muscle cells. Unlike an enzyme, a permease (as such proteins are called) effects no chemical change on its substrate. This ACh receptor was isolated in 1969 by Jean-Pierre Changeux, in Paris, from the electric organ of a fish. When purified it was seen as rows of rosettes under the electron microscope (Fig. 8.3). Each rosette is the end-face of a tube (ion channel) formed from five protein molecules arranged side-by-side. The ACh receptor is a small domain of amino acids shared by two of these protein strands (Changeux, et al., 1984).

The receptors of other neurotransmitters have since been isolated but not in such large quantity, e.g. the adrenergic β_1- and β_2-receptors have been purified to homogeneity and shown to retain their activity (Benovic, et al., 1984). All appear to be highly phosphorylated glycoproteins. Not all drug receptors are on proteins; some, as we shall see, are on nucleic acids.

Returning to Stedman's location of a drug receptor on an enzyme, it is strange that no extension of this phenomenon from pharmacodynamics to chemotherapy was made until 1940, when Donald Woods, in London, demonstrated the reversal of the antibacterial action of sulfanilamide (6.5) by p-aminobenzoic acid.

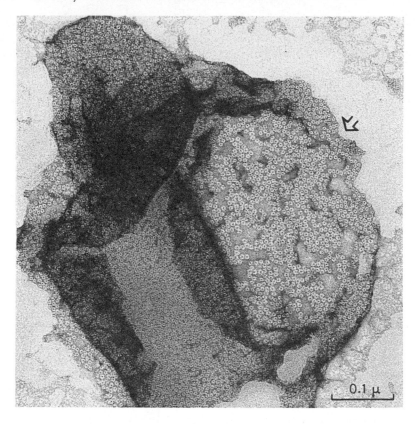

Fig. 8.3 Acetylcholine receptors in the massed permeases of the postsynaptic membranes of the electric organ of the fish, *Torpedo*. The centre of each rosette is a Na^+/K^+ channel, inside of which an ACh receptor is situated. (Courtesy of Dr. J. Cartaud, Paris).

This observation led to the isolation of dihydrofolate synthetase, the enzyme that converts *p*-aminobenzoic acid to the important coenzyme, dihydrofolic acid (*8.35*). The enzyme has a receptor site for this acid, and sulfanilamide fits the site very well. Hence the enzyme comes to equilibrium with either the natural substrate or the inhibitor preponderating, depending on the concentrations presented. Thus, when the sulfanilamide is in excess, the enzyme is blocked and no dihydrofolic acid can be made (Brown, 1962).

The many antibacterial drugs that appeared in the 1940s, each furnished with a sulfonamide group, provided one last hope for those who still believed that 'one chemical group controls one biological action'. However dihydrofolate synthetase can be antagonized by sulfur-free analogues of *p*-aminobenzoic acid, for example 4,4'-diaminobenzil (*8.36*) which is much more antibacterial than sulfanilamide (Kuhn, 1942). Moreover, many successful diuretic and antidiabe-

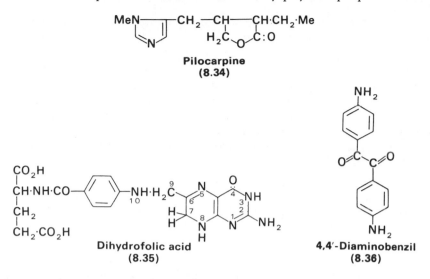

Pilocarpine
(8.34)

Dihydrofolic acid
(8.35)

4,4′-Diaminobenzil
(8.36)

tic drugs contain a sulfonamide group, but are not antibacterial. Once this was realized the 'chemical-group school' lost most of its support. People began to think that physical properties rather than the presence of a certain chemical group created the different kinds of pharmacological activity. Just how interpretations of structure–activity relationships switched to considerations of physical properties will be related in Section 8.3.

For further reading see Albert (1985, Chapter 2).

8.3 Important influences exerted by physical properties

The earliest indication that the biological activity of a drug could be linked to a physical property came at the start of the present century when Ernest Overton and Hans Meyer independently showed that narcotic* action depended not on the detailed structure of a molecule but on its lipophilicity. The latter property was measured by allowing the agent to equilibrate between olive oil and water. The ratio obtained was termed the partition coefficient (P). The more lipophilic the substance, the higher this ratio and the greater the hypnotic action (Meyer, 1899; Overton, 1901). This relationship held for the following chemical classes: hydrocarbons (aliphatic, aromatic, unsubstituted or chlorinated), alcohols, ethers, ketones, sulfones, amides and aliphatic nitrohydrocarbons, all of them non-ionizing substances.

Much of this early work was biologically evaluated by noting the minimal

---

* These authors wrote 'narcotic' to cover all the activities that we now characterize as hypnotic, general anaesthetic, and general biological depressant. More recently, the word is popularly applied to illicit drugs.

concentration that prevented tadpoles from swimming. Later octanol replaced olive oil as the non-aqueous layer in determining P. Table 8.1 lists a selection of hypnotics and general anaesthetics used (or, for ether and chloroform, formerly used) in human medicine. It will be noted that the log P values cluster mainly around 2, showing that these are moderately lipophilic substances favouring an oily environment over a watery one, by a factor of about one hundredfold. Note too the wide variety of chemical structures that can furnish the required physical property and hence the required pharmacological result. The membranes surrounding the brain favour accumulation of moderately lipophilic substances (p. 120); but how these act on the brain is not known. The selective swelling of sodium channels seems a likely explanation (Franks and Lieb, 1982).

Exciting as Overton and Meyer's results seemed at the time no wider application of them was realized. Forty years were to pass before further correlations of physical properties with pharmacological action were demonstrated.

However, in the 1940s my colleagues and I, working in the Universities of Sydney and Melbourne, quantitatively established the roles of ionization and chelation in the antimicrobial action of aminoacridines and hydroxyquinolines respectively. Interestingly, chelation is related to ionization to this extent: while ionization concerns the equilibria of the hydrogen cation, chelation concerns those of metal cations.

Table 8.1 Partition coefficients (P) of general anaesthetics and hypnotics used in human medicine (see Table A1 (p. 328) for coefficients of other substances). (After Hansch, *et al.*, 1968; Glave and Hansch, 1972.)

Drug	log P (octanol/water)
Halothane	1.81
Chloroform	1.97
Methoxyflurane	2.21
Diethyl ether*	0.77
Dipropyl ether	2.03
Ethchlorvynol	2.00
Barbiturates	
Ethyl, isoamyl (amobarbital, 'Amytal')	1.95
Ethyl, 1-methylbutyl (pentobarbital, 'Nembutal')	1.95
Allyl, 1-methylbutyl (secobarbital)	2.15
Ethyl, phenyl (phenobarbital)	1.42
Ethyl, 1-methylbutyl-2-thio (thiopental)†	3.00
Chlordiazepoxide ('Librium')	2.44
Diazepam ('Valium')	2.82

* Five times weaker an anaesthetic than dipropyl ether.
† Thiopental is an anaesthetic specialized for intravenous use.

While this work (which will be described below) was proceeding in Australia, another correlation with physical properties was being made by Bell and Roblin in Connecticut, USA who demonstrated that ionization and steric properties controlled the antibacterial action of the sulfonamide drugs. They showed that for these drugs to masquerade as *p*-aminobenzoic acid (PAB), thus blocking the enzyme dihydrofolate synthetase, the drug must possess close structural and electronic similarity to PAB. Any appreciable change in these physical properties altered the biological action, for the worse if the properties diverged too far, but for the better if they converged. The most important of the steric properties consisted of (a) a flat ring bearing a primary amino group situated para to a strongly electron-attracting group (here $-SO_2NH_2$), (b) the same distance between these two groups, as in PAB, and (c) the same molecular width. These features are shown here for PAB (*8.37*) and sulfanilamide (*8.38*, R = H) (Bell and Roblin, 1942).

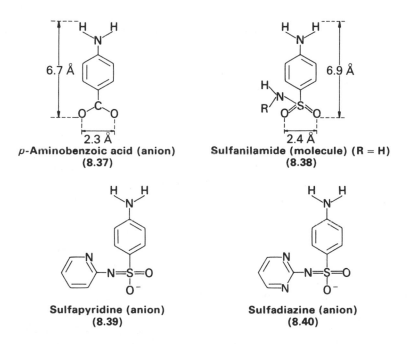

p-Aminobenzoic acid (anion)
(8.37)

Sulfanilamide (molecule) (R = H)
(8.38)

Sulfapyridine (anion)
(8.39)

Sulfadiazine (anion)
(8.40)

These authors at once saw an important difference between the two structures, namely that although PAB with its pK_a of 4.87 was 99% ionized as anion (at the human physiological pH of 7.3), sulfanilamide, with its pK_a of 10.43 was only 0.1% ionized. (For the influence of ionization on the action of drugs, and definition of pK_a, see Albert (1985, Chapter 10).) This difference was diminished by having an electron-attracting structure replace R in (*8.38*). The most versatile structure of this kind was seen to be a π-deficient heterocyclic ring. Figure 8.4

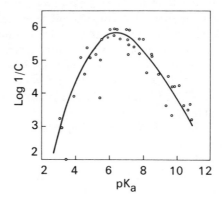

Fig. 8.4 How variation in the pK_a of a series of sulfanilamide antibacterial drugs affects the bacteriostatic action. Substances on the left are the more highly ionized (as anions) at the pH of the test (pH 7; synthetic medium; C = minimal inhibitory concentration). (Bell and Roblin, 1942).

shows how the antibacterial efficiency of sulfanilamide analogues reaches a maximum when the pK_a lies between 7 and 5 (67–99% ionized). Sulfapyridine (*8.39*), which had been introduced in England in 1939 and found clinically superior to sulfanilamide, was now found to have pK_a 8.43 (7% ionized). These data encouraged Bell and Roblin (1942) to proceed to sulfadiazine (*8.40*) which has pK_a 6.48 (86% ionized). (The increment is due to replacing the pyrimidine nucleus by the much more π-deficient (and hence more electron-attracting) pyrimidine nucleus.) This drug exceeded all previous sulfonamides in clinical efficacy and came to be considered the standard for sulfonamide antibacterials.

Returning to the Australian work on physical properties, we may take passing note that it was sponsored by the Australian Army during the Second World War. At that time the aminoacridines were much used to irrigate the deep, infected wounds sustained in the battles raging in the Southern Pacific Ocean. These drugs were specially valued for their selectivity, because they killed bacteria without harm to either leucocytes or abraded tissues; moreover the wounds healed rapidly. For this use, the Medical Directorate of the Army favoured proflavine (*8.41*) which stained everything intensely yellow. The Army wanted a non-staining equivalent, but above all it wanted to know the mode of action of these unusual antiseptics in order to use them with maximal efficiency. Our work in achieving these two goals opened up two perspectives in chemotherapy. It established the quantitative importance of ionization in the

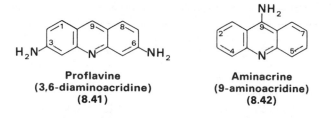

Proflavine
(3,6-diaminoacridine)
(8.41)

Aminacrine
(9-aminoacridine)
(8.42)

action of a drug and it led the way to recognition that a drug receptor need not be on a protein but could be, as here, on a nucleic acid.

At first it seemed puzzling that of the five possible monoamino acridines, two were highly antibacterial whereas three had little activity (Albert, Rubbo and Goldacre, 1941). At that time almost nothing was known about the ionization of heterocyclic bases therefore we began to determine the pK_a values of many examples from all the principal heterocyclic families and later we published the main rules that connect structure with basic strength (Albert, Goldacre and Phillips, 1948). Fortunately the correlation that we needed for our acridine work was found early in this seven year study. It turned out that 3-amino- and 9-amino-acridine had a resonance in the cation that was lacking from the neutral species and this made them very strong bases. This resonance is shown in (8.43–8.44). The other three aminoacridines could not, for reasons of valence, acquire this resonance and hence were not much stronger than the parent molecule, acridine – a weak base (pK_a 5.58). We called this amidine-like base-strengthening resonance 'the 4-aminopyridinium type of base-strengthening' because we first demonstrated it for 4-aminopyridine.

Table 8.2 shows how, depending on this resonance, mono- and di-aminoacridines can be highly ionized or poorly ionized at the pH of the antibacterial test. Those that are well ionized are highly antibacterial whereas those that are poorly ionized are feebly antibacterial.

We went on to show, using 102 different acridines and 22 species of bacteria, that the antibacterial action of aminoacridines increased with the proportion that was ionized at the pH and temperature of the bacteriostatic test. The nature of any non-amino substitutent, whether electron-attracting or electron-releasing, made absolutely no difference so long as it permitted at least 50% cationic ionization under these conditions (Albert, et al., 1945). Some examples are offered in Table 8.3.

As a result of this work, we were able to replace the Army's favoured deep-yellow wound irrigant (8.41) by the more selective and non-staining aminacrine (9-aminoacridine) (8.42).

Next we made several stepwise alterations to this molecule to discover the parameters of its efficacy. What we found was that any nucleus would do as well as acridine so long as the candidate was (a) basic enough to be ionized at least 50% at the pH of our test, and (b) had no less than 38 Å² of flat area.

Table 8.2 Dependence of bacteriostasis on ionization in aminoacridines.

Acridine	pK_a 20°C	Percent ionized as cation under test conditions (pH 7.3; 37°C)	Minimal bacteriostatic concentration (Streptococcus pyogenes, 48 h incubation in 10% serum broth)
Parent	5.58	2	1 in 10 000
1-amino-	6.04	2	1 in 10 000
2-amino-	5.88	2	1 in 10 000
3-amino-	8.04	75	1 in 80 000
4-amino-	4.40	<1	1 in 5 000
9-amino-	9.99	100	1 in 160 000
2,7-diamino-	6.18	3	1 in 20 000
4,5-diamino-	4.12	<1	1 in <5 000
3,6-diamino-	9.65	99	1 in 160 000
3,7-diamino-	8.11	76	1 in 160 000
3,9-diamino-	11.49	100	1 in 160 000

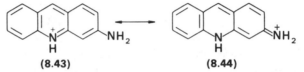

(8.43)   (8.44)

Cationic resonance that makes 3-aminoacridine a strong base

Table 8.3 Failure of electron-attracting or electron-releasing substituents to modify bacteriostatic action of aminoacridines (apart from their influence on ionization).

Acridine	Percent ionized as cation under test conditions (pH 7.3; 37°C)	Minimal bacteriostatic concentration (Streptococcus pyogenes, 48 h incubation in 10% serum broth)
4-amino-5-methyl-	<1	1 in 5 000
1-amino-4-methyl-	1	1 in 20 000
2-amino-9-methyl-	3	1 in 20 000
9-amino-2-methyl-	100	1 in 160 000
9-amino-3-methyl-	100	1 in 160 000
9-amino-4-methyl	100	1 in 320 000
2-amino-6-chloro-	<1	1 in <5 000
3-amino-9-chloro-	11	1 in <5 000
3-amino-6-chloro-	33	1 in 40 000
9-amino-3-chloro-	94	1 in 160 000
9-amino-2-chloro-	96	1 in 160 000
9-amino-4-chloro-	86	1 in 160 000

4-Aminopyridine and 4-aminoquinoline, although ionized enough, had too little flat area but when supplied with more of that property by inserting a coplanar substituent, as in 4-amino-2-styrylquinoline (*8.45*), the antibacterial activity returned. Moreover, the order of the rings comprising the acridine molecule was found to be relatively unimportant because many highly antibacterial amino-benzoquinolines and phenanthridines came to light. Not surprisingly our standard, 9-aminoacridine, was deprived of its activity by hydrogenating one of the outer rings, an operation that deleted flatness from one-third of the molecule.

Finally we boldly left the heterocycles behind and began to make basic anthracenes such as 2-guanidinoanthracene (2-anthrylguanidine) (*8.46*). This had enough of both requirements: ionization and flatness. To our delight it had the typical aminoacridine-like bacteriostatic properties, namely activity against a wide range of Gram-positive and Gram-negative organisms at high dilution, even in the presence of serum, without harm to phagocytes (Albert, 1944; Albert, Rubbo and Burvill, 1949). Here, just as with the antibacterial sulfonamides, the required biological action depends on the correct steric and electronic properties and not on the presence of a particular nucleus or substituent. Such a conclusion broke new ground but took time to be accepted as it is today.

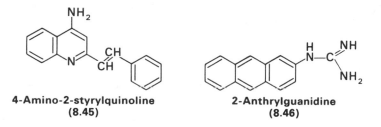

4-Amino-2-styrylquinoline
(8.45)

2-Anthrylguanidine
(8.46)

That aminoacridines were accumulated only by the nucleic acids of the living cell became known through their use in vital staining (Strugger, 1940). The reason for the necessity of molecular flatness became evident in 1961 when L. Lerman (Colorado) showed that aminoacridine molecules become 'intercalated'* into DNA by stacking between the layers of base pairs to which they cling by van der Waals forces supplemented by stronger ionic bonds to the phosphate ions of the DNA backbone (Fig. 8.5) (Lerman, 1961, 1964). The resultant increase of 20°C in the T_M ('melting temperature', i.e. temperature at which mutual coiling is halved) showed that the intercalation tends to inhibit the separation of the two strands and hence the normal functioning of the DNA (Chambron, Daune and Sadron, 1966). The picture was completed when J. Hurwitz and his colleagues in New York demonstrated that aminoacridines

---

* A word whose meaning had previously been confined to the insertion of the 29th of February into the leap year calendar.

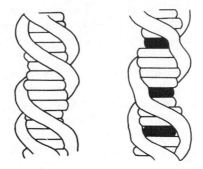

Fig. 8.5 Sketches representing the secondary structure of normal DNA (left) and DNA containing intercalated proflavine molecules (right). The helix is viewed from a remote point so that base-pairs and the intercalated acridine appear in edgewise projection; the phosphate deoxyribose backbone appears as a smooth coil. (Redrawn from Lerman, 1964).

injure bacteria by blocking the DNA template required by the polymerases that synthesize bacterial DNA and RNA (Hurwitz, *et al.*, 1962).

These studies of structure–action relationships in the aminoacridine series established that nucleic acids can be receptors. In fact the drug–receptor interaction was observable here in unusual detail much of it at the level of molecular biology. It is now recognized that nucleic acids are receptors for all the steroid hormones and many other kinds of drugs including the nitrogen mustards used in treating cancer as well as for many plant growth factors and several insect hormones.

Meanwhile another project had been handed to us by the Australian Army and once again some new general principles emerged. We had been asked to report on the mode of action of oxine (8-hydroxyquinoline) (*8.47*) which is strongly fungicidal as well as antibacterial. We began by making the six isomeric monohydroxyquinolines. We soon found that none of these isomers was able to chelate metals and none was antimicrobial. We formed the opinion that oxine was acting biologically by chelation, a mode of action unknown for any chemotherapeutic drug at that time. (A typical chelated product (with ferrous iron) is shown as (*8.48*). In this 1:1 complex the iron is unsaturated for oxine because, given more oxine, it can form the 2:1 complex.) To confirm our conclusion we blocked the chelating properties of oxine by methylating, in turn, the nitrogen and the oxygen atom. As expected the two products were neither chelating nor antimicrobial (Albert, 1944; Albert, *et al.*, 1947).

However we did not leap to the conclusion that oxine was removing a metal from the bacterium, very much as the antidotes dimercaprol and EDTA do from metal-poisoned patients. In fact oxine proved to be quite non-toxic for cells

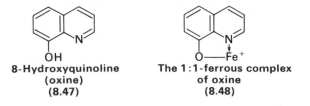

8-Hydroxyquinoline
(oxine)
(8.47)

The 1:1-ferrous complex
of oxine
(8.48)

provided that certain metals were excluded even in traces, namely *iron* for bacteria and *copper* for fungi. Clearly oxine does not function without a metal cotoxicant whose presence need only be accidental. This surprising conclusion was soon fortified by incubating *Staphylococcus aureus* in distilled water with oxine, with iron and then with both substances. Subsequent plating out on nutritive media showed that only bacteria that had been exposed to *both* oxine and iron were killed (see Table 8.4) (Albert, Gibson and Rubbo, 1953).

It soon became evident that drugs of quite different chemical structure, such as pyrithione (*8.49*), which is much used in the dermatology of the scalp, and sodium dimethyldithiocarbamate (*8.50*), a common agricultural fungicide, had the typical oxine mode of action. This action can be defined as the rapid killing of bacteria and fungi at high dilution, requiring the presence of either iron or copper, and preventable by a trace of cobalt (but no other common metal) (Rubbo, Albert and Gibson, 1950).

What was happening at the molecular level was revealed in Holland when Sijpesteijn and Janssen (1959) showed that these metal complexes catalysed the

Table 8.4 A metal co-toxicant is necessary for the bactericidal action of oxine, as shown by incubating in distilled water at 20°C and plating out after 1 h

Oxine 1/M	Ferrous sulfate 1/M	Growth (Staph. aureus)
nil	nil	prolific
100 000	nil	prolific
nil	100 000	prolific
100 000	100 000	undetectable

Pyrithione
(8.49)

$$Me_2N\cdot\overset{\displaystyle S}{C}\cdot SH$$

Dimethyldithiocarbamic acid
(8.50)

destruction of thioctic (dihydrolipoic) acid (*3.10*), the coenzyme of pyruvic oxidase. This chain reaction which is made up of successive oxidations is blocked uniquely by cobalt, as in non-biological situations. Thus thioctic acid appears to be the receptor for oxine-iron and related chelating combinations but so far few other examples of coenzymes acting as receptors have been discovered.

To summarize: drug scientists who had long and fruitlessly followed that seductive clue of 1869 began in the 1940s to realize how chemical structure is only secondary to the physical properties that the structure generates, and that these physical properties are the source of the observed biological activity. It became clear too that although a biologically-desirable action may be routinely available from one type of nucleus or substituent, it is usually available also from other nuclei or substituents. This new understanding vastly increased the possibilities for fruitful searching.

What are the most relevant of these physical properties? They are those that distribute the drug to the receptor and those that bind it to the receptor. In the last forty years three such properties have been most often correlated with the generation of biological activity. They are lipophilicity, electron distribution (as evidenced by ionization, chelation, or Hammett σ values) and a steric nature that is complementary to the receptor. Although, as has been known since 1900, a suitable degree of lipophilicity is the only physical condition necessary for generating hypnotic-anaesthetic action, all other types of activity require at least two of these three specified properties, in different proportions, to effect desired drug–receptor combinations.

Of the many attempts to quantify these relationships the most often used is one known as multiple regression analysis introduced by Corwin Hansch in California (Hansch, 1968). In this method the usual variables are (a) partition coefficients (P) from the system octanol/water, (b) the sigma (σ) and rho (ρ) values derived from Hammett's Linear Free Energy Equation (Hammett, 1970) and (c) Taft's steric factors (E_s) which are used to measure how much hinderance is exerted by a substituent on the adsorption of a nominated region of the drug on to the receptor. These variables are correlated in the following equation:

$$\log 1/C = -k(\log P)^2 + k_2(\log P) + k_3\sigma\rho + k_4 E_s + k_5$$

Let us look at three things: how this equation was put together, how it is operated and where it can be beneficially employed. C represents the lowest concentration that produces the observed effect. P, the partition coefficient, was defined on p. 175 and refers to octanol as the non-aqueous solvent. Hansch showed that the relationship between $\log 1/C$ and P is often parabolic. Consequently when the optimal degree of lipophilicity has been built into the molecule for the particular biological effect aimed at, it becomes counter-productive to exceed this value. An ideal substance is lipophilic enough to get into the membrane but hydrophilic enough to leave it on the far side; whereas a substance of very high P cannot leave the membrane. Hansch and Fujita (1964) had found that the following, simpler regression equation made a good fit for the partition/activity data on hypnotics:

$$\log 1/C = -k(\log P)^2 + k_2(\log P) + k_3$$

The square term tests the parabolic relationship of this simple regression equation which is easily seen to be the first part of the multiple regression equation given above.

In operation one uses only one half of one's series of compounds to find values of k, k_2 and k_3 by computer, employing the method of least squares. This provisional solution is tested by running the other half through the equation, with this difference: one must now use the various k values obtained from the first half instead of using the computer to find new coefficients. The r (correlation coefficient) calculated on the second set of results, should not differ appreciably from 1.0.

In a regression equation, each term needs at least five compounds to give statistical significance to its coefficients. In the simple equation there are three terms and hence 15 examples will be needed for the coefficient search and another 15 for the confirmatory test.

Hence to use the simple equation meaningfully a series of not less than 30 substances must be at hand for testing. However as the simple equation applies only to hypnotics and general anaesthetics, which many would regard as fairly well-solved problems, the use of the multiple regression equation is mandatory. This equation has ostensibly only 5 terms but, even so, 50 substances are needed for the results to have statistical significance. Here we can foresee practical limitations to the employment of regression analysis.

The new terms in the multiple regression equation are the two Hammett values multiplied together and the Taft steric factor. By working in a series where *rho* remains constant (say by confinement within the benzene or the quinoline series), *rho* may be dropped from the equation. The Taft factor permits of no such simplification. In fact the most cursory investigation warns us that not *one* steric term but a whole series of them is needed to describe the part of a drug that is to make effective contact with the active site (usually a cavity). Apart from flat molecules such as acridine, three Taft factors should be required to represent the three dimensions of a drug molecule.

In place of the Taft factor Hansch has sometimes obtained closer fits with molar refractivity, which can be applied either to a substituent or, by summation, to the whole molecule. Too often however, this descriptor tends to run parallel to another one, the partition coefficient, so that it may fail to inject new information into the analysis. Organic chemists often try to avoid use of a steric term by submitting a set of compounds closely similar in shape. However to proceed in this way severely limits what may be discovered. For a review of the origins of multiple regression analysis see Hansch, 1969, and for its development see Hansch and Leo, 1979. For more on this and other forms of QSAR (quantitative structure action relationships) see Albert, 1985, Chapter 16.

Multiple regression analysis has given some very useful results. It functions best in industry when a large series of closely related candidate drugs is on hand and a speedy indication is needed concerning what should be synthesized next. However for the purpose of finding scientific correlations among substances that are not closely related chemically, the biological situation is usually found to be more complex than such an equation can accommodate. For example the initial distribution of a drug need not depend on lipophilicity but on the use of facilitated channels that exist for the uptake of such natural products as sugars, purines, amino acids and even choline (p. 121). For these reasons those of a scholarly cast of mind, provided that they have the time and facilities, will continue to examine the connection between physicochemical properties and pharmacological action, in all their fine details and rewarding complexity.

In fact much steric and electronic information about receptors is available from sources other than regression analysis. For example, where the receptor is the active site on an enzyme, details (obtained by X-ray diffraction analysis) are often available from the Cambridge (UK) or Brookhaven (USA) crystal-structure databanks. In other cases one can usefully superimpose (on a transparent surface) scale drawings of all the drugs that act on the receptor. The shared features constitute what is called a 'hyper-molecule' to which the receptor should be complementary in outline and charge (Balaban, *et al.*, 1980). If an approximate image of the receptor can be generated on the screen of an Evans and Sutherland computer-graphics (computer controlled) Picture System the images of candidate drugs can then be applied in a contrasting colour. In this way the ability of the candidate to make a good fit may be judged (Blaney, *et al.*, 1982).

8.4 How one methyl group can significantly change the action of a drug

It is quite common to find a pair of closely related molecules where the first has a strong biological action whereas the other has none. How can two such substances which may differ in composition by only a single methyl group perform so differently in a biological test? In this Section a study of methyl groups will be made as examples of what are commonly termed 'chemically inert' groups. Yet these groups if suitably placed can profoundly change the chemical behaviour of molecules by well-understood steric and electronic effects. Their altered biological properties reflect these changes.

Steric influences

The steric effects introduced by small, inert groups are of two kinds. Some are evident even in aqueous solution whereas others require a surface for manifestation, as in enzyme reactions.

(a) *Steric influences on solubility.* It might be thought that the insertion into a given molecule of a methyl group would always lower solubility in water, because a methyl group is water-repelling. It usually does lower solubility but there are interesting exceptions. In order that a substance may dissolve in water the water molecules must be forced apart by breaking their hydrogen bonds. The lower alcohols, methanol and ethanol, readily do this because their hydroxyl group forms such a large part of each molecule and this group readily becomes hydrogen-bonded to water molecules. But in higher alcohols, the paraffinic side-chain becomes a more dominant feature: it cannot be accommodated in the interstices, it cannot force the water molecules apart and hence it tends to be squeezed out of the water, dragging the whole molecule with it. This explains the low solubility of the higher alcohols. Yet this effect can be considerably lessened by shifting the hydroxyl group to the centre of the molecule, as in tertiary amyl alcohol, which is consequently more soluble than its lower homologue, normal butanol (Ginnings and Baum, 1937). No less surprising, the 2-aminobutyric acids are more soluble than 2-aminopropionic acid (alanine), because of chain-folding.

Unusual solubilizing effects of methyl groups are found in the antibacterial sulfonamides, e.g. sulfadiazine (*8.40*), and in many other drugs of a similar degree of complexity and rigidity. In such molecules, any protruding C-methyl groups prevent strainless adsorption of dissolved solute (drug) on to the crystal-lattice of the solid phase. This anomaly displaces the final equilibrium in the direction of increased solubility (Gilligan and Plummer, 1943).

A methyl group can hinder addition of water across an adjacent double bond thus greatly increasing the lipophilicity of the substance, a property on which activity is apt to depend. Such addition of water is known as covalent hydration (Albert, 1976). Several naturally-occurring pteridines such as xanthopterin (*8.51*) which is present in the human kidney, are covalently hydrated, i.e. have become secondary alcohols. However the addition of a methyl group, as in (*8.52*), largely suppresses the hydration giving a less hydrophilic molecule. Many other natural products are covalently hydrated, a characteristic that can be suppressed by a neighbouring C-methyl group.

(b) *Steric influence on chelation.* The antibacterial action of 8-hydroxyquinoline (Section 8.3) is seriously decreased if a methyl group is inserted in the 2-position (Albert, *et al.*, 1947). This deactivation is most likely exerted through a steric

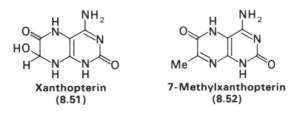

Xanthopterin   7-Methylxanthopterin
(8.51)   (8.52)

effect at the biological interface. Even in solution this substance (2-methyl-8-hydroxyquinoline) has lost its affinity for Al^{3+} (while retaining it for Fe^{3+}) because of the steric effect of the methyl group.

(c) *Steric influences on receptors and enzymes.* Most molecules that fit the muscarine receptor for acetylcholine have a quaternary nitrogen atom of which one substituent is a straight chain of five atoms in length. Addition of one more methylene group to this chain causes a dramatic loss of biological effect. At least two of the other substituents on the nitrogen atom must be methyl groups to achieve maximal action. If one of these is substituted by either hydrogen or ethyl, a sharp drop in activity takes place. On p. 100 we noted how the addition of a methyl group to the molecule of acetylcholine (6.2) to give methacholine (6.1) hindered hydrolysis of the molecule by acetylcholinesterase so strongly that the momentary pharmacological action exerted by ACh became a durable, and clinically valued, one. The biological effect of the vitamin thiamine (8.53) is very sensitive to addition or loss of a methyl group. When tested on pigeons, the activity drops to 5% if the methyl group is removed from the pyrimidine ring, and to less than 1% if the methyl group is removed from the thiazole ring. Finally if an extra methyl group is inserted into the thiazole ring, between nitrogen and sulfur, the vitamin action is completely lost (Schultz, 1940).

Sometimes a methyl group increases the biological effect of a drug by making it a poorer fit for a destructive enzyme. Thus amphetamine (7.24), which is 1-methyl-2-phenylethylamine, has a much more prolonged hypertensive effect than 2-phenylethylamine. This has been traced to the resistance of amphetamine to monoamine oxidase, the enzyme that quickly destroys the lower homologue (Blaschko, 1952). Similarly the action of corticosteroids and the steroid sex hormones can be intensified by inserting a methyl, or a fluorine, substituent – a steric device that has produced several clinically valuable drugs. Such seemingly inert substituents turn the steroids into poorly-fitting substrates for their natural destructive enzymes (Ringold, 1961).

Electronic influences

The methyl group is the commonest substituent that releases electrons no matter whether inductive or mesomeric mechanisms are operating.

(a) *Electronic influences on ionization*.* Because of its electron-releasing nature a methyl group, if attached to a nearby carbon atom, strengthens a base and weakens an acid. Also a methyl group attached to nitrogen, to give a secondary amine, is base-strengthening although most tertiary amines are weaker than secondary amines. Such changes in strength are usually less than one pK unit but can influence biological results if the pK falls within one unit of the pH at which

---

* For more on ionization *see* Albert and Serjeant (1984).

the biological test is made. When as usually happens one ionic species (e.g. the cation) is far more biologically active than another (e.g. the neutral species) this change in ionization can decide whether a substance is biologically active or not.

The triphenylmethane dyestuffs (*8.54*), which show a large increase in basic strength upon *N*-alkylation, illustrate how antibacterial action is correlated with ionization in this series as Table 8.5 illustrates. Thus antibacterial activity is virtually created here by the insertion of 'chemically inert groups'.

Although it is obvious that methylation of an acidic group must abolish its ability to ionize, the consequences of such a methylation in the barbituric acid series are particularly interesting. In aqueous solution, barbituric acid exists in the trioxo form (*8.55*) and forms the mono-anion by loss of a proton from *C*-5. It is

Table 8.5 Connexion between ionization and antibacterial activity in a series of triphenylmethane bases.

Substance	Formula	p$K_{equil.}$	Percentage ionized at pH 7.3	Minimal bacteriostatic concentration (*Staph. aureus*; 24 h at 37°C and pH 7.3)
Doebner's violet	(8.54a)	5.38	2	1 in 20 000
Malachite green	(8.54b)	6.90	28	1 in 80 000
Brilliant green	(8.54c)	7.90	80	1 in 1280 000

From Goldacre and Philips, 1949

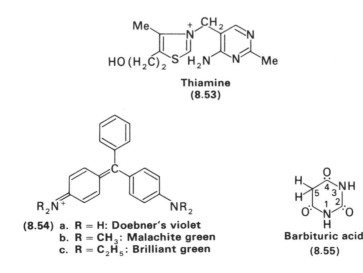

Thiamine
(8.53)

(8.54) a. R = H: Doebner's violet
b. R = CH$_3$: Malachite green
c. R = C$_2$H$_5$: Brilliant green

Barbituric acid
(8.55)

a fairly strong acid (pK_a 3.9). The insertion of two alkyl groups into the 5-position removes any possibility of an anion being formed in the 5-position. Consequently the anion is formed from N-3 but is much weaker. Thus barbital (5,5-diethylbarbituric acid) has a pK_a of 7.9 and hence is 10^4 times weaker as an acid than barbituric acid! The consequences of the insertion of these ethyl groups on the structure–activity relationship is momentous. A substance with a pK_a of 3.9 is completely ionized at pH 7.3, and hence unlikely to pass the blood–brain barrier. However when as in barbital the pK_a is 7.9 the substance is 80% non-ionized at pH 7.3, and hence passes through without difficulty.

(*b*) *Electronic influences on reduction–oxidation potentials.* The electrons released to the rest of the molecule by a *C*-methyl substituent lower the redox potential (E_0). As a result the affected substance becomes a more active reducing agent (and is more easily oxidized) than the unmethylated homologue. Redox potentials are used to record the equilibrium between oxidized and reduced forms.

An example of this lowering of E_0 is the insertion of a methyl group into the 2-position of 1,4-naphthaquinone which depresses the potential (by 76 mV) to 408 mV (Fieser and Fieser, 1935). In another example the reduction potential of NAD (p. 20) is -180 mV, a value so low that a substituted NAD of slightly lower potential could, most likely, not become reduced to its NADH. Any analogue that cannot be reduced in the living cell cannot act as a hydrogen carrier. It is apparently for this reason that 2-methyl-nicotinamide has no biological activity, even if the effect of the methyl group may be partly steric.

(*c*) *Electronic influences on reactions where a covalent bond is broken.* The electron-releasing effects of a methyl group described above were of an instantaneously-appearing character. Some time-dependent, i.e. kinetically controlled, effects will now be mentioned. Methyl groups, because of their electron-releasing properties, promote electrophilic substitution, e.g. they make neighbouring amino groups readier to be acylated or to form an azomethine (Schiff base). A methyl group also constitutes a side-chain that is conveniently biodegraded. Thus the metabolic oxidation of a methyl group to a carboxylic acid confers hydrophilic properties on a highly lipophilic molecule and leads to rapid excretion in the urine.

(*d*) *Solubility.* In an aromatic nitrogen-heterocycle such as pyridine replacement by methyl of the hydrogen atom in an –OH, –NH$_2$ or –C(:O)NH– group usually increases solubility in water dramatically. Thus 6-aminopurine (adenine) is soluble to the extent of only 1 part in 1100, whereas 6-dimethylaminopurine dissolves 1 in 120 (Albert and Brown, 1954); countless similar examples are known.

In conclusion it must be pointed out that this Chapter deals only with *activity*, which is the quality that makes a molecule more biologically active than a food. Yet activity can create only a poison unless selectivity is also incorporated. How selectivity can be introduced into a molecule, and what rules govern it, will be discussed in Chapter 9.

Further reading

For the biological effects of inserting chemically-inert substituents, see Albert, 1985, pp. 43–52.

Follow-up

Consider the traditional (and apparently unsinkable) phrase 'structure–activity relationships' (SAR) and discuss the extent to which the word 'structure' retains its original meaning. Could you think of a better phrase?

9

Selectivity: designing drugs without side-effects.

The three sources of selectivity

In Chapter 8 we saw how a biologically inert molecule could be redesigned to endow it with biological activity. However that would be only the first step in the creation of a useful drug because a biologically active substance remains only a toxicant (poison) until it is provided with selectivity also. In other words, it must be further designed to confine its action to the uneconomic cells (p. 101). The extent to which a drug can differentiate between economic and uneconomic cells is the measure of its selectivity. Toxicity in a drug is no drawback, in fact it is the very core of its usefulness. What is important is to arrange for this toxicity to be selective. The present Chapter lists and examines the properties from which selectivity can be derived.

Realization of the importance of selectivity dates from about 1911 when Paul Ehrlich introduced his chemotherapeutic index as the first means of measuring it (p. 111). Today the drug designer's goal is complete selectivity and this has been closely approached in several chemotherapeutic agents such as the penicillins, the antibacterial sulfonamides and several anthelminthics such as piperazine. However for some diseases the best available drugs still have only partial selectivity although current research is steadily improving on this position.

Since 1948 I have been seeking and publicly discussing the *principles* that can introduce selectivity into a biologically-active molecule. This search led me to conclude that three main principles govern this phenomenon:

1. *Comparative accumulation*, by choice of a toxicant that accumulates pre-ferentially in the uneconomic cells;
2. *Comparative biochemistry*, by choice of a toxicant that injures a biochemical process found only in the uneconomic cells;

3. *Comparative cytology*, by choice of a toxicant that interferes with a cytological feature peculiar to the uneconomic cells.

How these principles, singly or jointly, can establish selectivity in otherwise unselective toxicants will now be discussed under these three headings.

9.1 Selectivity through comparative distribution

Many substances that could be toxic for almost all kinds of cells can nevertheless be made highly selective by favourable differences in distribution. This applies even to the hydrogen ion (H^+) surely the simplest of all biologically-active agents. In the form of 10% sulfuric acid, it can safely be sprayed on emerging cereal crops to destroy weeds, as was discovered in France by Rabaté and confirmed in the University of California's field trials. Of course, sulfuric acid is injurious to the cytoplasm of both wheat and weed, but two factors restrain it from penetrating the cereal. Firstly the exterior of the cereal, a monocotyledon, is smooth and waxy whereas that of the weeds (mainly dicotyledons) is rough and absorbent; hence the acid runs off the former but is accumulated by the latter. Secondly the tender new shoot of the cereal arises from the soil and is protected by a leaf-sheath whereas the growing point of the dicotyledon is exposed and vulnerable because it forms the apex of the shoot. Hence the weeds die and the economic crop persists because of a selective action that depends entirely on distribution. (Unfortunately, acidification of the soil limits this type of weeding to a single season).

Human medicine provides many similar examples, notably the tetracyclines (e.g. *9.1*) which are, after the penicillins, the most frequently prescribed of all antibiotics. Franklin, working in Manchester, observed that the tetracyclines are accumulated by all bacteria whereas they hardly penetrate mammalian cells thanks to a difference in the cytoplasmic membranes of these two forms of life. As a result the synthesis of proteins by bacterial ribosomes is repressed and the bacteria die. Yet when both the economic and uneconomic cells were fractionated it was found that the ribosomes of the host were just as sensitive to these antibiotics as those of the parasites. However so selective is the distribution of these drugs that the tetracyclines do not normally reach the ribosomes in mammalian cells. Hence the high therapeutic index of these antibiotics (Franklin, 1971).

Selective partitioning is possible between the tissues of a single organism. In a rare example from anticancer therapy, 5-fluorouracil (*9.2*) is used by dermatologists to eliminate two malignant growths – basal and squamous cell carcinomas. So selective is this drug that patients are encouraged to rub a solution of it daily into the affected area. The eventual action is on thymidylate synthetase which is present in both healthy and malignant tissues. However the malignant tissue in this treatment is the only one to become inflamed. It finally disintegrates by necrosis and is replaced by healthy granulation tissue followed by new skin (Klein *et al.*, 1972).

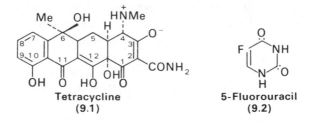

Tetracycline
(9.1)

5-Fluorouracil
(9.2)

Iodine, which is selectively accumulated by the thyroid gland, provides another good example of selective action through specific distribution. This concentration process is easily followed with radioactive iodine (^{131}I, half life 8 days) which is used for treating thyrotoxicosis. Depending on the dose this radioactive drug can be used merely to inhibit the excessive metabolism of the gland or it can be used actually to attack a tumour in the gland. The usual oral dose is only 10^{-12} g, yet 80% of this can be demonstrated in the gland soon after administration.

Cyanocobalamin (vitamin B_{12}), when injected intramuscularly, travels to the bone marrow and accumulates there after a dilution of 10^{10}-fold in the body fluids. Even a microgram, injected for treatment of pernicious anaemia, is enough to form new reticulocytes in the patient. This distribution process has been followed closely by using a specimen of vitamin marked with ^{57}Co (Schilling, 1953).

Griseofulvin (9.3), the antifungal antibiotic used in dermatology, after oral administration becomes selectively lodged in the patient's keratinized cells, namely the epidermis, hair and nails. There it blocks fungal mitosis; human cells suffer similarly so that the selectivity depends on the initial distribution (Gull and Trinci, 1973).

Selective distribution can be effected by size alone. When particles are inhaled, those above 5 μm in diameter remain in the nasal passages, whereas those of about 2 μm lodge in the larger bronchial areas. However particles must be narrower than 1 μm if they are to reach the smallest bronchi and the alveolar sacs as is necessary for effective medication by aerosol nasal sprays.

Remarkable selectivity has been attained in diagnostic agents. Organic compounds containing normal iodine (^{127}I) are used as radiopaques (X-ray contrast agents) in the radiography of the area in which each has been designed to accumulate. Thus the gall bladder and biliary ducts are specifically delineated by iopanoic acid (9.4) or the related substance, sodium ipodate, which is given orally. But for outlining the urinary tract diatrizoic acid (9.5) or its isomer iothalamic acid are given intravenously.

The safe and accurate diagnosis of diseases by the use of radiopharmaceuticals is the most important contribution that atomic energy has made to human health. For example gallium (^{67}Ga) specifically facilitates visualizing tumours in

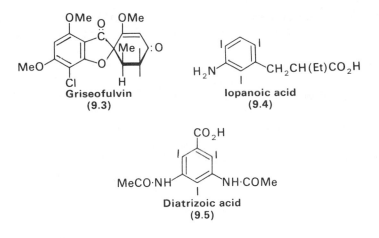

Griseofulvin
(9.3)

Iopanoic acid
(9.4)

Diatrizoic acid
(9.5)

the lymphatics; chromium (^{51}Cr) is specific for labelling erythrocytes; indium (^{113}In) is used to scan the lung (but it must first be adsorbed on particles of diameter 30 μm, a size that the blood capillaries of the lung specifically retain). Technetium ^{99}Tc (half life 6 h) is a powerful but safe emitter of soft gamma rays and is used in this way and also in simple solution to localize brain tumours which selectively accumulate it. Similarly, thallium (^{201}Tl) is used to locate damaged cells in the myocardium of a patient's heart. For more on the specificity of radiopharmaceuticals see Reynolds (1982).

It has already been indicated how a drug in transit from the site of administration to its specific receptor must cross several selectively permeable membranes (Section 7.1). Each membrane, because of its restrictive permeability, can make a contribution to the total selectivity. The apparent volume of distribution (V_D) (p. 119), coupled with the analysis of other withdrawn samples, enables the investigator to follow what is happening.

It is evident that the choice of a receptor as a target for a candidate drug has to be made at the start of the investigation (Section 7.2). Most human diseases offer a variety of such targets which may be associated with one another in parallel (most often in chemotherapy) or in series (most often in pharmacodynamics). As an example of linkage in series, drugs for controlling hypertension may be aimed at any one of the following five targets: (a) the central nervous system (e.g. clonidine), (b) sympathetic ganglia (e.g. pentolinium), (c) sympathetic nerve endings (e.g. propranolol (8.33)), (d) muscles of the arterioles (e.g. hydralazine (7.8), the organic nitrates) or (e) the causative angiotensin-forming enzyme (e.g. captopril).

In these preliminary choices as always in drug designing the close collaboration of chemists and biologists is essential. The more remote the chosen drug receptor is from the final regulating function the greater the likelihood of side-effects being elicited. Yet always to choose the ultimate regulating function as the target may by-pass helpful natural counter-regulating effects.

In between administration and arrival at the receptor the concentration of a drug often falls through operation of any of three factors – storage, inactivation or excretion, as recounted in Section 7.3. A close study of these losses will often indicate a point where selectivity is operating and can be heightened.

A new and related development is the self-cancelling drug – one that is automatically degraded after use and leaves behind only biologically-inert products. Such drugs do not depend on any enzyme for their destruction nor on any organ for their elimination. Because of the universal presence of water in the body, a self-cancelling drug disintegrates hydrolytically at whatever rate has been designed into its structure. This rate is obtained from consideration of Hammett sigma constants.

An outstanding example of a self-limiting drug is atracurium (9.6), which is valued as a muscle relaxant in general anaesthesia (Payne and Hughes, 1981). An average dose, given intravenously, is adequate for 30 minutes of surgery and can be renewed as necessary. In water it slowly undergoes a Hofmann degradation producing two inert substances by fission at the dotted line in (9.6). Other self-limiting drugs are being used in dermatology (Albert, 1985, p. 96).

The metabolic activation of a pro-drug, discussed in Section 7.4, provides many examples of selectivity, as exemplified by the urinary antiseptic methenamine (p. 140). Some self-converting pro-drugs which depend only on water for activation are coming into use.

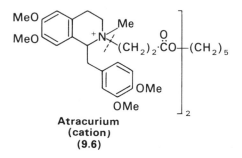

**Atracurium
(cation)
(9.6)**

It is in the study of quantitative aspects of distribution, particularly pharmacokinetics (Section 7.5), that the barriers to achieving selectivity can most reliably be detected and remedied. Every effort should be made to study the kinetics of a candidate drug's absorption, distribution, metabolism and excretion, all of which are rate-controlled. The chemical nature of any metabolites formed from these drugs needs to be ascertained, also whether any of them are biologically active. Such metabolic products are usually isolated by high-performance liquid chromatography and identified by mass spectrometry. These procedures and the use of isotopes were outlined in Section 7.3.

The studies of the pharmacokinetics of antibacterial sulfonamides by Nelson and O'Reilly (p. 149) illustrate how simple measurements on human volunteers can supply valuable data on selectivity, in a series of related compounds, leading to better prescribing practices and also to better drugs.

An interesting example of selectivity by distribution is provided by the schizonticidal antimalarial, chloroquine (9.7). When orally administered this drug has to penetrate the gastrointestinal membranes, then those of the erythrocyte and finally those of the plasmodial schizont inside these red cells. Chloroquine is a reasonably selective drug but not entirely without toxic effects on the patient. In seeking to improve it two questions arise: (a) how is this favourable distribution derived from the physicochemical properties of the molecule and (b) how are the patient-toxic effects derived, with a view to their elimination?

Propranolol (8.33), an example from pharmacodynamics, is a useful but non-selective β_1 and β_2-adrenergic blocker whose action is exerted on four organs: heart, the adrenergic nerves that terminate in blood vessels, bronchial smooth muscle and skeletal muscle. For treating angina an analogue was needed with specificity for β_1-adrenergic receptors, to confine the action to the heart. Metoprolol (9.8) is one of several simplifications of the propranolol molecule that are serving this end.

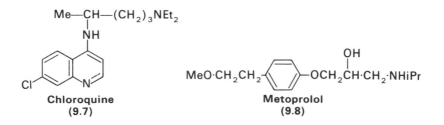

Chloroquine
(9.7)

Metoprolol
(9.8)

Such large chemical changes are not usually necessary. Even the smallest alteration in the molecule of a drug (such as inserting or just shifting the position of a single methyl group) often causes a sufficient change in distribution by altering the kinetic constant pertaining to one or more of the arrows in Fig. 7.1.

In the chemotherapy of cancer where many of the drugs are of only low selectivity their virtue is enhanced by physical means. Thus the cytotoxic agent can be infiltrated directly into the tumour. Intra-arterial infusion of a tourniquet-isolated limb represents another ruse for decreasing the body-volume in which the drug is distributed. Another strategy is to heat that region of the body where the anticancer drug is being perfused while cooling the other regions. The use of antidotes to sharpen the terminal edge of a perfusion of alkylating agent or methotrexate (suitable antidotes are cysteine and folinic acid, respectively) is successfully practised.

The restriction of a drug to its target area by mechanical means has been termed compartmentalization (Zaffaroni, 1974). By inserting a small piece of plastic, impregnated with the appropriate drug, a localized form of sustained release (p. 150) can be obtained e.g. for birth-control or to alleviate glaucoma in the eye.

9.2 Selectivity through comparative biochemistry

Of the three ways of introducing selectivity into a molecule, this is the one that has so far proved the most successful in developing clinically useful drugs. In the higher organisms increased efficiency is achieved by a division of labour, which is brought about by having a variety of organs and tissues (such as heart, kidneys, liver, blood, skin, nerves, muscle) to carry out the various essential functions without mutual interference. As a result certain enzymes tend to be concentrated in the tissues that require them. Thus arginase occurs mainly in the liver, alkaline phosphatase in the kidney, carboxylesterase and ribonuclease in the pancreas, β-glucuronidase in the spleen, glutamine synthetase in the brain and liver, while glucosamine phosphate isomerase is found mainly in the intestines (data from the rat, Dixon and Webb, 1979).

The organ-specific nature of so many enzymes indicates possibilities for devising selective pro-drugs, masked with a group that only the target tissue can remove; an example is fosfestrol USP (*9.9*). This drug (diethylstilbestrol diphosphate) remains biologically inert until hydrolysed by the acid phosphatase present in carcinoma of the prostate gland, but absent from healthy tissue. The liberated diethylstilbestrol effects regression of the tumour and this treatment is considered to be life-saving (Lambley and Ware, 1967).

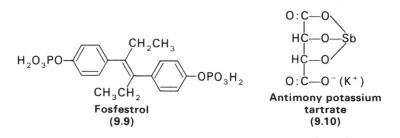

Fosfestrol
(9.9)

Antimony potassium
tartrate
(9.10)

Many examples are known where the enzymes that carry out apparently identical functions in dissimilar cells are themselves dissimilar. When the chemical differences between the two enzymes is small they are called isoenzymes but it can be quite large in which case we speak of analogous enzymes. The latter provide ideal opportunities for the incorporation of selectivity into a drug. An example is offered from the treatment of schistosomiasis (p. 114) with antimonial drugs. The phosphofructokinase (p. 36) of schistosome worms is much more easily inhibited by antimonials than is mammalian phosphofructokinase. In short these two enzymes form a pair of analogous enzymes. The therapeutic success of antimonials in the traditional treatment of schistosomiasis depends on blocking this enzyme selectively. This selectivity is illustrated by the use of antimony potassium tartrate (*9.10*) in Figure 9.1.

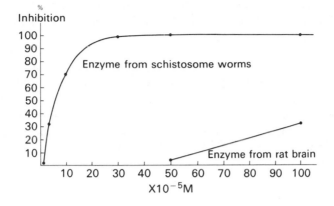

Fig. 9.1 Comparative inhibition of phosphofructokinase by antimony potassium tartrate, in parasite and host. (From Mansour and Bueding, 1954).

The rifamycins are antibiotics of which the slightly man-modified example known as rifampicin (rifampin) is much used in the treatment of tuberculosis. Because it is one of the most selective of all known antibacterial drugs it could be used in other infections were it not so expensive. However, it is valued for treating staphylococcal infections that resist penicillin. Rifamycins inactivate the β-subunit of the protein in RNA polymerase, but only in the analogue of this enzyme that bacteria depend on, for its mammalian analogue is completely unaffected (Tocchini-Valenti, Marino and Colvill, 1968).

A wealth of clinically useful drugs has been derived from analogous enzymes that centre upon dihydrofolic acid (*8.35*). Let us begin with dihydrofolate reductase (DFR), the enzyme that converts this vitamin to tetrahydrofolic acid which is in turn the parent of coenzymes that are indispensable for introducing a one-carbon substituent. If the formation of tetrahydrofolic acid is inhibited no more thymidine can be formed from uridine and no more purines can be biosynthesized. The organism affected in this way can no longer produce DNA by the purely synthetic route. It has indeed been fortunate in the treatment of man's infectious diseases that the DFRs constitute a family of analogous enzymes.

The first drug found to block DFR was aminopterin, made quite simply by changing the 4-oxo group of folic acid to a primary amino group. A more selective drug was obtained for treating human leukaemia by also inserting a methyl group in the 10 position giving methotrexate (*9.11*). This drug has been successfully used since 1950 in curing a cancer of the blood elements in young adults (acute lymphatic leukaemia). It also brings about a lasting cure in two other types of cancer: choriocarcinoma, a fast-growing tumour of pregnancy with normally a high death-rate, and Burkitt's lymphoma, a highly malignant form of cancer that affects African children (Farber, 1952; Zuelzer, 1964).

Chemically-altered folic acids such as methotrexate have no effect on bacteria and protozoa which are incapable of absorbing folic acid or its analogues. In the USA about 1950 G. H. Hitchings began systematically to simplify the structure of methotrexate (9.11) in order to obtain analogues that could penetrate into microorganisms. Each simplified product was tested on isolated DFR, so that the organism's barrier to penetration could not interfere with the test. Hitchings quickly found that both the glutamate and the *p*-aminobenzoyl regions of methotrexate could be eliminated, leaving the inhibitory power unchanged; also the pyrazine ring could be deleted from the pteridine nucleus. This left him with 2,4-diaminopyrimidine (9.12), a product that justified his hopes by being the first DFR inhibitor that could penetrate unicellular organisms (Wood, Ferone and Hitchings, 1961).

This knowledge enabled Hitchings to develop the powerful antimalarial drug, pyrimethamine (9.13) (Falco, *et al.*, 1951). This substance (2,4-diamino-6-ethyl-5, *p*-chlorophenylpyrimidine) has become the most widely used of all prophylactics against malaria. The lipophilic groups in the molecule favour its uptake by the tissues containing the malarial parasite, and they also increase the adsorption of the drug on to the dihydrofolate reductase by van der Waals forces (Baker and Shapiro, 1966). Dihydrofolate reductase, isolated from a malarial parasite *Plasmodium berghei*, has a molecular weight of 200 000, which is 10 times as large as those of analogous enzymes purified from mammals and bacteria.

Table 9.1 shows that the plasmodial enzyme is inhibited by pyrimethamine at a concentration about 2000 times lower than that which inhibits analogous mammalian enzymes. The concentration that inhibited the plasmodial enzyme

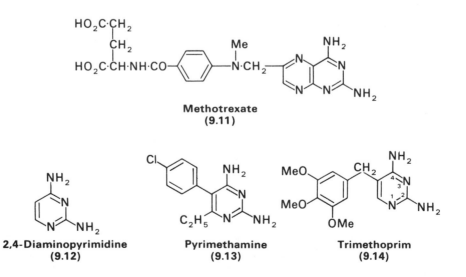

Methotrexate
(9.11)

2,4-Diaminopyrimidine
(9.12)

Pyrimethamine
(9.13)

Trimethoprim
(9.14)

Table 9.1 Concentrations ($\times 10^8$ M) of anti-folic drugs needed for 50% inhibition of dihydrofolate reductase, isolated from six sources. From Burchall and Hitchings, 1965; Ferone, Burchall and Hitchings, 1969; Jaffe and McCormack, 1967.

Substance	Human liver	Rat liver	Mouse erythrocyte	Pl. berghei	Tryp. equiperd.	E. coli
Pyrimethamine (9.13)	180	70	100	0.05	20	2500
Trimethoprim (9.14)	30 000	26 000	100 000	7.0	100	0.5
Methotrexate (9.11)	9	0.2	(not done)	0.07	0.02	0.1

corresponded to that achieved in human tissues after the usual prophylactic dose. These data established that the selective action of pyrimethamine in malaria is due to the extraordinary sensitivity of the enzyme in the parasite compared to the analogous enzyme in the host (Burchall and Hitchings, 1965).

It will be gathered from Table 9.1 that pyrimethamine is not selective for bacteria (exemplified there by *E. coli*) but is actually counter-selective. Further investigation showed that the DFR of bacteria is so different from that of either mammals or malarial parasites, that a different substitution pattern was required in the diaminopyrimidine matrix. Trimethoprim (*9.14*) was eventually discovered, an excellent antibacterial diaminopyrimidine. Table 9.1 shows that, compared with the excellent selectivities shown by trimethoprim and pyrimethamine, methotrexate exhibits a narrower range, even though there is no plasma membrane in this type of test to restrain its access to the enzyme.

Table 9.2 provides examples of the high selectivity that trimethoprim exerts against the dihydrofolate reductase of bacteria, both Gram positive and Gram negative types*, while leaving the analogous mammalian enzyme unharmed (Roth, Falco and Hitchings, 1962). It is noteworthy that these much-prescribed diaminopyrimidine drugs have been discovered by the exercise of scientific reasoning.

The therapeutic value of trimethoprim is often increased by prescribing it with a sulphonamide such as sulfamethoxazole (*9.15*), for reasons that will now be explained. Coenzymes are systematically built up from components that are moved along the enzymatic equivalent of a factory's production line, each stage of assembly being carried out by a different enzyme. This makes it worthwhile for the physician to prescribe two drugs, each of which inhibits neighbouring sites in this process. The arithmetic of this 'sequential blocking', as Hitchings termed it, is as follows. If the first of two enzymes is blocked to the extent of 90%, then only 10% of the partly completed factor reaches the next enzyme. If using a different drug one can also block this second enzyme by 90%, then only 1% of the partly completed factor emerges, and this is probably too little to sustain the life of the

Table 9.2 Effect of trimethoprim (*9.14*) on isolated dihydrofolate reductase. Concentrations (nM) causing 50% inhibition. From Roth and Cheng, 1982.

Source:	Mammalian liver		Bacteria		Ratio
Rat	1200		*Strept. faecalis*	0.96	1250
Ox	2400		*E. coli*	1.3	1840

* In 1884, Christian Gram, the Danish bacteriologist, discovered the strain that divides bacteria into two classes. The Gram negative bacteria, which have an extra outer layer, do not take the stain.

parasite. It may be asked why it does not suffice to use more of the first drug, to block the first enzyme by 100%. This is never done because dose–response curves are usually hyperbolic. Hence, increasing the concentration of a drug, beyond 90% inhibition, seldom leads to a worthwhile extra response. Instead it takes the dosage into that elevated area where side-effects often appear.

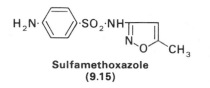

Sulfamethoxazole
(9.15)

In the sequence that we are considering, sulfamethoxazole blocks the incorporation of p-aminobenzoic acid into dihydrofolic acid, whereas the trimethoprim prevents the reduction of this pteridine to tetrahydrofolic acid. The combination of trimethoprim with sulfamethoxazole is almost universally known as co-trimoxazole* and is marketed under such trade names as 'Septrin', 'Bactrim' and 'Eusaprim'. It is a much used combination and is giving excellent results in bacterial dysentery, acute bronchitis and long-standing infections of the urinary tract, whether with Gram positive or negative organisms (Cattell, *et al.*, 1971). Combinations of pyrimethamine with an antibacterial sulfonamide (usually dapsone or sulfadoxine) are used in treating malaria (Richards, 1970).

A typical X-ray diffraction diagram of the active site of dihydrofolate reductase (derived from *Lactobacillus casei*) is shown in Fig. 9.2. The inhibitor methotrexate (*9.11*) and the essential coenzyme NADPH are shown bound to the active site at a resolution of 1.7 Å. The pteridine ring fits into a pocket lined by Leu-4, Ala-6, Leu-27, Phe-30 and Ala-97. The Asp-26 of the protein binds the amidinium ion formed from the N-1 and 2-NH_2 atoms in the drug, whose 4-NH_2 is hydrogen-bonded to the carbonyl groups of both Leu-4 and Ala-97. The nicotinamide portion of NADPH lies handy for delivering a hydride ion to position C-6 in the pteridine ring (Bolin, *et al.*, 1982). Other stereo diagrams, showing how differently trimethoprim sits in DFR from bacterial and mammalian sources, point to the molecular basis of selectivity (Matthews, *et al.*, 1985).

What may be regarded as the extreme case of the usual pair of analogous enzymes is encountered when one member of the pair is completely missing. Thus the-selectivity of the antibacterial sulfonamides depends on two deficiencies which reinforce one another to generate a high degree of selectivity. First mammals lack the enzymes needed to synthesize dihydrofolic acid and hence

---

* But in the USA as 'trimethoprim-sulfamethoxazole', a name that must be inconvenient for the prescriber.

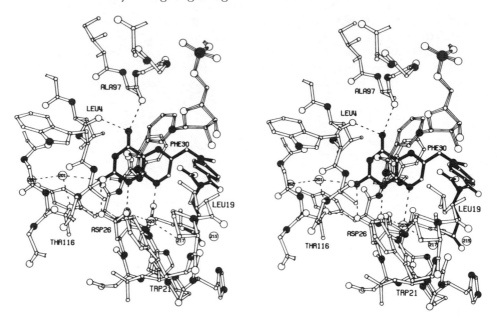

Fig. 9.2 Dihydrofolate reductase from *L. casei*, showing pteridine-binding site with an inhibitor, methotrexate (*9.11*), indicated by black bonds. The protein is indicated by open bonds and the NADPH coenzyme (only a portion shown) by striped bonds. Carbon atoms are represented by small (and oxygen atoms by larger) open circles and nitrogen atoms by blackened circles. Larger, independent circles represent fixed molecules of water (Bolin, *et al.*, 1982).

they tolerate these sulfonamides whose action on bacteria depends on their interfering with this synthesis (p. 173). Second bacteria lack the permease with the aid of which mammals absorb dihydrofolic acid from their diet.

A similar situation will now be described for malathion (*9.16b*) one of the safest of the organophosphate insecticides which act by inhibiting insect acetylcholinesterase. They phosphorylate a serine residue in this enzyme which is thereby inactivated. Malathion is a pro-agent which cannot carry out this phosphorylation until hydrolysed to malaoxon (*9.16a*) the actual toxicant. Fortunately the hydrolysing enzyme is not present in vertebrates, which go comparatively unharmed. An additional safety feature was built into the molecule of malathion. Mammals have abundant esterases that hydrolyse the ester (CO_2Et) groups to carboxylic acid groups, a type of structure which the kidney promptly eliminates. Again fortunately insects are poor in such non-specific enzymes.

The P : S to P : O change in insects is effected by microsomes, in the gut and the nerve cord itself. Table 9.3 shows how the mouse stands a high dose of malathion because it cannot readily convert it to the toxicant, malaoxon, whereas the cockroach and particularly the housefly are excellent converters.

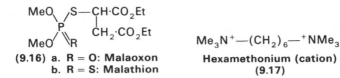

(9.16) a. R = O: Malaoxon
b. R = S: Malathion

$Me_3N^+ —(CH_2)_6 —^+NMe_3$

Hexamethonium (cation)
(9.17)

Table 9.3 Comparison of the toxicity of some phosphorus insecticides to mammals and to insects (LD_{50} in ppm w/w). From Kruegcr and O'Brien, 1959.

Species	Malathion	Malaoxon
Mouse (drug given l/p)	1590	75
Housefly	30	15
Cockroach	120	15

Striking differences in biochemistry are not often found between a malignant tumour and its tissue of origin. Nevertheless several cancers lack an enzyme which is abundantly present in the parent tissue. Thus some strains of human leukaemia cells lack the enzymes for synthesis of L-asparagine, although this is necessary for their metabolism and growth. When asparaginase is injected, the patient's pool of this amino acid can be depleted without causing him great distress. In the cancer wards drug-resistant lymphoblastic leukaemia of children responds well to this treatment (Levy and Boiron, 1969). Pyrethrins, which are much used insecticides, are harmless to man who detoxifies them rapidly with non-specific oxidases that insects lack (Yamamoto, 1970).

In the foregoing we have considered several examples of a metabolite and its antagonist, the structure of which differs from that of the metabolite by a small but effective change. Examples are *p*-aminobenzoic acid (*8.37*) and sulfanilamide (*8.38*); also dihydrofolic acid (*8.35*) and methotrexate (*9.11*). Such relationships are usually competitive at the active site of the enzyme. That is to say if *x* molecules of metabolite are antagonized by *y* molecules of analogue, then 10 *x* molecules of metabolite require 10 *y* molecules of analogue to give the same biological endpoint, and so on. It has been found very useful to record the index of inhibition for such pairs. This index is defined as the ratio of the number of molecules of the analogue to those of the metabolite when 50% inhibition has been achieved. This ratio, which will vary with the test species, expresses the relative affinity of analogue and metabolite for the appropriate receptor. However when the site of action lies behind a biological membrane the ratio includes a hidden term for differences in the penetrative ability of the two substrates.

The index of inhibition is obtained by dividing the dissociation constant of that inhibitor (K_i) by the appropriate Michaelis-Menten constant (K_m). These are found as follows:

$$K_i = [E] [I]/[EI], \quad \text{and} \quad K_m = [E] [S]/[ES]$$

where [E] is the concentration of the enzyme, [I] is that of the inhibitor, [EI] is that of the complex that they form, and [S] is the concentration of the substrate. The smaller the inhibitory index the more efficient the inhibitor. That for the antagonism by sulfanilamide of p-aminobenzoic acid in streptococci is 300, a rather large but still useful figure. At the other end of the scale lies the index of 0.0001 for the antagonism by methotrexate of dihydrofolate (measured on its free reductase). Values somewhere in between these extremes are more commonly met.

Although it is not difficult to make inhibitory metabolite analogues it is rather uncommon to find ones that are selective. Either one must find a metabolite that is important in the uneconomic species but unimportant in the economic species, *or* discover a pair of analogous enzymes (one in each species). Alternatively one can seek an analogue that is taken up in greater quantity by the uneconomic species (Section 9.1). Although many successes have been achieved in chemotherapy through these strategies, the receptors for the human body's neurotransmitters have proved to be just as rewarding, because they occur as various sub-types. Thus concerning the receptors for acetylcholine, tubocurarine (*8.25*) acts at the junction between nerve and voluntary muscle, hexamethonium (*9.17*) at the parasympathetic ganglia, and atropine (*8.27*) at the postganglionic nerve endings. These are all inhibitors but specific agonists are also known classified as nicotinic or muscarinic (p. 168).

The relative complexity of the structures of nicotine and muscarine has cost many years of guessing how they could mimic acetylcholine. However these traditional classifiers survive considerable simplification. Thus the N-pentyltrimethylammonium cation (*9.18*) is as active and selective as nicotine and eight times as active as the natural neurotransmitter acetylcholine. Similarly the specificity of muscarine is available in as simple a compound as methacholine (*6.1*). As always, antagonists tend to have higher molecular weights than the agonists. This is clearly seen in the higher homologues of the agonist *9.18*; for example N-dodecyltrimethylammonium cation is purely antagonistic (Paton, 1961).

In Section 8.1 we saw how a large number of clinically useful drugs have been derived by paying attention to the selective nature of the sub-types of neurotransmitter receptors. This facility is as available for norepinephrine as for

$$Me_3N^+C_5H_{11}$$

**Pentyltrimethylammonium
(cation)**

(9.18)

acetylcholine receptors and is being extended to dopamine, serotonin and GABA receptors (see Albert, 1985, Chapter 12).

9.3 Selectivity through comparative cytology

Of the three principles that can confer selectivity comparative cytology is the least explored but many think it to be the most promising.

It is an everyday observation that the different forms of life differ greatly in their external structures and this is also the case internally. Plants differ from animals by having photosynthetic devices and they also have walls around all cells. Animals differ from plants by having nerves and muscles. Many herbicides, such as simazine (*9.19*) and diuron (*9.20*), exterminate weeds by interfering with the photosynthesizing organelles (chloroplasts), a structure lacking in animals who are consequently not endangered while grazing near treated areas. Again systemic insecticides, which are usually organic phosphates such as dimethoate (*9.21*), are taken up from the soil by plants completely unaffected by their presence which spells death to all insects who bite the stems or leaves.

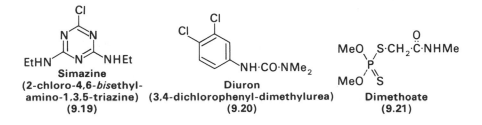

Simazine
(2-chloro-4,6-*bis*ethyl-amino-1,3,5-triazine)
(9.19)

Diuron
(3,4-dichlorophenyl-dimethylurea)
(9.20)

Dimethoate
(9.21)

Turning from complete organisms to their tissues, we note that the organization of plant and animal cells into a variety of tissues makes a valuable division of labour possible. The many, often conflicting, chemical reactions that take place simultaneously in cells require many isolated compartments constructed from membranes of selective permeability. These membranes comprise up to 80% of the dry weight of animals (O'Brien, 1967).

Organs and tissues are able to perform specialized functions only because they are made up of highly differentiated cells, each kind adapted to a particular task. Examples are the nerve, muscle and epithelial cells. Cancer cells develop from normal cells by progressive loss of differentiation. As a result, they undergo mitosis faster, and make DNA in excess amounts. The aim of a great many anticancer drugs is to interrupt the mitotic cycle as selectively as possible. Analogues of the natural purines and pyrimidines are much used for this purpose. An alternative cancer therapy tries to restore differentiation to the cancer cells, a research topic now being actively explored, e.g. with the retinoids related to vitamin A.

The various widths of different synaptic gaps provide excellent opportunities for selectivity. Let us consider adrenergically innervated smooth muscles. Across the wide gaps (80–400 nm) characteristic of nerve–blood vessel junctions, nerve stimulation releases a concentration of norepinephrine which, even at its peak value, tends to be close to the threshold concentration. In such tissues, decreasing the amount of transmitter, either by depleting the vesicles (e.g. with reserpine) or by interfering with its release (using, e.g., bretylium), can easily interrupt neurotransmission to the involuntary muscle. On the other hand, these two types of drug have little effect on tissues in which this gap is small because the peak concentration of norepinephrine may normally be 100 times the threshold concentration. Examples of such tissues are the nictitating membrane, the vas deferens and the sphincter papillae, all of which have a gap of about 20 nm only. The lack of inhibitory action of prazosin (an alpha-adrenergic blocking drug used to lower blood pressure) on the 'narrow gap' tissues, follows from this (Burnstock and Costa, 1975).

From 1940 onwards the application of the electron microscope to cells showed that division of labour, already noted for organs and tissues, occurred also at the sub-cellular level (see Fig. 3.1).

Vulnerability to selective toxicants is particularly evident in bacteria whose small size compared to eukaryotic cells leaves no space for a nucleus or for even one mitochondrion. In place of a nucleus the chromosomal DNA is gathered into a strand attached to the plasma membrane. Again the entire plasma membrane has to function as a mitochondrion breaking down nutrients and storing the energy as ATP. Thus the exposed position of the nuclear and mitochondrial functions contrasts sharply with the membrane-protected situation of these functions in the cells of higher organisms. The selectivity of the aminoacridines against bacteria in wounds (p. 178) depends partly on bacterial nucleic acid being so much more accessible but also on its consisting of closed loops, for which intercalating agents like the aminoacridines have a particular affinity. Similar selectivity shown by the 8-hydroxyquinoline antibacterials (p. 182) depends on the exposure of mitochondrial functions in bacteria.

Although bacteria have numerous ribosomes these are structurally different from those in eukaryotes (higher organisms). One sign of this difference is that they sediment at 70S (Svedberg units) instead of the usual 80S. Moreover the two halves of bacterial ribosomes (unlike those of eukaryotic ones) are easily separated by withdrawing the magnesium ion that unites them. In this way, two smaller particles (30S and 50S, respectively) are formed. Fig. 9.3 illustrates the fact that many drugs that are selective antibacterials, because they inhibit protein synthesis in bacteria much more than in man, owe this selectivity to the fact that they inhibit one or other of the bacterial ribosome fragments without displaying affinity for human ribosomes. Thus the aminoglycoside antibiotics such as gentamicin bind to the 30S unit exclusively whereas erythromycin and chloramphenicol bind only to the 50S unit. Note that the tetracyclines which bind equally to 30S and 80S material in isolated ribosomal fractions do not reach the 80S human material under therapeutic conditions on account of a highly selective distribution effect (p. 192). In passing, note the counter-selective effect of emetine and cycloheximide which bind to eukaryotic, but not to prokaryotic, ribosomes (these two drugs are now little used).

The plasma membrane offers another site for selective attack. Three classes of agents are known that destroy the bacterial plasma membrane: the phenols, the large cations and the polypeptide antibiotics. Their selectivity is not great enough to permit parenteral use in man but they are much used for cleaning fresh wounds and for treating skin infections. Chloroxylenol (9.22) and the bi-phenol hexachlorophene (10.7) are the most used of the phenolic antiseptics but suffer from inactivity against Gram negative organisms. Chlorhexidine (9.23) is one of the best large cations, a series that also includes benzalkonium chloride and cetrimide (cetyl trimethylammonium bromide). Chlorhexidine, which acts rapidly on both Gram negative and Gram positive organisms, is much used for pre-operative sterilization of surgeons' hands. Polypeptide antibiotics, of which polymyxin (9.24) is the most used, play a useful part in dermatology but are too nephrotoxic for internal use.

The plasma membrane of fungi becomes leaky on contact with polyene antibiotics, such as nystatin (9.25) whose name derives from New York State where it was discovered. It is used locally and orally to overcome fungal infections particularly those of *Candida*. Systemic infections with more virulent fungi are treated intravenously with the related drug, amphoteracin. This antibiotic is effective in fungal infections that, prior to introduction of this drug, were almost invariably fatal. In addition amphoteracin is being increasingly used in patients whose immune system is in suspense and who, as a consequence, can die from an otherwise innocent fungal infection. The polyene antibiotics act by penetrating the plasma membrane and coming to rest next to the phytosterol molecules, making a disruptive fit. Bacteria remain unaffected as their membrane contains no sterols. Mammals are reasonably protected because their

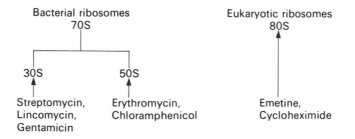

Fig. 9.3 Selective binding to ribosomes of several inhibitors of protein synthesis.

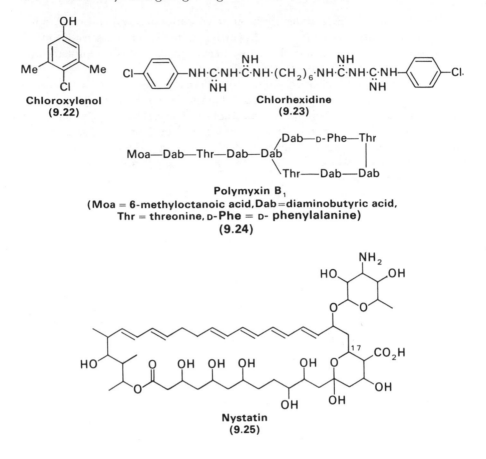

Chloroxylenol
(9.22)

Chlorhexidine
(9.23)

Polymyxin B₁
(Moa = 6-methyloctanoic acid, Dab = diaminobutyric acid,
Thr = threonine, D-Phe = D- phenylalanine)
(9.24)

Nystatin
(9.25)

plasma membranes contain cholesterol not phytosterol. Nevertheless the selectivity of these antibiotics is incomplete and good, systemic antifungal drugs are still being sought (Dennis, Stead and Andreoli, 1970).

In human pharmacodynamics the aim is not to injure the plasma membrane but to change its permeability. Diuretics such as hydrochlorothiazide (*8.6*) change the permeability of kidney tubules. This effect is confined to the upper part of the rising distal segment where resorption of sodium ions is inhibited by the drug. Another example of pharmacodynamic use is afforded by cromolyn sodium (sodium cromoglycate) (*9.26*), the prophylactic against attacks of asthma. This drug acts by preventing the immunoglobin designated IgE from rupturing lymphocytes and mast cells of the lungs. As a result the intensely irritating eicosanoid, leucotriene, is not liberated (Johnson, 1978). Cromolyn is not effective orally and has to be inhaled as a dust.

Finally we should consider the bacterial cell wall – a structure absent from the animal kingdom. The continuous web that holds this wall together is known as murein. It is a cross-linked polymer of acetylmuramic acid (*9.27*) with pentapeptide side-chain (e.g. *9.28*) attached in the 7'-position. Lederberg (1957) showed that bacteria are under high osmotic pressure (this can amount to 20 atmospheres for some Gram positive organisms). The function of the cell wall which is a network with no permeability barrier is to protect the bacteria from bursting. Any drug which can prevent the polymerization will ensure that the bacteria burst as soon as they begin to grow and need to synthesize some more cell wall.

The penicillins, most used of all antibacterial drugs, irreversibly block the polymerase by covalently acylating its active site. The lactam group of penicillins is a highly selective acylating agent, selective enough not to attach any other cellular constituent. Tipper and Strominger (1965) saw the penicillins (*9.29*) as structural analogues of D-alanyl-D-alanine (*9.30*) which the polymerase uses as a recognition group on the monomer. Alternative but somewhat similar hypotheses are under consideration.

The original penicillin, known as benzylpenicillin (*9.31*), is still much used. For special purposes (such as inertness to drug-degrading organisms, or extension of the bacterial spectrum to include Gram negative types), semi-synthetic (or 'man-finished') penicillins are available, in which the R of (*9.31*) can be, for example as in (*9.32*).

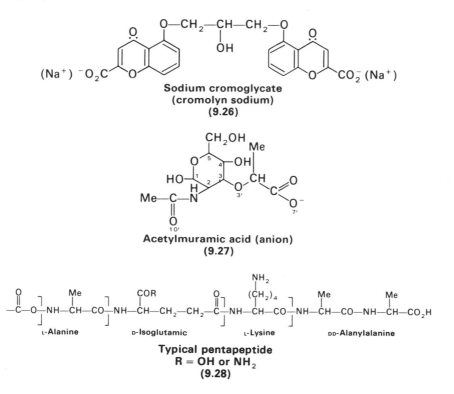

Sodium cromoglycate
(cromolyn sodium)
(9.26)

Acetylmuramic acid (anion)
(9.27)

L-Alanine   D-Isoglutamic   L-Lysine   DD-Alanylalanine

Typical pentapeptide
R = OH or NH$_2$
(9.28)

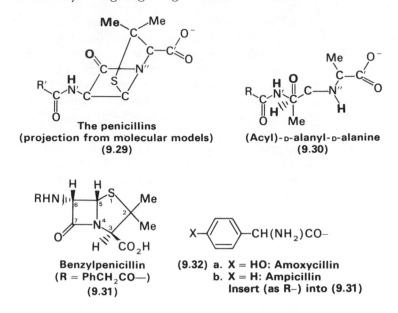

The penicillins
(projection from molecular models)
(9.29)

(Acyl)-D-alanyl-D-alanine
(9.30)

Benzylpenicillin
(R = PhCH₂CO—)
(9.31)

(9.32) a. X = HO: Amoxycillin
b. X = H: Ampicillin
Insert (as R–) into (9.31)

Further reading

Albert (1985, Chapters 5 and 14).

Follow-up

Attempt a five page essay outlining the general approach by which chemists or biologists, working alone or together, could develop a lead compound to improve its selectivity to the point where it could be considered a candidate drug for trials. (As used here, lead rhymes with feed and not with fed. It implies a newly discovered substance of promisingly high activity but insufficient selectivity).

Poisons

'I never cook anything until I've washed my hands'
(*saying attributed to Lucrezia Borgia (1480–1519)*))

10

Introduction to Part Three: Poisons as foreign substances

The review of selective toxicity (namely safe medication) that formed Part Two of this book is balanced in this Part Three by a discussion on unselective toxicity (namely poisoning).

The question 'Is this substance a poison? springs lightly to the tongue of administrators, legislators and the general public. It is a natural question but there is no simple answer.

Paracelsus as we have seen (p. 1) taught that all substances were poisonous if the dose were large enough. To answer the question we need to ask: (a) are people likely to come in contact with the substance, (b) if so, at what concentration and (c) does it cause a harmful effect at that concentration? Only those substances which carry a high risk of producing harmful effects at a likely encountered dose are properly designated poisons; the same substance may be a food, a medicine, or a poison depending on the circumstances. Hence it is impossible to compile a list of all known poisons unless it includes all known substances, including foods! As we have seen (p. 46) even water is poisonous and fatalities still occur when the 'water cures' of alternative medical practice have been pushed too hard.

From this introduction it follows that this Part Three, although boldly headed 'Poisons', will deal mainly with circumstances in which commonly encountered substances can become poisonous. The two chemicals that most often kill individuals accidentally, carbon monoxide and hydrocyanic acid, are constantly being generated (at a low concentration) by the human body. Indeed if we were not constantly generating hydrogen cyanide it seems that our leucocytes would be very inefficient slaughterers of invading germs (p. 243).

10.1 Intentional poisoning

This topic will be divided into poisoning (a) at the level of the State, and (b) at the level of the individual, although some intermediate examples would fit either category.

Poisoning at governmental level

Although many toxic substances were known in both ancient and medieval China, it appears that they were not used in State executions (Needham, 1954). Again the Bible records no instance of intentional poisoning, although poisonous plants grew in Palestine such as the hemlock (Hosea, 10:4) and the gourd (2 Kings, 4:39). Could it be that, from the most ancient times to the present century, poisoning was considered too unspectacular an end for a criminal, and preference was given to methods that implanted a lesson in the minds of the witnessing public?

What appears as a solitary exception is consonant with all we know of the great humanizing effort of Ancient Greek civilization. Political prisoners in the Athenian Democracy were executed painlessly, while conversing with friends by drinking the juice of hemlock (*Conium maculatum*). In the Spring of 399 BC, this punishment was allotted to Socrates, the philosopher, who consequently died of cardiac arrest (Burnet, 1911). Soon afterwards Greece lost its sovereignty and more barbarous methods of capital punishment dominated the scene for the next two millenia.

The death penalty for crime is much less used today but is still in force in many countries. In the United States about two dozen States have retained it, while strictly limiting the offences for which it can be used. Here we are concerned only to record the chemical methods used for execution. Nevada was the first State to legislate for lethal gas (hydrogen cyanide, for pharmacological properties see Section 11.1) in 1921. It is now the only permitted method in Arizona, California, Colorado, Maryland, Missisippi, Missouri, North Carolina, Oregon and Wyoming.

In May 1977, Oklahoma became the first US State to require that the death sentence be effected by a lethal injection, defined as 'Continuous intravenous administration of an ultrashort-acting barbiturate in combination with a chemical paralytic agent'. Nevada switched to this method followed by Idaho, New Mexico and Texas (Bedau, 1982).

History records how from time to time those in power have introduced widespread poisonings, not as deserved punishments but for political gain, sorry examples of 'Man's inhumanity to Man'.

The Renaissance, in almost explosive flowering of learning in fifteenth century Italy, produced a richness of innovation and enquiry that led to questioning of the traditional moral code. The more unscrupulous of the reigning princes took advantage of this situation to further their intrigues. Outstanding among them were the Borgias whose poisonings of political rivals became as frequent as their many physical killings. The head of the Borgia family, Pope Alexander VI (1431–1503), arranged poisonings of at least three cardinals according to Onofrio Panvinio (1530–1568) who, in more settled times, chronicled the lives of the Popes in his book, *Epitome Pontificium* (Burckhardt, 1929).

Of Alexander's children, a son Cesare (1475–1507) retained both a hangman and a poisoner on his staff. Alexander's daughter Lucrezia (1480–1519), although portrayed as a poisoner in Victor Hugo's novel and hence in Donizetti's opera, is considered by historians to have been an innocent dupe of her father, who had her wedded at the age of 13, re-married at 18, and again at 20, always to advance his political aims. Her sole connexion with poison seems to have been the presentiment that Alfonso of Aragon (her second husband, a year younger than herself) whom she dearly loved, would be murdered by poisoning. To avoid this fate she personally cooked all his meals. (In the end Cesare Borgia had him strangled in bed). The Borgias were said to use, as their toxicant, a tasteless white powder which took many hours before it acted (Avery, 1972), a description that suggests arsenious oxide.

During the Second World War (1939–1945), the Nazi Government of Germany implemented their inhumane genocidal policy by killing about 6 million of their citizens and prisoners, most of them Jews but also many gypsies, pacifists and communists. This was accomplished mainly by gassing with hydrogen cyanide. The first gas chamber was installed in Poland in the Spring of 1942. Later a larger one at Birkenau (Brzezinka) near Auschwitz (Oswiecim in Polish) was used to kill 2000–3000 people at a time, a process which took 20 minutes from sealing to re-opening (Kuper, 1981; Ferencz, 1979). Auschwitz was the site of a large armament factory and those who were (or became) physically unable to work in it were sent to be gassed. In Auschwitz alone at least 2.5 million human beings were killed in this way as Camp-Commandant Höss testified at the Nuremburg trials (International Military Tribunal, 1947). There were six other HCN gassing camps, some of them in Germany. In the Auschwitz Museum one can now see photographs and plans of the gas chambers and crematoria, reproduced in Müller (1979).

'Poisoning by persuasion' may best describe the following examples. In the late 1970's a certain reverend Jim Jones took his flock, the California- based 'Peoples' Temple', to Guyana on the north coast of South America where, in the jungle near Port Kaituma, they set up a model hamlet named Jonestown. Towards the end of November 1978, after a previous rehearsal, their 47-year-old paranoic leader, persuaded the trusting adherents to drink a solution of potassium cyanide and chloride from paper cups while their babies had this solution syringed on their tongues. Escapees reported that it took about 5 minutes for each person to die. The Guyanian police later found about 900 corpses at the site in relaxed postures (Anon, 1978).

The suicide in 1893 of the famous composer Pyotr Tchaikovsky (*b.* 1840) was, as the Soviet scholar Alexandra Orlova revealed in 1981, exacted from him by a court of the School of Jurisprudence in St. Petersburg, because of an indiscretion in aristocratic circles. What terminated his life was not, as officially stated at the time, cholera but (almost certainly) arsenic (Brown, 1980).

Grigori Rasputin, the peasant monk who wielded much influence over the Tsar and Tsarina at the court of Nicholas II, was assasinated late in December 1916 at the age of 44 while Russia was suffering a series of defeats on the German front in the First World War (1914–1918). A party of noblemen who attributed Russia's misfortunes to this monk, persuaded Rasputin to visit the Palace of the Tsar's nephew-in-law, Prince Yusupov, where they regaled him with cakes and wine, to both of which a Dr Lazovert had added white powder from a box of supposed potassium cyanide. Seemingly the original contents had taken up carbon dioxide from the air, and the stronger carbonic acid (pK_a 6.35) replaced the weaker hydrocyanic acid (PK_a 9.22). In the event the sturdily-built fellow suffered no harm and so was killed by shooting (Minney, 1972; Fulöp-Miller, 1927).

The last six months of the Second World War in Europe saw many induced suicides among the German leaders. Field-Marshal Erwin Rommel, who directed Germany's North African and Normandy ('D-Day') campaigns, and Field-Marshal G. von Kluge, both of them suspected of pacifism and of complicity in the abortive attempt on Hitler's life (July 20th, 1944), were persuaded by emissaries from Berlin to swallow poison in October, 1944 (Ruge, 1974). As the fortunes of war declined for Germany, capsules of potassium cyanide (referred to as KCB) were mass-produced and made available to officers and highly-placed government officials in Berlin. Finally, in April 1945, when the invasion of Berlin ended the war in Europe, Hitler's companion, Eva Braun, accepted his advice to swallow cyanide, after which der Führer killed himself with a revolver shot (Ryan, 1966).

Chemical warfare is a much more overt form of government-decreed poisoning. It is not a new phenomenon because the medieval Chinese used to lead toxic fumes (apparently sulfur dioxide) down a hose into enemy vessels during naval battles (Needham, 1954). Chemical warfare surfaced again during the First World War, in April 1915, when the German Army sent the first, choking clouds of chlorine, downwind across no-man's-land, into the Allied trenches near the Belgian city of Ypres (Haber, 1986). This weapon was soon superseded by the more insidious but devastating 'mustard gas' (*10.1*) [bis (2-chloroethyl)sulfide] which caused blistering of the skin, chronic respiratory impairment and often permanent eye damage. In all there were more than a million casualties.

To be effective chemical warfare needed an element of surprise. Once the allied forces had acquired protective clothing and antidotes, the attacks ceased. In general high explosives were judged to give a better return for resources expended. Towards the end of that war, the Americans invented lewisite (*10.2*) [dichloro-2-(chlorovinyl)arsine] which caused vesication, respiratory distress and death in experimental animals; however it was never used in the war.

The Second World War saw the creation in Germany of powerful acetylcholinesterase inhibitors, commonly referred to as 'nerve gases'. These arose from a
search by Gerhard Schrader for new insecticides (Schrader, 1963). The most
potent of these nerve gases were the phosphate esters sarin (*10.3*), tabun (*10.4*)
and soman (*10.5*), all of which produced immobility followed by death
(Saunders, 1957). High stockpiles were accumulated in Germany. All three
esters would appear to be equitoxic (~ 0.01 mg/kg), but each represents a step in
(a) better penetration of protective clothing, and (b) insusceptibility to reversal.
It was held that no antidote could save a person who had been exposed to soman.
As it happened no chemical weapons were used in the Second World War.

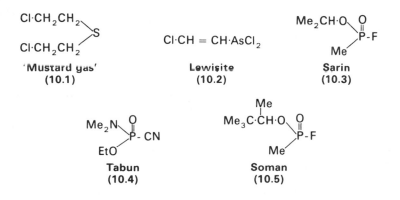

In 1925 most of the world's Nations signed the Geneva Protocol that outlawed
use of chemical weapons. The subject seemed forgotten until 1981 when the
United States accused the Soviet Union of supplying its ally, Vietnam, with
'yellow rain' for use against defenceless people in Laos and Campuchea. If true,
this would also have been a violation of the UN Biological Weapons Convention
of 1972. Specimens of the 'rain' yielded tricothecene (a toxicant formed in
fungus-infected grain stored under tropical conditions). Most investigators think
that 'yellow rain' consisted mainly of bee faeces contaminated with a little
tricothecene (Hay, 1983; Anon., 1986; Palca, 1986a).

Chemical warfare re-emerged in March 1984 when the Secretary General of
the United Nations despatched an international team of specialists to the Middle
East. They found that Iraq had recently used mustard gas in its war against Iran
(Ember, 1986). On March 12th, 1986, the Security Council of the United
Nations reported that a similar team had just found renewed use of mustard gas
by Iraq.

The current situation is that the Soviet Union, the United States, and France
(reputedly in descending order) are known to possess stocks of chemical weapons,
and the United States has considered production of binary weapons. These
would carry two relatively harmless chemicals that combine to form a lethal
substance when the shell that contains them is fired.

Poisoning at the level of the individual

Here we must dwell though only briefly on murder, suicide and euthanasia, when achieved by toxic means.

Personal murder whether for revenge or gain has tended to be more frequent at those times when the State is taking life freely or when great international tension exists. It is likely that in these circumstances life may seem less precious than before. However, in choosing his means, the individual prefers secretive ways whereas the State tends to the spectacular.

The intending murderer often acquires his poison by pretending that he has pests to dispose of. Thus Geoffrey Chaucer (1343–1400) in his Canterbury Tales tells of a youth who asks an apothecary for rat poison with which he kills companions (The Pardoner's Tale). Commentators point out that this story reflected real life at that time and afterwards for many centuries. In the early 1940s, when thallium acetate was a favoured rodent poison in Australia, it was much favoured for murder, the source of which was revealed by the accompanying epilation. Today when cinema and television illustrate so often, and so exactly how to shoot a victim, but hardly ever how to poison him, murder seems to be swinging from poisoning to physical violence.

In *suicide* the nature of any poison used tends to follow a current fashion which may be unconsciously propagated by the news media. However poisoning has yielded some ground to physical methods in recent decades (McClure, 1984). Suicide has to be distinguished from the 'self-poisoning' of young people who wish to draw attention to their circumstances without actually courting death (Walsh, 1984).

Euthanasia, a word derived from the Greek *eu* (good) and *thanos (death)*, is conceding to the hopelessly ill and for reasons of mercy the *right to die* if they so wish it. Though favoured in ancient civilizations few contemporary nations have given it a legal status. In spite of this official discouragement it is possible at least in the great teaching hospitals of industrialized countries to terminate a life that is already at the terminal stage, e.g. by the disconnection of support apparatus or the injection of insulin. This action can be initiated by the physician-in-charge of the case only after wide and appropriate consultations.

Euthanasia is sometimes initiated by the patient or his close relatives ('mercy killing') although this is entirely illegal and subject to abuse. There are indications that the insistence of some patients on smuggling the illegal drug laetrile to their bedside had euthanasia rather than cure as its goal (p. 65). A physician's case for freeing euthanasia has been clearly stated by Barnard (1980).

10.2 Accidental poisoning

Accidents constitute, after cardiovascular events and cancer, the commonest cause of death in industrialized countries. Although traffic incidents contribute a large proportion of these fatalities, domestic and industrial accidents also bulk large and of these poisonings play a prominent part. In the USA (population 236 million), in 1982 there were 4733 deaths from accidental poisoning whereas 28 242 people died from suicides (all kinds). Only 198 iatrogenic deaths were recorded. The corresponding figures for Britain in 1984 were 48, 519 and 4 respectively out of a population of 56 million (World Health Organization, 1985).

Domestic poisoning

Common protagonists of toxic episodes in the home are children who apparently swallow prescribed medicines and household cleaners. It is a matter of observation that the parent who usually witnesses only the tail-end of this event is more disturbed than the child. It is current practice not to apply treatment unless the child exhibits symptoms (Morley, et al., 1986). In any case, the parent should telephone the Poisons Information Centre or the casualty (emergency) department of a local hospital for advice, giving the name and amount of material swallowed. Usually it turns out that the child has not swallowed more of the material than his body can cope with. In England (population 47 million) there were in 1982 97 420 hospital admissions for poisoning of which 430 died. However only one in 10 000 cases of child poisoning resulted in death. The adult medicines that most often poisoned children were ferrous sulfate, aspirin, the benzodiazepines and the tricyclic antidepressants. Of household agents the most often lethal were the hydrocarbons, white spirit and kerosene (Morley, et al., 1986). The problem can be avoided by keeping potential toxicants where no child can reach them.

For further reading on management of accidental poisoning see Vale and Meredith, 1985.

Poisoning in the workplace

Whereas a patient undergoing therapy is protected from overdosage by his supervising physician, the agricultural or industrial worker has historically been at greater risk. Gradually and mainly in the present century the risk has decreased very much thanks to the conjoint action of three influences: (a) a growing sense of responsibility among employers, (b) representations from the worker-financed trade unions and (c) supervision of the workplace by a State-controlled inspectorate. Dangers range from a mild, acute or chronic toxicity to utter disaster but the latter is fortunately rare.

Chronic toxicity arises when a foreign substance is absorbed (more often by inhalation than through the skin) in larger daily amounts than the body can detoxify or eliminate, excellent though its capabilities usually are (see Section 7.3).

In the United Kingdom, introduction in 1974 of the Health and Safety Work

Act (HSWA) provided legislation for the safety of all who work with chemicals. It clarified the duties of both employers and employees for ensuring safety, also the obligations of a supplier to his customers. This Act also set up a Health and Safety Commission (HSC) through which the public can register its voice. This Commission also publishes 'Occupational Exposure Limits' for noxious, but essential, chemicals encountered in the workplace, e.g. for asbestos, carbon disulfide, acrylonitrile, ethylene oxide, isocyanates, lead, styrene, trichloroethylene and vinyl chloride. In the USA the Occupational Safety and Health Act of 1970 set up an Occupational Safety and Health Administration (OSHA) which issues similar limits and has been given the legal power to enforce them. Similar regulations operate in Continental Europe.

It is current practice not to ban a toxic substance if it is irreplaceable for making a completely safe product. Instead the toxic hazard is carefully assessed and the worker protected accordingly. For example when it was established about 1975 that vinyl chloride produced the rare tumour angiosarcoma of the liver, the first thought was to ban the substance that it was used to make, namely the harmless and much-used plastic, polyvinylchloride. An international debate took place as a result of which it was decided to continue to manufacture the product, but to impose rigid limits on the exposure of factory workers who either made or handled the monomer (Reeves, 1981). Even before imposing these rules only 50 cases of this rare tumour had ever been found among vinyl chloride workers and now there should be none.

How are the toxic hazards of the workplace assessed? Usually by integrating information from the following sources: epidemiology in the workplace, mutagenicity tests, tests on laboratory animals, studies of metabolic alteration of chemicals, and structure–action relationships. More about these sources can be found in Section 13.1. This information is combined with studies made in the workplace of (a) the level of toxic material created by current manufacturing practices and (b) the allowable flexibility in manufacturing conditions within which the safe limits must be reached. In almost all industrialized countries the Law specifies the threshold concentrations for each commonly-used toxic substance, for short exposure (10–15 min) and maximum exposure (8 h) (Laing, 1986).

(a) *Disasters.* From time to time chemical factories have sustained explosions with release of toxic fumes. A series of such disasters occurring in a recent decade precipitated a new round of legislation. This series was initiated by Flixborough (1974 in England) followed by similar incidents in Holland (1975) and at Manfredonia (1976) on the Adriatic. Whereas poisoning played only a minor part in these events it came to the fore in the explosions of Sèveso (1976) and Bhopal (1984). In Britain the Control of Industrial Major Accident Hazards (CIMAH) Regulations were introduced in 1984 to help prevent such disasters. Parallel legislation was enacted in Continental Europe and the USA.

The incident at Sèveso (near Milan in the North of Italy) occurred in July at the ICMESA factory which made only one product: 2,4,5-trichlorophenol. This was done by hydrolysis of 1,2,4,5-tetrachlorobenzene with sodium hydroxide. The trichlorophenol has two large-scale uses (a) to make the selective bactericide hexachlorophene (*10.7*), and the herbicide, 2,4,5-trichlorophenoxyacetic acid (*10.6*) ('Agent Orange', p. 250). ICMESA, a subsidiary of the Swiss firm Givaudin, required this phenol for conversion to hexachlorophene. This hydrolysis has a long history of causing violent explosions, first in the Monsanto plant (in 1949 at Nitro, in West Virginia), then at the BASF plant in Germany (1953) (see Goldman, 1973 for injuries). The next explosion took place at the Philips-Duphar plant (1963 in The Netherlands), followed by one in the Coalite works (1968 in Derbyshire, England) (Renzoni, 1977; Hay, 1982). One can only wonder what unique virtues the users saw in the bactericide or the herbicide that would justify this long list of explosions and risk another one.

Even when this hydrolysis goes smoothly, it generates a small percentage of a toxic byproduct, popularly known as dioxin or TCDD (*10.8*), but correctly named 2,3,7,8-tetrachlorodibenzo-*p*-dioxin. It is particularly unfortunate that whenever this reaction gets out of hand a higher percentage of dioxin is produced. The Sèveso explosion ejected about 240 g of dioxin (Hay, 1982), thus exposing the largest population so far to the highest recorded concentration.

Wilson (1982) called dioxin one of the most toxic of all man-made chemicals because the TC_{50} for rabbits is only 115 μg/kg. It proved carcinogenic in rats and mice but only if they were dosed daily for two years, which is most of their lifetime; also it was teratogenic in mice (Poland and Knutson, 1982).

Although laboratory animals are much used to predict, approximately, the toxicity of numerous chemicals in man, there are some remarkable exceptions. For instance norbormide a commercial rat poison does no harm to nearly 30 other species of mammal including man (Albert, 1985). Dioxin seems to display some such species specificity because, nearly 40 years after the first explosion, there seem to have been few ill-effects in the human species, apart from chloracne, a temporary facial eruption long known in workers exposed to chlorinated lubricants. Ten volunteers in Pennsylvania allowed 7.5 mg of dioxin to be applied to a one square inch of the back. Eight of these men developed chloracne which had disappeared in 4–7 months, but no other effect could be detected (Hay, 1982, p. 135).

At Sèveso no one died and no lasting injury has been reported in spite of a reprehensible 17 days' delay in evacuating the nearby inhabitants (Cattabeni, Cavallaro and Galli, 1978; Dagani, 1981; Wilson, 1982). Yet so strongly had the sensational news media implanted a myth that all children being carried would be born deformed, though none were, that many expectant mothers procured abortions (Hay, 1982, p. 215). Holmstedt (1980) pointed out how much less toxic dioxin seems to be to man as compared to rodents. In four decades since the West Virginia explosion took place no excess cases of cancer were detected among those exposed. Let us hope that this will also be true of the Sèveso explosion.

Further evidence that human exposure to dioxin is not necessarily disastrous is

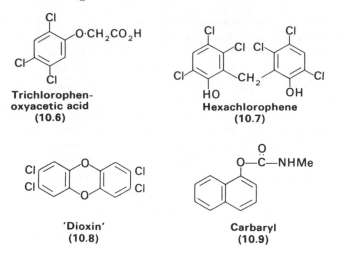

Trichlorophen-
oxyacetic acid
(10.6)

Hexachlorophene
(10.7)

'Dioxin'
(10.8)

Carbaryl
(10.9)

provided by recent investigations of a civic blunder effected in 1971. Scientists form three Institutes, including the US Federal Centers for Disease Control, Atlanta, examined 154 people who had lived for an average period of 3 years in a Mobile Home Park (near St Louis, Missouri) where soil was contaminated with dioxin. This happened when waste oil containing dioxin was sprayed over the surrounding ground 'to control the dust'. Even in 1983 when the contamination was discovered up to 2200 ppb of dioxin were recorded on the site. The health of these people was compared with that of 155 others who also lived in Missouri but had no exposure to dioxin. No difference could be found between the two groups by physicians who looked into miscarriages, birth defects, cancer and liver disease. The exposed population however did show slight impairment of the immune system in laboratory tests but were considered to be as fit as the controls (Hoffman, *et al.*, 1986).

It is worth recalling that the half life of dioxin in the rat is only 31 days (Poland and Knutson, 1982), and humans might be expected to lose it reasonably fast too. For further reading see Poland and Kimbrough, 1984; Coulston and Pocchiari, 1983; Safe, 1986).

The most devastating of all factory explosions occurred in December 1984, at Bhopal in Central India. The plant, operated jointly by an American firm (Union Carbide) and the Indian Government, regularly made large batches of the insecticide carbaryl (*10.9*), a pesticide strongly recommended by the UN Food and Agricultural Organization for its Integrated Pest Management programme (p. 248). For this synthesis methyl isocyanate (MeN = C = O) was prepared in quantity. The explosion followed accidental entry of about half a tonne of water into a tank that was storing this isocyanate, part of which underwent a heat-evolving polymerization. As a result about 28 tonnes of unchanged methyl isocyanate (b.p. 37 °C) were propelled into the densely populated surroundings. More than one million inhabitants had to seek first aid, and about 2500 died. Survivors complained mainly of two long-term effects: (a) chronically watering eyes and (b) breathlessness from lung injury. While there is no reason to expect either cancer or birth defects from this chemical, the problem of long-term disability remains, and recompense is being negotiated in India (Jayaraman, 1986).

A completely different type of explosion took place on the 26th of April, 1986 at Chernobyl, in the Ukranian Republic of the Soviet Union. This was by far the most serious nuclear-energy accident that the world has experienced. Although the force of the explosion killed only two people, and 29 more died from *acute* radiation injury, about 200 others received a highly damaging dose of radiation, as revealed by gastrointestinal injury and inhibition of the formation of new blood cells. The prevailing winds carried radioactive dust in a Northwesterly direction, across Poland to Sweden, though without manifest harm. The accident created tremendous international concern at the time. There were some who foretold that the 50 000 people who were evacuated from areas near the explosion site would show a greatly increased incidence of cancer in 20 years' time.

This gloomy surmise is not supported by careful studies of the much more directly irradiated populations, totalling 80 000, who survived the atomic bombings of Nagasaki and Hiroshima in August, 1945. Looking back over the last 40 years, observers note that the principal form of cancer to emerge was leukaemia, and that this came to a peak seven years after the explosions and then fell away.

Indeed, compared to laboratory animals, the repair of injured genetic information in man is remarkable. Schul, Otake and Neel (1981), reporting for the Radiation Effects Research Foundation (Hiroshima and USA), describe their study of the survivors. Despite the intense irradiation of the two bombed cities, investigations continuously carried out over 34 years revealed no heritable defects. In short parental exposure conferred no statistically significant mutations on the offspring and pregnancies followed a normal course, all compared to a matched population from a non-irradiated area.

That a nuclear war would be the most inhumane of all catastrophes cannot be denied, and is something to be avoided at all costs. However the statement that it would cause 'Millions of cases of cancer and birth defects' (Sagan, 1985) seems wide of the mark, nor do the dark prognostications of P. R. Ehrlich (1984) have quite the ring of scientific objectivity. An alternative view is provided by the 1984 report of the Commission of Radiological Dose Assessments and Biological Effects. This Commission, set up by the International Council of Scientific Unions' Scientific Committee on Problems of the Environment (SCOPE) calculated that, in the event of nuclear war, 'The long-term increase in genetic and carcinogenic effects on humans, from global fallout, is of the order of one per cent of the natural incidence, and should be considered a second-order effect' (Knox and Shapiro, 1986).

The principal products from explosion of an uranium pile are strontium (^{90}Sr), caesium (^{137}Cs) and iodine (^{131}I). The strontium isotope, which can enter bone by the calcium-uptake pathway, has a half life of 28 years, during which time its decay produces some yttrium (^{90}Y) which emits β-radiation more powerfully, so that bone sarcomas could result. The caesium isotope has a long half life but is fairly rapidly eliminated from the human body. The iodine isotope has a half life of only 8 days and is a familiar drug, much used in diagnosis and treatment of hyperthyroidism.

Long before man learnt how to split the atom he stood at risk from natural radioactivity. One disastrous example occurred during the First World War among the women who painted luminous marks on optical instruments that servicemen needed to use in the dark. Using a paint containing radioactive mesothorium these workers strove after good definition by frequently pointing the brushes between their lips. No ill effects were foreseen but many of these women died young, from leukaemia and bone tumours (Aub, *et al.*, 1952).

Such incidents apart, man has always been exposed to natural radiation from several sources yet he has evolved and prospered and is now surviving for more years than ever before. None of us can escape the irradiation of potassium, the element that drives nerves and muscles. Containing 0.012% of the isotope ^{40}K, potassium continuously emits both β- and γ-rays and has a half life of over a billion years. If we stand in the open air cosmic rays constantly if mildly assault us with their γ-radiation*. If we retreat into a building the natural radiation of dense building materials such as brick and concrete assails us, and it is not at all clear what can be done for protection (Anon., 1986b).

Whether a threshold exists below which further radiation does us no harm, is one of the most controversial issues of our times and not easily resolvable (Saunders, 1986). Other areas of public anxiety include the disposal of waste from atomic piles and the fear of accidental discharge of nuclear weapons.

Environmental

The earth's atmosphere has never been clean. It has suffered constant pollution from natural sources such as volcanoes, subterranean gases, hot boron springs, fumes from decaying animals and vegetation, smoke from spontaneous forest fires, windblown dust and salt spray. This pollution was to some extent neutralized by the purifying activities of plant life, the air, and the ocean, which conferred benefits through oxidation, dilution, dispersion, settling and adsorption. This equilibrium was changed when man appeared on the scene most

* Cosmic radiation furnishes us with about 0.30 millisieverts a year and total natural radiation for those living near sea level adds up to about 2 millisieverts a year for each person. A limit for one who works with radiation is 50 millisieverts a year. The sievert (Sv), the unit of radiation received, equals 100 rem (a formerly-used unit). Radiation emitted is measured in becquerels (Bq) but formerly in curies (Ci): (1 Ci = 3.7×10^{10} Bq).

particularly after the industrial revolution began. Gradually the natural system proved unable to cope with the new high loadings and the level of pollution began to rise. The curiously named Alkali Act of Victorian England was a pioneer attempt to control the emission of acid from factory chimneys.

Today most pollution eminates from the combustion of solid and liquid fuels, from abrasion of motor car tyres and brakes and from incinerations at the domestic, commercial and industrial levels. Also from open-cut mining, from factories (including power plants), from the dust of unmade roads and eroded farms and particularly from motor-vehicle exhaust which provides carbon monoxide, unburnt hydrocarbons, the oxides of nitrogen and, indirectly, ozone.

This deteriorating situation is countered by legislation. There is widespread agreement that the wastes of Industry form a threat both to health and to the natural pleasantness of the environment. Although industry is the principal wealth generator of human society and furnishes much of what makes contemporary life so enjoyable, industrial enterprise will not be able to survive let alone flourish unless its operations are acceptable to the society within which it renders services. To this end the various industrialized nations have introduced legislation whose enforcement controls an environmental situation that was threatening to get out of hand.

In Britain for example a Department of the Environment has been created to oversee such issues as the supply of pure water, the discharge of smoke, solid-waste disposal, the treatment of sewage and discharges into rivers. Its policies are implemented through Town and Country Planning regulation at the level of local government. In addition dumping at sea and the toxic hazards from some agrochemicals are handled by the Ministry of Agriculture, Fisheries and Food; and the Health and Safety Executive controls miscellaneous factory emissions and enforces its standards through the Industrial Air Pollution Inspectorate. The Department of Energy has the powers to control pollution arising from energy raising.

These are highly divided responsibilities but they are unified under the Control of Pollution Act (COPA) 1974 which is even empowered to control noise. The Health and Safety at Work Act (HASWA) 1974 was strengthened in 1983 by introduction of the Health and Safety (Emissions into the Atmosphere) Regulations. Similarly the Control of Pollution Acts of 1974 and 1984 regulate discharges into land (landfill) as well as into both inland and coastal waters. The passage of chemical wastes from the point of origin to the site of disposal is carefully monitored.

The situation is more difficult in Continental Europe where some nations have little water to drink other than the rivers that carry industrial and domestic effluent from other nations. This situation demands effective cooperation. To this end the World Health Organization has been asked to draw up guidelines to assist drafting legislation. The elimination of mercury, cadmium and carcinogens from drinking water was a particular goal. The WHO's Regional Committee for Europe, at their 55th session in Amsterdam (1985), noted that chemical pollution caused by more than 60 000 different substances, including industrial wastes and agricultural chemicals and fertilizers, was a serious threat to Europe's water supply. It added that a major effort in this direction was needed to carry out research, issue guidelines, establish monitoring stations and reach international compliance.

Whereas in Britain the policy of regulation has always been cooperative and based on reasoned persuasion; Vogel (1986) sees the USA pattern as rather confrontational. The Environmental Protection Agency (EPA) is constantly improving environmental quality by the exercise of the strong legislative powers that have been built into it. It oversees the generation and disposal of chemical waste and counters pollution of streams and lakes. It has on occasion imposed fines of over one million dollars and is also able to close down uncooperative plants. It finds that much contamination of streams arises from landfills, underground storage tanks, over-application of pesticides, septic tanks and spills of oil and chemicals. A *cause célèbre* arose in the Love Canal incident at Niagara Falls, NY. The local government wanted this disused waterway filled in and a local chemical firm were pleased to oblige with their accumulated sludges which were rich in chlorinated hydrocarbons. Later the municipality built on the reclaimed site; but the increased rate of miscarriages and birth defects made them decide to evacuate all pregnant women living near this canal and all children under two years of age (Anon., 1978a; Hay, 1982).

The EPA also administers the Safe Drinking Water Act (1974) which was further strengthened in 1986. Standards (threshold values) are issued for many likely pollutants. The Toxic Substances Control Act (TSCA) of 1976 enabled EPA to draw up a list of all toxic substances manufactured by, or used in, US industry. Furthermore it enabled this agency to obtain Premanufacture Notices from firms who desire either to manufacture or import a new industrial chemical, and to supply evidence of its comparative toxicity. The agency can then ask for further tests to be performed or it can prohibit the substance because of an unreasonable risk to human health or to the environment.

A most valuable chemical-transportation emergency response centre (CHEMTREC) is run by the Chemical Manufacturers Association to answer queries about handling spills from trains and trucks that carry toxic chemicals across the United States. CHEMTREC receives about 150 calls a day; about 10% of the spills require evacuation of local households (Anon., 1985b).

The ship *Vulcanus II*, ready to service the whole world, is a floating incinerator. It is prepared to call at any port, collect chemical wastes and burn them at sea, for a charge made by its owners Chemical Waste Management. On land, high-temperature incinerators which are usually rotatory kilns provide a more immediate alternative. However there is often difficulty in finding sites for these burners (human nature being what it is the NIMBY (not in my back yard) principle may intrude).

All of this worldwide activity to restore purity to the environment requires increased availability of trained scientists, from chemists and toxicologists to occupational physicians. This rapidly growing demand presents tertiary educational institutes with challenges to provide the relevant courses. Much of the future improvement of the environment will depend on the intuitiveness and inventiveness of chemists in developing syntheses alternative to those presenting hazards.

Culpable negligence

If accidental poisonings are defined as those that take place in spite of the exercise of reasonable care, some examples remain where indifference to the welfare of human beings was the precipitating factor. This grey area is encountered most often when preventive measures would be expensive and the need for them easily dismissed from the mind. A common form of culpable negligence is to site a factory, particularly one that employs a hazardous process or produces toxic emissions, in a district or country where regulations are less exacting than in the parent area. Those who make such a decision are not necessarily criminal for they may think that the local regulations are unduly severe. Another form is to unload toxic wastes in areas where they contaminate the local atmosphere, shoreline or even the drinking water.

One form of culpable negligence is the export, to countries that lack banning legislation, of drugs whose toxic side-effects have caused them to be banned at home. The rather severely named book *Corporate Crime in the Pharmaceutical Industry* (Braithwaite, 1984) provides several instances. For example physicians in the United States were well informed that the antibiotic chloramphenicol, when used for treating diarrhoea may cause severe, and often fatal, aplastic anaemia, yet the manufacturers exported this product to Central America without any such warning. A United States Senate Subcommittee noted this evidence and also recorded that the warnings were not being given in Italy or Spain either (1976: US Senate Subcommittee Reports 15359 and 15385–6). Again the sedative drug thalidomide was promoted in West Africa in the 1960s as being completely harmless, although its teratogenic (birth-defect producing) properties were known, and the drug banned, in Europe and North America (Knightley, *et al.*, 1979).

Although manufacturers now exercise more care in their extraterritorial promotions, much clinical testing of candidate drugs is arranged in foreign countries when regulations in the manufacturing country would make this more difficult.

Asbestos is a mineral with carcinogenic properties which were first demonstrated, by J. C. Wagner in 1956, among those who mined it in South Africa. In the 1960s E. C. Hammond of the American Cancer Society and I. J. Selikoff of the Mount Sinai School of Medicine, showed that workers who had used asbestos in their insulation tasks for 20 years were more subject to lung cancer than other members of the public. In spite of these warnings the asbestos companies continued to promote the uses of this basic magnesium silicate fibre. In 1971 asbestos became the first material to be regulated by the newly-formed Occupational Safety and Health Administration (OSHA). In 1982 many people suffering from asbestos-related diseases filed lawsuits against the largest supplier of asbestos in the USA, the Manville Corporation, which responded by going into bankruptcy in August, 1982 (Zurer, 1985). The carcinogenic properties of asbestos will be discussed in Section 13.1.

What could be classified as culpable negligence has often been associated with the practice of unorthodox medical treatments (unorthodoxy is defined as the rejection of what has been scientifically established). The danger of 'alternative therapies' is that they are rooted in mistaken beliefs of the past, beliefs discredited by the advance of knowledge. A recent investigation found that much of the attraction that unorthodox medicine exerts is derived from the long time that its practitioners spend with each patient. This latitude stands in contrast to orthodox medicine whose general practitioner is rushed off his feet by the pressure of appointments, examination of the patient, despatching specimens to the pathologist, referrals to specialists, arranging hospitalization, writing countless certificates, and many other duties inherent in the web of patient-care of which he has become the centre (British Medical Association, 1986).

That patients often respond to unorthodox treatments (the BMA report continues) is a manifestation of the placebo effect (defined in Section 7.6, p. 154). 'In considering the propriety of applying remedies to accurately diagnosed conditions that ordinarily resolve without medical intervention, we are satisfied that witholding unnecessary medication in these circumstances is advantageous'. This arrangement releases the physician to concentrate on those who are seriously ill, while absent molecules are caring for elusive symptoms.

Culpability arises especially when placebos are employed in serious diseases such as cancer, heart disease or potentially lethal infections which the unorthodox practitioner has neither the training to recognize nor the means to benefit. A particular menace is presented by herbal treatment. 'Despite herbalism's pure and harmless image, some herbal remedies give rise to adverse reactions' (British Medical Association, 1986). The Law which has a low regard for herbal remedies does not require them to be standardized, although it rigidly controls the strength and purity of all orthodox medicaments. Thus herbs come to the market over or under their average strength according to soil and season; in this way dangerous overdoses can be prescribed. Much illness has arisen in this way from the herb comfrey (*Symphytum officinale*) which is prone to cause severe liver damage from the pyrrolizidine alkaloids that it contains (Roitman, 1981; Mattocks, 1986). This herb also causes liver cancer in rats. Poke root (*Phytolacca americana*), prickly ash bark (*Xanthoxylium* spp.) and sweet flag root (*Acorus*) are also dangerous (Shellard, 1986). For sassafrass see p. 84. Extract of mistletoe (*Viscum album*), which has been promoted in Western Europe since 1921 as an unorthodox cancer remedy, has caused much liver necrosis (Harvey and Colin-Jones, 1981). The section on laetrile in this book (p. 65) may usefully be read at this point.

For further reading on all aspects of poisoning, see the end of Chapter 10.

10.3 The principles of toxicology

Toxicology is the study of adverse effects of substances on living creatures, particularly man. Not only drugs, but nutrients and purely destructive chemicals (including pesticides) come under its care. Toxicology is practised by scientists of several different orientations. First, there are the descriptive toxicologists who devise tests to find what risk a nominated chemical substance may pose. Some others are mechanistic toxicologists who try to discover the molecular basis of an adverse effect. Next come the regulatory toxicologists whose task is to determine if the risk inherent in a nominated substance is low enough to allow it to be used in medical treatment or in crop protection. Such investigators obtain the evidence necessary to decide if a candidate drug satisfies existing regulations, or else needs some special regulation. Related to this work is that of the forensic toxicologist, well versed in the medico-legal aspects of poisoning and trained to assist at a postmortem. There is also the clinical toxicologist, medically qualified, who is occupied with the diagnosis and treatment of poisoned patients. All of these investigators depend on tests made on laboratory animals.

Mice and rats are the most-used laboratory animals and the median lethal dose (LD_{50}), as defined on p. 111, is one of the values for which they are most frequently required. This value (in g/kg body weight) is usually obtained by administering, either orally or intra-peritoneally (to groups of, say, five mice) a dose that is expected to lie in the lethal range; similar groups simultaneously receive somewhat larger and smaller doses. The percentage response (which may be death or any other nominated pathlogical result) is read daily up to (usually) five days. To obtain the LD_{50}, the final response is plotted against the logarithm of the dose or, more conveniently, against the dose plotted on semilogarithmic paper, as in Fig. 6.4. From such plots, the LD_{50} can be read by inspection. However, for greater accuracy and meaning, the response is better converted to probits (units of deviation from the mean) which, when plotted against the dose as before, give a straight line. From this plot, the LD_{50} is found by simply dropping a line from the point where the probit is 5 (i.e., 50% mortality) on to the dose ordinate.

Autopsies (postmortem examinations) often follow these tests, and can indicate the nature and site of the intoxication. It is a matter of common observation that some toxicants give steep, and others gentle, slopes in such linear plots. Those that produce a steep plot tend to retain much of their toxicity when the dose is lowered – an adverse property which must be emphasized in reports.

For some tests animals other than rats and mice may be specified, particularly ferrets, rabbits and dogs. The value of ferrets is that they are non-rodents yet small and economical. The larger animals, which for reasons of economy have to be used more sparingly, are usually subjected to small doses that are increased at intervals during, say, two weeks, and the nature of any toxic effects are recorded. Environmentalists use fish as experimental animals in assessing the effect of chemicals on rivers and lakes.

Acute-toxicity trials give little information relevant to chronic toxicity, where cumulation often becomes important. When subacute toxicity trials are required they are usually performed on rats and dogs, in parallel, for about three months followed by postmortem examinations of organs and tissues. Chronic (or long-term) toxicity studies, when required, usually last from 6 to 24 months. The use of chronic tests to assess carcinogenicity is discussed in Section 13.1. Other chronic tests are devised to report on possible sensitization, or on teratogenicity (causation of birth defects).

The general toxicological information provided by a LD_{50} is usually supplemented by more specific tests on particular organs, tissues or cells, whose vulnerability is often indicated during the LD_{50} trials.

The question is often asked, to what extent do toxicological data, such as those obtained from LD_{50} tests, transfer meaningfully from laboratory animals to man? Although body weight (as in these g/kg results) is valuable for comparing different substances in experimental species, it must be borne in mind that man can be up to ten times more sensitive. When body weight is replaced by body surface area, toxic effects in man and in experimental animals usually correspond (Klaassen, 1985). Also, as indicated in Section 7.5 (p. 144), the blood level (in mg/ml) at which a biological effect occurs in a laboratory animal usually corresponds with what is found in man.

Testing for toxicity is in many ways more difficult than testing to optimize a candidate drug in order to improve its selectivity for two reasons. Firstly, drug improvement is concentrated on optimizing a single well-defined response, whereas toxicological testing must search for every response that could be injurious to the test animal and, by inference, to man. Secondly, for perfecting a discovery, the pharmacologist is provided with a collection of candidate drugs, all chemically or physically related to one another, whereas the toxicologist (particularly in Government laboratories) has only the submitted compound. Thus, when he observes a toxic effect, he has no opportunity to see how this develops or recedes in response to small changes in the molecular structure.

Distribution of poisons

The distribution of toxicants in the human body follows much the same patterns as that of drugs, as outlined in Chapter 7, and the kinetics are amenable to the same mathematical treatment (Section 7.5). Improved instrumentation and measuring techniques, introduced in the 1960s, have greatly extended range and delicacy of toxicological studies because they facilitate the determination of the very small concentrations in which toxicants, and their metabolites, usually occur.

Half life of toxicants

Many poisons have longer half lives than would be acceptable for a drug (typical figures for drugs are in Table 7.2). Thus $t_{0.5}$, in man, for mercuric chloride is 60 days, truly a long period but still exceeded by that of the insecticide DDT (*10.10*), for which $t_{0.5}$ is 3.7 months (Hathway, 1984). Yet some of the commoner and more dangerous poisons have very short half lives because they immediately combine with haems on whose moment-by-moment functioning our lives depend. As with drugs, the eventual toxic effect of a poison usually arises from its occupying a receptor designed for some normal biochemical process. The chief difference is that whereas drugs are being designed to be more and more selective, i.e. for man's welfare, a typical poison is unselective or even counter-selective. This distinction is not meant to exclude the classification (as poisons) of drugs, and even foods, consumed too liberally!

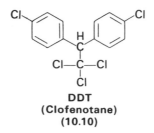

DDT
(Clofenotane)
(10.10)

Toxicants have access to the same metabolizing and excreting mechanisms as drugs do, as discussed in Chapter 7. The majority of present-day agricultural chemicals, and many industrial chemicals, occasion no harm thanks to these pathways of degradation and elimination. However, highly lipophilic substances, such as the chlorinated hydrocarbons, particularly the poorly volatile ones, find their way into the body's adipose tissues from where they are slow to move. A few foreign substances, harmless in themselves, can become toxic through chemical changes wrought by the body's metabolizing enzymes (see Table 7.1 and related text on p. 136). Methanol, hexane, benzene and benzidine are examples of biologically-inert material transformed into toxicants by the action of the liver (see Sections 11.2 and 13.1). A few other substances such as ethanol and paracetamol exhibit toxicity only when taken in overdoses which saturate normal detoxifying mechanisms.

Symptoms of poisoning in man

We are at risk of being poisoned mainly from two sources: the air we breathe and the food we eat, which are treated further in Chapters 11 and 12 respectively. Quite the commonest symptoms of mild poisoning are unexplained excitement or tiredness, indicative of interaction with the central nervous system.

Here we shall first review local poisoning, where the targets lie outside the human body, and then proceed to systemic poisoning where the targets are within the body. What is considered inside, and what outside, was defined on p. 15.

Local poisoning affects principally the skin, eye, and the cells that line the gastrointestinal tract and the respiratory tract. Irritating substances tend not to reach the general circulation but become spent at the first site of contact, either by dilution or by covalent reaction.

The outer layer of the human skin (the stratum corneum, or horny layer) offers great resistance to water-soluble substances, though not to liposoluble ones. Lying outside this general rule, a few quite simple substances can disorganize the stratum corneum so that its protection is lost and a deep wound results that can heal only slowly. These exceptions include formic acid, hydrogen fluoride and sodium hydroxide. Surprisingly, concentrated sulfuric acid causes little harm if wiped off fairly promptly. Keratolytic agents, such as trichloroacetic acid and a whole range of phenols, are used in dermatology to remove warts and other keratinized growths in an orderly manner. Mustard gas (*10.1*), a potent bifunctional alkylator of DNA, was mentioned on p. 218 for its vesicant properties. Tear gases, as used in riot control, cause stinging pain in the eyes followed by profuse lachrymation. Common examples are bromoacetone, chloroacetophenone (mace), acrolein, and *o*-chlorobenzylidenemalononitrile (CS) *.

The human respiratory tract is powerfully irritated by sulfur dioxide and nitrogen peroxide (N_2O_4). Chlorine and phosgene ($COCl_2$) produce, in addition, an oedema which arises from a permeability change that allows water to pass from injured tissues into the air spaces. This produces difficulty on breathing, cyanosis, foaming from the mouth and death by (actual) drowning. Irritation of the gastrointestinal tract produces nausea, vomiting and diarrhoea.

Turning to systemic poisoning we note that for those poisoned by stimulants of the central nervous system the following four (progressive) stages can be observed:

(a) restlessness, tremor, sweating, and exaggerated reflexes
(b) confusion, hyperactivity, accelerated breathing
(c) delirium, elevated temperature and bloodpressure
(d) convulsions, coma, and eventual collapse.

Contrariwise those who have been subjected to depressants tend to pass through the following five stages:

(a) arousable somnolence
(b) semicomatose but withdrawing from painful stimuli
(c) fully comatose and not withdrawing from stimuli
(d) most reflexes failed

---

*Lachrymators act by inhibiting enzymes that depend on a mercapto group (–SH) for activity (e.g. hexokinase). A lachrymating agent is an electrophile that combines covalently with the mercapto group in one of two ways. If it has an active halogen, it alkylates the –SH group by simple substitution but if it has a reactive double-bond, as in acrolein (CH_2=CH·CHO), the nucleophilic –SH group adds itself across this bond (Dixon, 1948).

(e) respiratory depression with cyanosis or circulatory failure.

The blood cells constitute another common site for poisoning in man, whether acutely (as with carbon monoxide, hydrogen sulfide or hydrogen cyanide) or chronically (as with benzene, chloramphenicol or those anticancer drugs that attack the bone marrow).

Less frequent sites for attack by systemic toxicants are the liver, kidneys, lungs and heart. Patients with liver or kidney disease are at special risk when exposed to toxicants. Heavy consumption of ethanol, over the years, eventually produces hepatotoxicity, sometimes fatal. Carbon tetrachloride and aflatoxin (from fungus-infected foods) also cause severe liver damage which sometimes proceeds to cancer. The mushroom *Amanita phalloides*, when eaten in mistake for edible mushrooms, causes serious liver damage. The polypeptide antibiotics, such as polymyxin, cause too much kidney damage to be used internally, whereas the aminoglycoside antibiotics, such as gentamicin, may safely be used systemically provided that the patient's kidney function is monitored. Heavy metal cations, also, attack liver and kidneys (see p. 270).

The rat poison, Antu, which is 1-naphthylthiourea (*10.11*), acts on the capillaries of the human lung, and produces drowning by pulmonary oedema. The herbicides, diquat and paraquat (*10.12*) also attack the lungs. These are systemic poisons because they reach their site of action through the bloodstream, whereas chlorine and phosgene (above) are local poisons because they reach the site directly through the airways. The glycosides isolated from *Digitalis* or *Strophanthus* are beneficial in cardiac insufficiency but excess elicits death through cardiac arrest.

Bone tissue (as distinct from bone marrow) and muscle (other than the heart) are rarely targets for poisons.

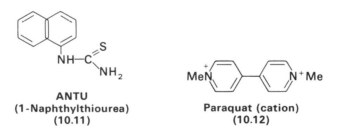

ANTU
(1-Naphthylthiourea)
(10.11)

Paraquat (cation)
(10.12)

The treatment of poisoning

Contemporary treatment of poisoned patients is much more conservative than formerly. While it is important to know the name of the toxicant that the patient has encountered, treatment is focused mainly on countering the symptoms, because these can vary greatly with both the patient and the dose. The guiding principle has become 'Treat the patient, not the poison'. An important exception is made for hydrogen cyanide poisoning where the antidote must be given promptly (p. 243).

Maintenance of respiration and circulation are paramount in the treatment, and hence the patient usually fares better if hospitalized at once. In acute poisoning the principal aims are to prevent absorption and hasten elimination. Emesis is usually indicated, effected by an injection of apomorphine or a draft of ipecacuanha syrup, which produce vomiting in about 5 and 15 minutes, respectively. Apomorphine, because it is a respiratory depressant, must not be used when the toxicant is a sedative.

Emesis is counter-indicated if the patient has swallowed hydrocarbons, or central nervous system stimulants, or strong acid or alkali, and should be replaced by the slower treatment of gastric lavage. In this method water or saline is forced down a tube inserted through the patient's mouth; after a small delay the stomach contents are retrieved with the aid of syringe, and these actions are repeated many times.

The next item in the treatment is usually activated charcoal (about 50 g in a glass of water). It is a non-specific detoxicant, working by adsorption, and may be given by gastric tube if the patient is comatose. The neutralization of acids or alkalis has given way to a policy of dilution in which the patient is fed a great deal of milk or even water (Rumack and Burrington, 1977). Saline cathartics, such as magnesium sulfate, are used in poisoning by hydrocarbons (e.g. kerosene), or when the patient has not been seen until the stomach contents have had time to move along (Rumack and Lovejoy, 1985).

The excretion of poisons in the urine is often hastened with a diuretic, such as furosemide. Because ions are more rapidly eliminated by the kidneys than neutral species, the pH of the urine can often be usefully altered. Thus acids, such as barbiturates and the non-steroid anti-inflammatory drugs, including salicylates, are eliminated faster if the urine is made alkaline with intravenous sodium bicarbonate. How well this can work is exemplified by the clearance of phenobarbital as shown in Fig. 10.1. Peritoneal dialysis or the more demanding but much more efficient haemodialysis (passage of the patient's blood through a charcoal column), are used to remove poisons that have only a small volume of distribution, a term defined on p. 119.

Follow-up

Select a pattern of thought that is parallel (or opposed) to the following, and develop it.

'For thousands of years man has been reckless in his treatment of the environment. A glance at the map will reveal immense deserts created by thoughtless deforestation, even in the ancient world, to build ships, and thereafter, in addition, to make charcoal for winning iron from its ores – a practice that continued up to the comparatively recent advent of coal mining. The erosion and

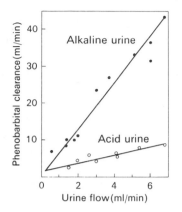

Fig. 10.1 Increased excretion of phenobarbital (pK_a 7.4) in the dog by raising the pH from 5 to 8. (Adapted from Waddell and Butler, 1957).

despoliation that followed these human adventures made many areas of our earth most unpleasant to live in and much of it quite uninhabitable. In the present century the headlong growth of industry and industrial energy-production have added an extra burden of pollution to air and water. Nowadays, there are popular movements emotionally urging rejection of industrial activities. Yet, their motto 'Back to Nature' is but a daydream based on ignorance of the immense needs, yet limited resources, of humanity. The production and distribution of materials, such as food, clothing and medicines, underlie any decent standard of living for the millions of people who inhabit our earth, so many of them in wretched circumstances. Emotional rejection of industrial activity is a threat to the health and prosperity of all human beings.

The solution to these problems is for man to learn how to deal with modern methods of production in such a way that the valuable facets are fully developed, while negative aspects are reduced to an acceptable level. In achieving this goal, it is heartening to see increased support being given to creation of a body of scientists, trained to deal rationally with these difficulties' (Condensed from Ariëns, et al., 1976).

Further reading

General toxicology
Klaassen, 1985; Klaassen, Amdur and Doull, 1985; Ariëns, Simonis and

Offermeier, 1976; Timbrell, 1985; Hodgson and Guthrie, 1980; Reeves, (1981).
Biological testing for toxicity
Gorrod, 1981; Li, 1985; National Academy of Sciences (1956–1959) – five
volumes of results: 1 general, 2 antibiotics, 3 insecticides, 4 tranquillizers and 5
fungicides.
Isolation and chemical analysis of toxicants
Moffat, 1986; Stewart and Stolman, 1960.
Clinical toxicology and occupational hazards
Turnbull, 1985; Brown and Savory, 1983; Gosselin; 1984.
Compilations of toxicological data
Sax, 1984; Sittig, 1985; Baselt, 1982; Lewis and Tatken, 1980.
Periodicals
Ecotoxicology and Environmental Safety (Academic Press); Environmental
Toxicology and Chemistry (Pergamon Press).

   An ON-LINE toxicology and retrieval system TOXNET, accessible to users
of MEDLARS (Medical Literature and Retrieval System) is compiled by the US
National Library of Medicine. TOXNET has two components, (a) the
Toxicology Data Bank includes 4100 toxic substances, and (b) the Hazardous
Substances Data Bank, broader in nature, includes environmental fate, US
government regulations and standards (thresholds), monitoring, analysis and
safe handling.

11

Poisons absorbed through lungs or skin

An introduction to the study of poisons as provided in the previous Chapter may stimulate interest in looking more closely at the commoner toxicants. Examples will be divided between Chapters 11 and 12 as follows. Poisons that enter the body through the mouth, as in eating or drinking, are allocated to Chapter 12 whereas those which enter through lungs or skin are dealt with here. The distinction is not a fundamental one, because the final actions are usually systemic not local. Yet the separation practised here has relevance to two most humane questions: How did the poison reach the individual and how could it have been prevented?

11.1 Absorbed through the lungs as gases and particles: environmental pollution

Although this title has immense scope we shall limit this discussion to the entry of a foreign substance from the environment into the human body. Not for us the thinning of the ozone layer, the melting of polar ice caps, acid rain. (Radiation was discussed in Section 10.2). In spite of these limitations we shall not lack important and exciting things to discuss, dealing with the lungs before the skin because they are the more permeable.

The architecture of the lungs is such as to allow for the transmission of foreign substances in either direction. The bronchial tree (the airways) which is to be thought of as outside the body is lined with selectively-permeable epithelial membrane which transmits lipophilic, non-ionized substances through the unselective lining of the capillaries, with which they are in intimate contact

(Schanker, 1978). The capillaries, which are connected through veins to the main circulatory system of the body, are definitely inside the body. The lungs also contain metabolically-active cells capable of many of the oxidative, reductive and hydrolytic reactions already described for the liver (p. 126). For more on pulmonary uptake and metabolism of xenobiotics see Bend, Serabjit-Singh and Philpot (1985).

Oxygen

For discussion of a selection of common poisons we cannot do better than to begin with oxygen, a highly toxic substance to whose chemical reactivity the human body has become comfortably adapted, so long as the concentration is maintained at about 20%. Yet it is only by our constant repair of oxygen damage, minute by minute, that we are able to tolerate this toxicant and enjoy its benefits. This equilibrium, no longer an easy one when excess of this poison is imposed, neatly illustrates what is meant by a threshold dose.

Of all known substances oxygen best illustrates the Paracelsian doctrine. In moderation it is an indispensable nutrient for us, as discussed on p. 8. At a higher concentration it has well-established medical uses (p. 162). Finally, exposure to pure oxygen can reveal its essentially poisonous nature. The chemical reactivity of oxygen arises from the peculiar structure of this element, in which each atom sports an unpaired electron (revealed by the molecule's paramagnetism). These free electrons confer a type of unsaturation that produces an unusual pattern of selective chemical reactivity.

The toxic effect of pure oxygen was unwittingly demonstrated by Antoine Lavoisier who had been the first to establish the role of this newly-discovered element in animal respiration. Lavoisier observed that guinea-pigs, maintained in pure oxygen under a bell jar, died before all the oxygen was consumed – a happening that he mistakenly attributed to carbon dioxide poisoning. That was in 1785 but subsequent workers included a tray of soda-lime and obtained the same result. Lavoisier's experiment was carried out just four years before the French Revolution began – a disturbance during which this scientist, universally admitted to be the father of modern chemistry, was to lose his head.

The first systematic study of oxygen toxicity was made by another Frenchman, Paul Bert, in 1874 who concluded: 'L'oxygène, à trop haut dose, est donc un agent mortel pour toutes les espèces animales' (Bert, 1878). This scientist's results have provided a firm basis for oxygen therapy, diving, aviation and space medicine.

The biochemical basis for oxygen toxicity is the conversion of lipids to lipo-peroxides. These inflict three kinds of injury: (a) oxidation of –SH groups in enzymes, (b) destruction of glutathione and (c) disruption of membranes (Chance and Boveris, 1978). An earlier hypothesis that oxygen toxicity was caused by the superoxide anion radical ($\cdot O_2{}^-$) has been disproved (Hathway, 1984, p. 196). An example of an enzyme rendered useless by oxidation of its mercapto (sulfhydryl) group is the aminophosphoribosyl transferase used in the biosynthesis of purines in man (Itakura and Holmes, 1979).

Before discussing the symptoms of oxygen poisoning in man, we need to note how workers in that field record pressure in ATA (atmospheres absolute). One ATA is 1.013 bar, or 1.033 kg/cm², or 14.7 lb/in² and shows a gauge pressure of zero.

As no prophylaxis or treatment for oxygen damage in man is known, care must always be taken not to exceed recommended pressures. Most of the rules have been learnt from experiments on healthy human volunteers, usually in naval establishments. Such subjects, exposed to pure oxygen at 1 ATA developed, after a latent period of about 6 hours, some coughing and chest pains which became progressively worse with further exposure. Symptoms diminished when the subjects returned to breathing air but bronchopulmonary irritation persisted for several days. The record period for exposure to 1 ATA for man is 110 hr. In hospital wards it has been found that therapeutic inhalation of 80% oxygen (with 20% nitrogen) can be tolerated by adults for 12 hr after which extreme irritation in the chest is complained of, and further exposure has brought pulmonary congestion and eventually atelectasis (lung collapse) (Miller and Winter, 1981).

Premature infants are usually treated with high concentrations of oxygen, which formerly often led to retinal detachment and blindness. This is now avoided by monitoring the arterial oxygen pressure which is more relevant to these cases than the inspired pressure.

Central nervous system toxicity is seen, in adult volunteers, only at high pressures of oxygen such as 3 ATA. Sweating, vertigo and vomiting are the first symptoms, followed by convulsions in less than one hour. No subject had any permanent injury if decompressed before convulsions set in. In fatalities from excess of oxygen, the cardiovascular and respiratory systems are seen to be profoundly damaged. Ultrastructural inspection reveals that many different loci are affected, particularly the mitochondria, cell membranes and the cell nucleus. For more on oxygen toxicity see Balentine (1982).

Carbon monoxide

Of all accidental deaths by poisoning carbon monoxide causes the largest number. There are two contributing factors – the widespread generation of this gas and its complete lack of odour. Carbon monoxide deaths often occur when a fire breaks out in a hotel, the sleeping victims being gassed into unconsciousness long before they are at any risk of being burned. Another source of mass deaths from this gas is 'temperature inversion', a meteorological event in which hot fumes are inhibited from rising. Under these conditions, because carbon monoxide is a common constituent of flue gases from boilers (steam-raising and power-generating) and industrial processes (e.g. smelting; converting coal to coke), whole local populations have been extinguished, particularly in cloud-covered valleys. There are many factory emissions that exacerbate bronchitis or sting the eyes or nose, such as sulfur dioxide, hydrocarbons, nitrogen oxides and dust, but these seldom kill, whereas carbon monoxide does. The lethal 'afterdamp' that follows blasting in mines, is carbon monoxide.

Turning to the domestic scene we find carbon monoxide in the exhaust gases of automobile traffic, often drawn into the living space by fans. Faulty exhaust pipes are apt to channel this gas into the interior of cars. In the home poorly ventilated gas-fired ovens and fireplaces cause many deaths because, even when the gas supply lacks carbon monoxide, much of this substance is formed when combustion is inefficient. In many small towns and villages any reticulated gas is often 'coal gas', rich in carbon monoxide.

Carbon monoxide poisoning is essentially asphyxiation because the gas molecules become attached to haemoglobin at the site normally occupied by oxygen – a site for which the toxicant has about 250 times greater affinity. As a result as little as 0.07% of carbon monoxide in the inspired air can inactivate 50% of the blood's haemoglobin which it converts to the useless carboxyhaemoglobin. The first symptoms occur when about 10% of the oxygen-carrying capacity of the erythrocytes (red blood corpuscles) has been inhibited, and take the form of a feeling of tightness across the forehead, slight headache, and swelling of superficial blood vessels. At 20% inhibition, the headache becomes more severe and the temples often throb. In the 30–40% range collapse occurs, often after vomiting, and death is to be expected at 60%. Ironically the victims display a healthy looking, rosy countenance.

The human body continuously produces low concentrations of carbon monoxide by oxidation of the methene bridges, when recycling haem (White, 1970). This is not enough to diminish appreciably the blood's oxygen-carrying capacity but heavy smokers have 5–10% of their haemoglobin tied up in this way. Passive smoking, which can arise from sharing transport, an office or a bed with smokers, soon produces measurable levels of carboxyhaemoglobin. More on the adverse effects of smoking will be found on p. 298 (carcinogenesis) and p. 311 (dependence).

Because the combination of carbon monoxide with haemoglobin is reversible, prompt use of artificial respiration supplemented by oxygen therapy can save lives. A common effect of steady exposure to small amounts of carbon monoxide is premature coronary heart disease (Petersdorf, *et al.*, 1983, p. 1303). For more on carbon monoxide poisoning see Hathway (1984).

Hydrogen cyanide

Hydrogen cyanide is one of the most powerful and rapidly-acting of poisons and many people exposed to 270 ppm, or more, have died within a few minutes. It is a highly volatile liquid (b.p. 26°C) with a characteristic sweetish odour yet, because of the low molecular weight (27), many people cannot smell it*. Although it bears the synonymous names hydrocyanic acid and prussic acid it is only a weak acid (pK_a 9.2) and easily displaced from its salts by the carbon dioxide of the atmosphere.

Hydrogen cyanide is much used as a fumigant to rid ships and warehouses of rodents, and to fumigate citrus trees. In industry, aqueous solutions of the sodium salt are used for recovering gold from weak ores, to case-harden steel, to polish metals and in electroplating. The waste effluents, rich in cyanide, are usually detoxified by chlorination. The gasification of coal, whether performed underground or in retorts, evolves substantial amounts of hydrogen cyanide. Dilute solutions of hydrocyanic acid, sometimes in the form of the pleasant-tasting cherry-laurel water, were formerly used to control nausea and vomiting.

The molecular basis for the toxic action of hydrogen cyanide is reaction of the cyanide anion with iron in (the ferric form of) cytochrome oxidase, in all mitochondira. This brings the normal flow of electrons to a sudden halt and thus puts an end to the body's utilization of atmospheric oxygen. As a result the respiratory centre in the brain rapidly becomes paralysed, leading to hypoxic convulsions and then death by respiratory arrest. The heart survives a little longer. The risk of cyanide intoxication from glycosides present in otherwise wholesome foods was outlined in Section 4.3. Many deliberate cyanide poisonings are briefly referred to in Section 10.1. When a salt, such as sodium cyanide, is swallowed, the time of death may take anything up to an hour depending on whether the stomach is in an acid phase or not. Hydrogen cyanide is rapidly absorbed through the skin but sodium cyanide is not.

Because hydrogen cyanide is a rapid poison, an antidote must be administered at once. While the standard solution of sodium nitrite and sodium thiosulfate is being given intravenously, the patient should inhale amyl nitrite for about 20 seconds. The purpose of the sodium nitrite is to create a large pool of ferric iron, which it does by oxidizing some of the blood's haemoglobin to methaemoglobin which binds cyanide tightly and harmlessly as cyanomethaemoglobin. The sodium thiosulphate, with the help of the widely-distributed enzyme rhodanese, converts the cyanide to the less toxic thiocyanate ($CN^- \rightarrow SCN^-$). Concomitant administration of oxygen if available intensifies these antidotal effects which, even without oxygen, have saved many lives. Alternative antidotes are 4-dimethylaminophenol (to replace sodium nitrite) and dicobalt edetate (Co-EDTA). Hydrogen cyanide, because of its low molecular weight, penetrates the usual charcoal-filled gas masks but a specially designed mask is available. For more on the pharmacology and toxicology of hydrogen cyanide see Way (1981).

Disastrous though encounter with an excess of hydrogen cyanide may be, we must bear in mind that it is a normal, and apparently essential, component of the

---

* The odour of both hydrogen cyanide and benzaldehyde have traditionally been described as 'like that of oil of bitter almonds' (in which they both occur), yet they do not smell like one another!

human body. In our phagocytes, glycine is steadily chlorinated by myelo-peroxidase, with concomitant liberation of HCN which is thought to play a part in the defence processes (Stelmaszynska and Zgliczynski, 1981). Hydrogen cyanide is excreted in the expired air of all healthy people (Boxer and Rickards, 1952), and in larger amounts by cigarette smokers.

Synthetic polymers

It may seem a far cry from these three toxicants (oxygen, carbon monoxide and hydrogen cyanide) to the upholstery and fittings of aircraft. About thrity years ago synthetic polymers began to replace wood, rubber and the natural-fibre fabrics in the manufacture of partitions, furnishings, sound and electrical insulation, foam mattresses, and packing materials. In spite of their lightness and other advantages these polymers carry an overriding disadvantage: they all evolve large volumes of toxic gases, quite suddenly, through thermal pyrolysis. In an accidental fire they contribute to the hazard, not by catching alight as wood does, but by emitting dense clouds of carbon monoxide, hydrogen cyanide or hydrogen chloride. It is recorded that 80% of the victims of such fires die from these fumes without being touched by fire. For example fires on board aircraft killed 119 passengers by hydrogen cyanide in Paris, in 1973, and 303 pilgrims died similarly in Saudi Arabia in 1980 (Weger, 1983).

Urea-formaldehyde polymer, which is much used for foams and for insulations suddenly releases a large volume of HCN at 450°C, without igniting and phenol-formaldehyde polymer (bakelite), which is used to make solider items, releases carbon monoxide at 300°C, again without igniting. Polyvinylchloride, when heated, evolves great clouds of hydrogen chloride. The maximum permissible concentration of inhalable poisons in the workplace is exemplified by the US Code of Federal Regulations (1985), which stipulates the following allowable average concentrations as maxima during an 8 hour shift in a 40 hour working week:

Carbon monoxide	50 ppm
Hydrogen cyanide	10 ppm
Hydrogen chloride	5 ppm.

Some may be surprised that HCl should rate so badly, seeing that the human stomach tolerates a pH of 2.0 (1 g of HCl in 2700 ml of water). However hydrogen chloride inflicts pulmonary injuries for which no treatment is yet known and from which recovery is slow. For further information on the toxicity of smokes from polymers see Alarie (1985).

Hydrogen sulfide

Hydrogen sulfide, like hydorgen cyanide, kills people by inhibiting their cytochrome oxidase. Concentrations of about 200 ppm irritate the respiratory tract and, on longer exposure, produce pulmonary oedema. Immediate death has often followed exposure to 1000 ppm. Although the rich, ripe odour of this gas may cease to be sensed after a short exposure, stinging of the eyes (felt at 50 ppm) remains as a reliable warning (HM Stationery Office, 1969).

Hydrogen sulfide poisoning is a common industrial hazard in chemical works, mines and sewage-treatment plants; also in pits where skins and other animal tissues are soaking. Such poisoning occurred also in inorganic chemical teaching laboratories before Bunsen's traditional separation of cations as sulfides was replaced, e.g. by the benzoate method. Particularly at risk are men in charge of those barges which carry H_2S-evolving sludges downstream for dumping. A man who falls into the bilge receives an even higher concentration of this toxicant than that which made him collapse into it.

City air

This is an amenity that becomes less attractive when beset by smog, a word coined in 1905 to describe a fog intensified by smoke and fumes. The darkest smogs arise in cold, damp climates; but warm, sunny climes produce quite another kind, defined as 'a photochemical haze caused by the action of solar ultraviolet radiation on an atmosphere polluted with hydrocarbons and oxides of nitrogen from automobile exhausts'. Heavy air pollution promotes an excess of deaths in very young and very old people, as well as those who suffer from chronic chest complaints. However atmospheric pollution does not contribute appreciably to cancer according to statistical analyses made by Richard Doll (1977), a view supported by Kaplan and Morgan (1981).

Classic examples of 'killing fogs' include the December 1930 episode in Belgium's highly industrialized Meuze Valley near Liège. It lasted for 5 days and led to 63 excess deaths. The valley town of Donora, near Pittsburg, which smelts iron and zinc, was immersed in fog for 6 days in 1948. Of its population of 14 000, 6000 went down with acute respiratory seizures and 20 died. In November 1966 the busy traffic of New York City was paralysed by fog and the State Governor made a Declaration of Emergency. The abundance of sulfur dioxide and particulate matter resulted in 168 excess deaths and very many more people were temporarily incapacited.

These events pale into insignificance alongside the five day London fog of November 1952 which caused more than 4000 excess deaths within two weeks and a tremendous harvest of the acutely ill. Long-term exposure to less polluted air is recognized as a potent factor in chronic bronchitis. Such considerations led to the British Clean Air Act of 1956 which set limits to emission of sulfur dioxide, carbon monoxide and particles from factory flues, power-plant chimneys and domestic fires. The USA followed with the Federal Clean Air Act of 1963. Europe, Canada and Australia have similar legislation. Cities now look brighter than before and the air is blander to breathe. The US Federal Motor Vehicle Air

Pollution Control Act was passed in 1965 and other countries have similar legislation.

A special problem exists in Southern California where geography (horsehoe-shaped ranges facing a sea partial to on-shore winds) creates huge stagnant pools of air. In such a setting the exhaust emission of unburnt hydrocarbons and nitrogen oxides react, in strong sunlight, to produce ozone which irritates eyes, nose and throat. The chemical mixture also creates an opaque, white land-hugging cloud, impairing visibility.

In the home, oxides of nitrogen, generated above the gas flames of cooking stoves, have been found responsible for excess respiratory illness in children under the age of two.

For further reading on the pollution of air see Perkins (1974), Krier and Ursin (1972) and the five volumes of Stern (1976).

Formaldehyde

Formaldehyde has long been used in the manufacture of mouldable resins (plastics) and even longer by enbalmers. In recent years one heard complaints that this pungent one-carbon molecule was polluting the home environment. The situation arose mainly through a technique of insulating a house against winter's cold by blowing beads of urethane-formaldehyde resin between the inner and outer cladding. In some cases where the resin had been incompletely cured (i.e. reacted) air in the rooms was contaminated with as much as 5 ppm of formaldehyde which tapered off in the first few weeks to almost zero. Nevertheless a minority of occupants proved to be hypersensitive to this gas and experienced irritation in throat and chest even at concentrations lower than 1 ppm. Other items that sometimes brought a similar complaint were low-cost furniture and even complete mobile houses made from particle board, a composite of sawdust and plywood bonded with a formaldehyde resin, or even from traditional timber joined with a formaldehyde-resin adhesive.

While this situation was being remedied, the more dread-spreading sections of the news media claimed that the exposed householder ran great risk of contracting cancer. Now it is true that 1% of rats, experimentally exposed to 6 ppm of formaldehyde throughout their lifetime, developed squamous cell carcinoma of the nasal cavity, however mice did not. Moreover an exhaustive study by the US National Cancer Institute of 26 500 people who had worked with formaldehyde for 20 years or more found little to link this chemical with human cancer (Anon., 1986a). For further reading on the toxicology of formaldehyde see Turoski (1985) and Starr and Gibson (1985). For discussion of species differences in carcinogenesis tests see Section 13.1.

Mineral dusts

The pneumoconioses (Gk *konis* a dust) are diseases characterized by fibrous malformations in the lungs. They are brought about by dust accumulated during normal breathing in dust-laden atmospheres. Some dusts, notoriously coal, silica and asbestos, are much more fibrogenic than others. The causation is not completely understood but a repeated mincing action of hard, sharp particles seems to play a leading part.

Coal miners' pneumoconiosis takes a severe toll in every nation where coal-mining is an important industry. In spite of the application of protective measures it can be seen radiographically in about 12% of all coal miners, with lower figures for those who work with soft (bituminous) coal and higher figures for those who win the hardest coals (anthracite), who may average 50% incidence after 20 years work. The lungs fill with small, rounded opacities (fibrositis), there is shortness of breath on the least exertion and further mining work is precluded (Cochrane and Moore, 1980). Coalminers are further disadvantaged by accidents in which they are narcotized to death by large pockets of methane (firedamp), or meet a quicker end from the carbon monoxide (afterdamp) remaining after methane explosions.

Silicosis (stone-workers' pneumoconiosis) affects those who blast and quarry stone, particularly granite, and those who work at stone-cutting, roadmaking and abrasives. In silicosis, fibrotic masses in the lungs tend to be larger than those developed by coal miners. In spite of legislation and protective equipment, silicosis remains a major occupational hazard; for example 3 million workers are at risk in the USA. Those who have to tunnel through rock in a confined space are often invalided by silicosis in as little as 10 months and many of them die in less than two years without further exposure. The more fortunate, who work in a lower concentration of stone dust, usually last about 20 years before being invalided out of their work. Tuberculosis is a common complication.

Asbestosis, discussed on p. 229, arouses more public interest because it can be (but seldom is) contracted in office and home. Of the three dusts, coal, silica and asbestos, only the latter is associated with cancer and not in high proportion.

For further reading on illnesses caused by dusts see Dauber (1982), International Labor Office (1983) and Petersdorf, et al., (1983).

Agrochemical sprays

The frequent presence of three kinds of pests in crops (insects, fungi and weeds) necessitates regular spraying. While many of us may yearn for more biological methods of control these are remarkably slow in coming forward and we may have to make do with the selectively toxic agents for a long time yet. The synthetic organic insecticides came into use in the late 1940s replacing lead arsenate and other non-selective non-biodegradable poisons. The new agents, though not as selective or biodegradable as was desired, offered, from the very nature of their simple organic molecules, tremendous opportunities for improvement in these two qualities. In fact steady research has effected great improvements and is being maintained. The nature of this research is to find new substances that are effective in the field yet non-toxic to man, to pollination and to insects, birds and fish.

An early triumph of this research was replacement of the original, insufficiently selective organophosphate insecticides by safer analogues such as malathion (*9.16b*) (p. 204).

The average citizen expects of agrochemicals that, having done their duty in the fields, they will not turn up in the food on the meal table. This aspect is discussed in Section 12.1. The FAO and WHO agencies of the United Nations are delighted at the increased crop yields that use of the new agents has brought about, as well as the value of these agents in controlling insect vectors of many grave diseases such as typhus, malaria, filariasis, and trypanosomiasis. However our present task is to consider the effects of pesticides on those who apply them in the fields and who are at risk of absorbing them through lungs and skin.

Spraying of crops is conducted either from the air or the ground. The former method is reserved for really large holdings. The owner usually places an order by telephone with the licensed operator who uses a light aircraft. They agree on a date but adverse weather can interfere with the plans. The owner's responsibility is to clear the nominated area of people and herds before spraying begins and for a safe period after. On the whole such arrangements have worked well although occasionally the wrong field gets sprayed *.

Spraying from the ground can be a more precise operation but demands a large, skilled workforce. The expense of conscientious work has sometimes been avoided by using untrained operators who can unknowingly be put at great risk. Many countries have legislated for compulsory use of masks, frequent laundering of clothing, and ready availability of hot showers but, sad to say, culpable negligence (p. 229) is not unknown. The very nature of crop-spraying requires it to take place in remote country areas where the arrival of Government inspectors is necessarily rare. Nor are the spraymen always blameless. Experience has shown that no matter how strongly protective clothing is urged on them, some will cast it aside when hot weather makes its wearing almost unbearable. Much illness has resulted from such non-compliance. It is only fair to add that the majority of farmers, contractors and spraymen are sensible and cooperative.

The cooperation of farmers is also needed for another matter: taking care not to spray unnecessarily or inappropriately; such errors of judgment have led to the emergence of resistant strains of insect. Indeed so widespread is resistance today that the world's output of food is seriously threatened. The United Nation's Food and Agricultural Organization responded to this situation in 1976 by devising a charter known as Integrated Pest Management (IPM). This aims to control resistance and prevent the poisoning of pollinating insects, insect-eating birds and fish. It asks all adhering countries to use, as far as possible, only the insecticides contained in its main list, all of them biodegradable. It also draws

---

* A most bizarre case of mistaken identity occurred in January 1979 (summer) when about 200 people were sprayed with insecticide from a plane, in an open-air cinema in Gippsland (Australia). The justifiably furious audience complained of irritated nose and eyes, but no lasting disability followed.

attention to the immense insecticide-sparing help that can be had from attention to season, rainfall, temperature and timing. Emphasis is given to the need of using only the least possible amounts of insecticide, to space the spraying as far apart as possible, and to use only those insecticides that are known to work on the *identified* infestation, coupled with close monitoring of any residues before marketing the crop (Metcalf, 1980).

Under the IPM plan the main list is restricted to the following five insecticides: trichlorofon (metrifonate) (*7.36*), malathion (*9.16b*), carbaryl (*10.9*), methoxychlor (*11.1*) and the inorganic substance, cryolite (sodium aluminofluoride). A supplementary list of insecticides for specialized purposes consists of dimethoate (*9.21*), diazinone, dicofol (*11.2*), chlorpyrifos, lindane (hexachlorocyclohexane), endosulfan, phosphamidon, methomyl, camphechlor, and three pyrethroids – deltamethrin (decamethrin), permethrin and fenvalerate.

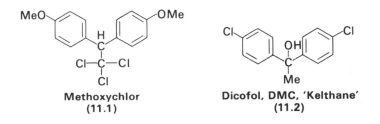

Methoxychlor
(11.1)

Dicofol, DMC, 'Kelthane'
(11.2)

Implementation of the IPM plan calls for tighter Governmental control. This may be regarded adversely by sections of the democratic communities, not least by the farmers who by nature are highly self-reliant people. What is happening is exemplified by the Food and Environmental Protection Act of 1986 which in Britain provides for a large force of trained inspectors, ready to advise, demonstrate and report. Commendably the pesticide manufacturers, so often the butt of public abuse, are firmly supporting this Act (Anon., 1985c).

It seems worthwhile to dwell a little on the chlorinated hydrocarbons, often the subject of popular debate. To begin with it is worth noting that DDT* (*10.10*) and pyrethrins have the same molecular mode of action. As Holan (1971) showed both families of insecticides owe their activity to *wedge-shaped* molecular features which prop open the ion-channels of cold-blooded creatures, leading to chaotic nerve action. The main difference is that the pyrethrins are biodegradable whereas DDT is not. However many biodegradable analogues of DDT are now known and two of them, methoxychlor (*11.1*) and dicofol (*11.2*) are much used. The original pyrethrins, extracted from Dalmatian daisy flowers, were weak, expensive and rapidly spoilt by sunlight – disadvantages which gave DDT a head start for it is inexpensive and light-resistant.

---

* DDT has the WHO International Non-Proprietary Name (INN) of clofenotane but it is also called dicophane in the UK and chlorophenethane in the USA.

For his discovery of the insecticidal action of DDT, Paul Müller was awarded the 1948 Nobel prize in Medicine. Agricultural uses assumed equal importance. By increasing crop yields, DDT's insecticidal action played an important part in alleviating extra need for food and clothing in an ever-expanding world population. However in 1962 the fear arose that DDT constituted an ecological hazard and many countries banned its use in agriculture or limited it to particular crops (such as cotton) where no adequate substitute existed, as was done in the USA in 1972.

That DDT was harmful to fish, whose bones became deformed, and to large birds, whose eggs became fragile (examples of altered calcium biochemistry) was well established. There were also fears that it would harm man through accumulation in the liver. Many substances, such as vanadium, accumulate in the liver throughout life without apparent harm. In a rather bold experiment Hayes, Durham and Cueto, (1956), of the US Public Health Service, fed 35 mg of DDT each day (i.e. 200 times the highest average dietary intake at that time in the USA) to human volunteers for 18 months. None of these brave subjects developed any symptoms related to DDT. Even more to the point was the careful medical examination of 35 men who had experienced from 11 to 19 years of exposure to DDT dust in the Montrose plant in California, where most of the DDT used in the United States had been produced continuously since 1947. No ill-effects (including signs of cancer) were found in these men, each of whom was storing, in fat and liver, up to 80 times as much DDT as the average member of the American public (Laws, Curley and Biros, 1967; Warnick and Carter, 1972).

Discovery of the insecticidal action of DDT was followed by the marketing of other chlorinated hydrocarbons, of which the chlorinated cyclodienes (notably aldrin, dieldrin, heptachlor and chlordane) suspected of being carcinogenic in man, were eventually banned. Their insecticidal action, although derived from nerve-injury, did not depend on the Holan wedge, as DDT and the pyrethrins do. In the field the chlorinated cyclodienes conferred symptoms of headache, nausea, vomiting, excitement and collapse, all of which vanished rapidly when the fieldworkers were removed to uncontaminated air. Here as elsewhere little can be learnt about long-term toxicity from observation of short-term effects.

So far we have been looking mainly at insecticides. While the spraying of fungicides has caused little concern, some herbicides have attracted widespread publicity. An unfortunate situation arose in Vietnam in the 1960s after American Army helicopters sprayed defoliants to rob the jungle of its obscuring darkness and allow ground troops to see and pursue the enemy. The most-used defoliant, called Agent Orange, consisted principally of 2,4-dichloro- and 2,4,5-trichloro-phenoxyacetic acid (*10.6*), substances long used in agriculture and thought to be harmless to man. Unhappily such large quantities were required and in such haste, that *crude* material was shipped from the USA containing a small proportion of TCDD (*10.8*), popularly known as 'dioxin'. The properties of this highly controversial substance are summarized on p. 223.

Several years after they had returned to civilian life groups of Vietnam veterans began to attribute persistent feelings of lassitude and instablity of mood to exposure to Agent Orange. The few who had developed cancer attributed this also to the exposure, while others blamed the exposure for birth defects in their children.

In 1979 the US Congress requested a study to settle these questions of causation. The enquiry was allotted to the Centers for Disease Control (CDC) in Atlanta, Georgia. As it happened CDC had already begun a study of its own in which 2000 men who had served in Vietnam were being compared with a like number whose military service had been elsewhere (Palca, 1986). By November 1985, CDC had drawn up plans to examine two cohorts, each of 6000 veterans, half of whom claimed to have been exposed to Agent Orange whereas the other 6000 said that they had not. However the US Office of Technology Assessment rejected this new project on the grounds that no verifiable measure of exposure existed. Certainly it was a matter on which Army records held no data. One thing is certain: defoliation does not take place until many hours after spraying is complete. Hence the majority of combatants could not have been exposed to TCDD (a non-volatile substance of m.p. 325°C) through the lungs, but may have absorbed it through the skin, depending on how much each body contacted.

While these official enquiries were wending their unhurried way, the seven firms who supplied the defoliant to the Army offered an *ex gratia* payment in 1984 of $180 million to the veterans (Anon., 1985d). Even if we put on one side the question of whether any physiological basis exists for the veterans' claims, it remains clear that many of them suffered anguish from the public rejection that affected all who took part in an (eventually) unpopular war.

While American veterans were reporting their symptoms the Australian and New Zealand soldiers who had fought alongside them in Vietnam did so too. The report of the *Royal Commission on the Use and Effects of Chemical Agents on Australian Personnel in Vietnam* was tabled in Federal Parliament (in Canberra) on August 23rd, 1985. It concluded that the exposure of Australian servicemen in Vietnam to Agent Orange and related chemicals was unlikely to have caused any long-term health problems, including cancer, and birth defects in the offspring. This Commission had arranged a study of 8500 infants with birth defects carefully matched with the same number of controls. It reported that the babies with birth defects were no more likely to have a Vietnam veteran for a father than the healthy babies. It also reported that cancer in these soldiers was no greater than in the general male population. The Government accepted this report but the veterans remained unhappy.

Independently the Commonwealth (of Australia) Institute of Health, in a retrospective study of 46 166 national servicemen, found that the 19 209 who had served in Vietnam (with an average of 11.6 years of post-Vietnam service) had a lower mortality rate, and a cancer rate no higher, than among the others (Australian Veterans Health Studies, 1984). However, because cancer is so prevalent in any population a small increase may not have shown (see also

Section 13.1). These cancer data will be looked at again after 20 years of post-Vietnam service.

The birth defects reported by the Vietnam Veterans' Association of Australia were mainly of teratogenic nature (Australian Senate Standing Committee on Science and the Environment, 1982). MacPhee and Hall (1985) think it extremely unlikely that exposure of the *male* partner, about 5 years before the birth of the affected children, could produce teratogenic birth defects. The offending substance would require prolonged storage in the father's body and then transport to the foetus *in utero* at precisely the right moment, and in the right amount, to produce a birth defect rather than a spontaneous abortion (Pearn, 1983). Similar conclusions were reached in parallel studies of civilian spraymen in the USA (Townsend, *et al.*, 1982), and in New Zealand (Smith, *et al.*, 1982).

Since the last use (1970) of Agent Orange in Vietnam we have become more aware of sources of TCDD (*10.8*) in civil life, such as from the combustion of polyvinylchloride in municipal waste. A week-long symposium on *TCDD in the Environment* concluded 'Although more and better data are being compiled steadily on dioxin in the environment, the question of whether it poses a hazard remains a subjective one, and one on which there is still no concensus' (American Chemical Society, 1985). The US Environmental Protection Agency has developed a mobile incinerator 'to send the solution to the problem'. Upon request it travels interstate to burn TCDD wastes at 1200°C in its rotary kiln. For more on the risks presented by Agent Orange and dioxin, see Gough (1986).

Prominent among other chlorinated substances that have provoked discussion are the polychlorinated biphenyls (PCBs) such as *11.3*. These were formerly used as the dielectrics in transformers, also as heat-transfer agents and as lubricants for hot-running machinery (even for electric razors). It has been calculated that the United States produced half a million tonnes of PCBs before manufacture was banned in 1977. Their proven carcinogenicity to laboratory animals aroused concern for human safety, particularly because levels in the food chain were increasing. Moreover PCBs have been shown to move across the transplacental barrier in the pregnant rat, injuring the foetus, and also to move across the transmammary barrier in the lactating rat, injuring the neonate (Allen and Norback, 1977). Epidemics of human poisoning by accidental ingestion of polychlorobiphenyls have occurred in Taiwan and the Fukuoka region of Japan (Masuda, *et al.*, 1982; Hay, 1982). In 1968, in Fukuoka prefecture 1684 people developed a skin rash (chloroacne, p. 223) through their rice-bran cooking oil becoming contaminated with PCBs which were, in turn, contaminated with

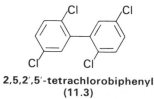

2,5,2′,5′-tetrachlorobiphenyl
(11.3)

5 ppm of tetrachlorodibenzofuran which has a similar structure to dioxin (*10.8*) and similar biological properties.

11.2 Absorbed through the lungs as vapours of solvents

Because we encounter them everywhere, in the home, the street and in the workplace, organic solvent vapours deserve this separate section so that (a) we may become more aware of their prevalence and (b) we can note which ones are particularly poisonous.

Most organic solvents are depressants of the central nervous system. In spite of great structural diversity they are highly lipophilic members of the Overton-Meyer series (p. 176) and hence resemble the general anaesthetics. Exposure to their vapours brings drowsiness, confusion and eventually unconsciousness. Transferred to fresh air the bemused subject usually makes a quick recovery.

Situations where solvent vapours occur

Here are examples of the many situations where solvent vapours daily contaminate the air we breathe.

(*a*) *Home.* In the home we encounter fumes that arise from the re-painting of rooms, from the use of adhesives and cements in hobbycrafts or the laying of plastic tiles, from fabric cleaners (spot removers), from furniture-, floor-, and metal-polishes, bath cleaners and cigarette-lighter fluid. In the bedroom a splash of cologne, lavender, bay rum or other 'toilet water' provides the embellisher with a generous inhalation of ethanol or isopropanol*. Moving into the garden for some fresher air we encounter exterior house-painting, lawnmower exhaust fumes, the solvents used in car cleaners and accessory fluids, some garden sprays (e.g. white oil) and (for those who repair their cycles) volatile rubber solvents. Without moving a step we inhale neighbours' fumes from burning household wastes and garden clippings, and also the greasy smoke from barbecues.

(*b*) *Office.* In the office the fumes of correcting fluid are inhaled at close range and to these the volatiles from adhesives can add an unwelcome quota. Unfortunate indeed are those who endure office re-decoration and house painting in the same week!

(*c*) *Industry.* In the trades and manufactures, exposure to solvents has increased greatly in the last quarter century. Where the businesses concerned are large ones they attract enough Government inspection to safeguard the health of the

---

* This is not an innocuous practice. Seven patients prepared with 'alcohol' when undergoing long-term haemodialysis, became dependent on ethanol vapour and suffered withdrawal symptoms (De Santo, 1975).

workers. However small businesses, especially cottage industries or backyard manufactures and businesses transferred to low-cost countries, do not always work under this advantage.

Examples of solvent-vaporizing trades are house- and building-painting and the spray painting of objects in factories, from automobiles down to toys. Associated trades are paint-stripping and tile cleaning. The solvents that are generally regarded as safe (a relative term of course) for these tasks are ethanol, butanol, acetone and toluene as well as carefully selected chlorinated hydrocarbons*. Particularly unsafe are methanol, benzene and other chlorinated hydrocarbons. In the building industry, modern technology makes good use of adhesives based on volatile solvents.

Metal degreasing, that essential step before electroplating, requires a non-flammable solvent with a heavy vapour suitable for use at its boiling point in an open vessel. Only chlorinated hydrocarbons meet these specifications. In recent years there has been a shift to safer types. Dry cleaning of garments has similarly switched from trichloroethylene to trichloroethane.

Agricultural workers encounter hydrocarbons in pesticide sprays and other volatile solvents in adhesives, such as those now used to join huge plastic sheets that are employed to consolidate dykes and embankments. Extraction with solvents (water, carbon dioxide, chlorinated hydrocarbons) has become established in the food industry, as in the preparation of 'instant' coffees. International specifications exist for limiting any residual solvent in the products.

The clothing industry (including shoes and hats) has a long tradition of working with adhesives and has unwittingly exposed operatives to solvent-linked illnesses. In the manufacture of textiles carbon disulfide is irreplaceable for making viscose (rayon), a fabric demanded by purchasers all over the world. Carbon disulfide presents a considerable health hazard as well as being so inflammable that contact of its vapour with a hot pipe will set it ablaze. The viscose industry has a long tradition of safety practices.

Volatile solvents are much used in the printing industry and in various aspects of commercial art. However it must be in the synthetic organic chemicals industry that the largest amounts of volatile organic solvents are to be found. It is the very essence of performing an organic synthesis that the reacting chemicals should be presented to one another in solution.

Hazardous solvents

Before proceeding to a discussion of some particularly hazardous solvents we should note that even the best tolerated of organic solvent vapours affect all

---

* Chlorinated solvents that are generally regarded as safe are 1,1,1-trichloroethane (methyl chloroform), b.p. 74°C, and tetrachloroethylene, b.p. 121°C. The last-named is also used in the oral therapy of hookworm infections. Solvents more likely to produce liver damage are dichloromethane (methylene chloride), trichloromethane (chloroform), tetrachloromethane (carbon tetrachloride), trichloroethylene ('Trike'), and tetrachloroethane (see p. 256 for the biological basis for this damage).

human processes that require judgment and coordination, such as driving a vehicle or operating machinery.

(a) *Aliphatic hydrocarbons*. The aliphatic hydrocarbons for the most part generate the least noxious of solvent vapours. The three principal types of these hydrocarbons are marketed as petrol (motor fuel, gasoline, benzine), white spirit (mineral turpentine) and kerosene (kerosine, paraffin). They are all prepared by fractionating crude petroleum (mineral oil) followed often by pyrolytic cracking and catalytic reforming. To meet the physical rather than the chemical specifications of end-uses, these liquids tend to be complex mixtures of straight- and branched-chain paraffins with various proportions of *cyclo*aliphatics (naphthenes), alkenes (olefins) and small amounts of aromatic hydrocarbons. Petrol contains mainly C_4 to C_{12} hydrocarbons and usually has a boiling range of 40–200°C, of which half boils at about 110°C (the octane range). White spirit usually has the boiling range of 130–220°C whereas kerosene, said to be the C_{10}–C_{16} cut, rich in dodecane, boils between 175 and 325°C.

The vapours of these hydrocarbons sensitize the myocardium of the human heart to normally circulating epinephrine so that ventricular fibrillation results. Higher concentrations of these vapours produce respiratory failure by depressing the central nervous system. Workmen, while cleaning storage tanks have often met their death which, in the case of petrol, can be instantaneous.

Relatively safe as the above hydrocarbons are, if handled with ordinary caution, there is one petroleum component that has exceptional toxicity. This is normal hexane (*11.4*) which has b.p. 69°C and is the main constituent of a favourite laboratory solvent known as 'light petroleum' or 'pet ether' of b.p. 60–80°C. The insidiously dangerous nature of *n*-hexane was first observed in Japan when 93 workers who were making sandals were poisoned by the hexane-containing glue (Iida, Yamamoto and Sobue, 1973). Beginning with a decrease in nervous conduction, the fingers and toes soon lost both sensibility and motility. These workers, when removed to a clean atmosphere, recovered completely after several months.

Hexane neuropathy consists of a central as well as a peripheral degeneration of myelinated nerve fibres. The molecular basis is an oxidation of hexane by the P-450 cytochrome oxidase system of liver (p. 130) to hexan-2-one (methyl butyl ketone) (*11.5*) and then to the real toxicant, hexane-2,5-dione (*11.6*). Other 1,4-diketones act similarly whereas 1,2- and 1,3-diketones are innocuous (Spencer, *et al.*, 1980). There is evidence to suggest that hexane-2,5-dione condenses with the ε-amino group of lysine residues in the main protein of nerve fibres, to produce a structure (*11.7*) that leads to mechanical disorganization (De Caprio, Olajos and Weber, 1982).

(b) *Aromatic hydrocarbons*. Though these are normally well-tolerated they have an unrepresentative and highly toxic member in benzene. Although the acute effect is only a CNS depression common to most solvents, two very severe chronic

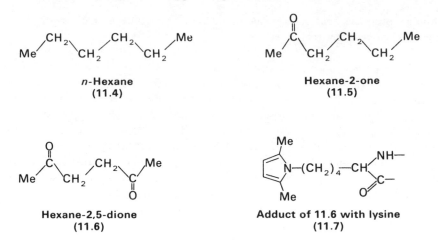

n-Hexane
(11.4)

Hexane-2-one
(11.5)

Hexane-2,5-dione
(11.6)

Adduct of 11.6 with lysine
(11.7)

effects were brought to light by epidemiological studies on workers in tyre and shoe factories. Many excess deaths were found, from leukaemia and aplastic anaemia in equal amounts (McMichael, *et al.*, 1975; Aksoy, Erdem and Dincol, 1974) It was then found that bone-marrow cells are attacked in an early stage of development. These pathological events followed the arylation of DNA which is thought to be effected by an epoxide such as (*11.8*) and formed by the cytochrome P-450 system in the liver (p. 130) (Greenlee, Sun and Bus, 1981; Tunek, *et al.*, 1978). Be that as it may, the major metabolite is 1,2,4-trihydroxybenzene (pyrogallol). Toluene causes neither leukaemia nor aplastic anaemia.

(*c*) *Chlorinated solvents.* Of these, the most pathogenic seems to be carbon tetrachloride, formerly used to treat hookworm infestation in man, and not yet

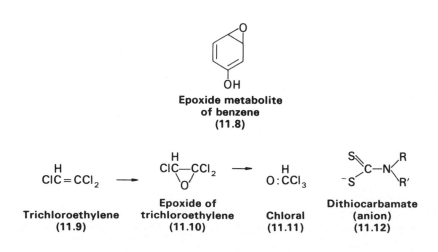

Epoxide metabolite
of benzene
(11.8)

Trichloroethylene
(11.9)

Epoxide of
trichloroethylene
(11.10)

Chloral
(11.11)

Dithiocarbamate
(anion)
(11.12)

completely replaced as a fire extinguisher, as a dry cleaning solvent, or as a vermifuge for farm animals. The liver converts carbon tetrachloride to the free radical $^{\bullet}CCl_3$ (Slater, 1966) which attacks lipids and proteins of the endoplasmic reticulum, and protein synthesis ceases (lipids undergo induced peroxidation of the double bonds). The patient presents with symptoms of hepatic and renal insufficiency, often dying from the latter. Whereas liver necrosis caused by a single dose of carbon tetrachloride is completely repaired in a week, continuous dosage results in the repair work being taken over by connective tissue – the start of cirrhosis. For further reading see McBrien and Slater, 1982 and Hathway, 1984, p. 198.

The most hepatoxic and nephrotoxic of other commercially-available solvents are chloroform and 1,1,2-trichloroethane. Chloroform may owe its toxicity to formation of phosgene ($COCl_2$) (Krishna, Pohl and Bhooshan, 1978). Dichloromethane (methylene chloride) has a low boiling point (40°C) which provides the user with abundant vapour. It was long used as a paint stripper. Dichloromethane raises the level of carboxyhaemoglobin (p. 242) in the human bloodstream by forming carbon monoxide as follows (Kubic and Anders, 1975):

$$CH_2Cl_2 \rightarrow H{\cdot}COCl \rightarrow CO$$

Trichloroethylene (*11.9*), which used to be self-administered to women in childbirth (under supervision) forms an epoxide (*11.10*) in the human body – a product which seems to be rapidly and harmlessly disposed of as chloral (*11.11*) (Hathway, 1984, p. 101). When death occurs in factories from the use of this or another chlorinated solvent, it is usually because the victim, overcome by the fumes, falls unconscious, vomits, inspires his vomitus and so dies by drowning before his plight is noticed.

Many halogenated hydrocarbons are carcinogenic in mice but usually not in rats nor (as far as is known) in man. These differences indicate different metabolic pathways, a problem often encountered in studies of carcinogenicity and discussed in Section 13.1. (See also p. 297 for vinyl chloride, a carcinogenic gas).

(*d*) *Methanol.* This is outstandingly the most dangerous of the alcohols yet depresses the CNS far less than ethanol does. Instead it produces irreversible blindness through exposure of the retina to its oxidation product, formaldehyde, which the eye cannot convert to the harmless formate anion (Kini and Cooper, 1962).

(*e*) *Carbon disulfide.* This reacts with amino groups of tissue proteins to form dithiocarbamates of the type (*11.12*). This reaction is thought to be the source of its irreversible neurotoxicity exerted through the strong copper-binding properties of dithiocarbamates (O'Dell, 1976).

(*f*) *Acetone and toluene. Elevation of mood* is obtained by anyone who inhales the vapours of plastic cement (glue) or lacquer thinners. Such vapours, often a mixture of acetone and toluene, induce exhilaration through depressing inhibitory centres of the CNS, but somnolence follows. Many deaths, following cardiac arrhythmias, stem from this practice. In 1986 New Zealand initiated a new police charge – 'driving under the influence of glue'. Voluntary inhalation of aerosol-propelled products is associated with long-lasting brain damage. For the toxicology of solvent abuse see Hayden (1976); Sharp and Carroll (1978). Cigarette smoking is discussed on p. 311.

11.3 Absorbed through the skin

The human skin is a less common port of entry than the lungs but not a negligible one. It is designed for excretion, and although it has some ability to absorb, no absorption is necessary for the body's health. Indeed the skin's outer layer is designed to provide a barrier against uptake of foreign substances. This outer protectant is the stratum corneum (SC) or horny layer. It consists of about twenty layers of dead cells, piled on one another and, in the horizontal plane, overlapped like shingles on a roof. It averages about 10 μm in thickness. The continuity of the SC is interrrupted by sweat pores, fat-secreting pores and hair follicles, but none of these permits more penetration than the SC itself. Underneath the SC lies the living, highly vascularized, epidermis whose outer cells replenish those of the SC as the latter wear away.

Thus the SC is the barrier to permeability and the junctions between its cells are waterproofed with a waxy material known as sebum. Organic solvents (ethanol excepted) remove this wax and hence increase permeability. In general the skin is far more permeable to lipophilic than to hydrophilic substances. When the SC is injured, as by an abrasion, cut or rash, its function as a barrier is lost. Even regular exposure to plenty of hot, soapy water or to synthetic detergents removes sebum. Then the skin begins to crack and dehydrate, a condition that is often the prelude to painful infections or to chemical dermatitis. In a milder way, simple friction, by mechanically separating the scales of the SC, aids penetration.

The absorptive properties of the skin (of which the average 70 kg, adult male has about 1.8 m^2) varies according to the site – being highest for the scrotum, somewhat less for the scalp, still less for the abdomen, and least for the palms and soles. For experimental purposes the best approximation to human skin is that of the pig or guinea-pig.

The skin has a metabolic capability similar to that of the liver (p. 127) but much weaker. Steroid sulfatase and β-glucuronidase have been located in the adult human skin.

In dermatology drugs are often driven into the skin by what is called *occlusion*, namely the site of application is covered by a waterproof dressing which, by humidifying the horny layer, makes it swell and become more permeable. Some poorly volatile solvents (such as propylene glycol and particularly the controversial dimethyl sulfoxide) are able to separate the scales of the SC and thus increase its permeability. The great difficulty under which dermatology labours is how to use these devices (or even simple rubbing) to increase the penetration of a medicine into the skin without driving it through into the bloodstream. Certainly it is unsafe to allow a wound to have contact with any dose of a drug larger than the established safe parenteral dose (Schaefer, Zesch and Stüttgen, 1982).

Currently, much interest is being taken in the application of drugs to the skin to achieve systemic effects, whenever a destructive first-pass metabolism (p. 119) can be avoided by these means. It can also prolong the effect of a drug that is short-acting when given orally. The most often prescribed example is nitroglycerin ointment (2%) applied to the patient's chest for treating angina pectoris. The effect of one application persists for about 3 h, whereas oral dosage provides only a brief action. Another example is the application of hyoscine in a plaster affixed to the ear to ward off seasickness.

Salicylic acid

Salicylic acid ointments, 10% in strength and applied daily for many years, are much used to suppress chronic skin conditions from dandruff to psoriasis. Yet this treatment often causes chronic gastritis, singing-in-the-ears, irregular heartbeats and even permanently impaired hearing. Infants have been found to develop acute poisoning with salicylic acid salves as weak as 0.5% if these are left on the skin for a day.

Hexachlorophene

Hexachlorophene (*10.7*) passes through the human skin apparently without harm in adults but children have often died from it when burns were treated with a 3% solution of this antiseptic. Also many new-born babies, similarly treated, have developed neurological symptoms and convulsions, leading in some cases to death. Many such mishaps have led to a more restrained use of this antibacterial (Curley, 1971; Goutières and Aicardi, 1977).

Lindane

Lindane (gamma-hexachlorocyclohexane) which has been extensively used to rid children of lice or scabies caused convulsions in those patients who had been too liberally treated with it (Anon., 1977a). Penetration of insecticides through the adult skin was investigated by Feldman and Maibach (1970, 1974) and by Simpson and Shandar (1972) who found that it was substantial enough to increase the risk that inhalation presents to field workers.

Mercury

Of the inorganic poisons mercury probably causes the most steady intoxication through the public's fondness for freckle-removing creams containing amino-mercuric chloride ($Cl \cdot Hg \cdot NH_2$ – 'White Precipitate'), which are usually applied daily, year after year. Typically they increase the usual mercury content of healthy skin (about 30 ppm) to about 500 ppm, and urinary excretion goes up from 10 μg to 1 mg in a 24 hour collection, accompanied by symptoms of salivation and disturbance of sleeping (Marzulli and Brown, 1972).

Boric acid

When applied to the napkin area of infants in traditional medicine this produced symptoms ranging from simple vomiting to circulatory collapse and death. The American Academy of Pediatrics successfully campaigned against this 'granny knows best' practice, and the European Economic Community limits the boric acid content of talcs to 5% and uses the label 'not to be used for babies'.

Lead

The traditional dermatological preparations of lead such as the acetate and oleate were found not to enter the circulation whereas tetraethyl lead (the fuel additive) passes easily through the skin and is found in blood, liver, kidney and lung (Laug and Kunze, 1948).

Further reading

Amdur (1985) and Seinfield (1986); atmospheric pollution.
Petersdorf, *et al.* (1983, pp. 1524–1532); poisoning through the lungs.
Schaefer, Zesch and Stüttgen (1982), supplemented by Gibaldi (1984); on the structure and permeability of skin.
Nater and De Groot (1985); unwanted effects of cosmetics and drugs on the skin.
Worthing's handbook (1987) gives the composition of all pesticides.
'Entoma' of the Entomological Society of America (1981) gives the same for insecticides.
Hutson and Roberts (1986); a multivolume work on pesticide biochemistry and toxicology.

Follow-up

Make a list of possible environmental pollutants omitted from this chapter – such as the perfluorinated hydrocarbons (former pressure-pack propellants) or the chlorinated hydrocarbons (e.g. methyl chloride) – that seem to be biosynthesized in isolated places from naturally-occurring materials or else arise in the chlorination of unifiltered (but not of cell-free) drinking water. Evaluate anything that the literature has to say about possible hazards to man from these substances.

12
Poisons absorbed through eating or drinking

Poisons that occur naturally in foodstuffs, such as goitrogens in cabbage, methanol in pineapple and hydrogen cyanide in many staple foods, were dealt with in Section 4.3. Here we shall look at those much more avoidable poisons, namely the contaminants introduced into food during farming, marketing or meal making. Of all sources of contamination by far the commonest is infection by microorganisms.

For the most part contaminated foods do not reach the consumer in highly industrialized countries because of the conscientious and sophisticated inspection and analytical services maintained by the Departments of Health. On the other hand developing countries are often at risk from lack of this costly infrastructure. Many of them lack either the finance or the technical knowledge to choose, say, an insecticide that is effective (on a particular crop growing under local conditions) and yet can be depended on not to leave a residue at harvest time. Fortunately such countries can be helped by the Food and Agricultural Organization of the United Nations, in Rome.

12.1 Contaminants introduced during farming

For animal farming the principal topics for discussion are infections, toxicants and growth promoters. For plant farming the main heads of discussion are fungal toxicants and pesticide residues.

Animal farming

At first sight it may seem odd to be discussing infectious organisms in a book devoted to 'The behaviour of foreign substances in the human body'. However the infections which we shall be considering are associated with a release of toxin. The vibrio (a bacterium) that causes cholera would give little trouble did it not secrete a toxin that stimulates the epithelial cells of the small intestine to manufacture an immoderate excess of (otherwise beneficial) cyclic adenosine 3',5'-monophosphate. This precipitates an osmotic chaos in which highly contagious fluids gush effortlessly from the bowel.

(a) *Transferrable infections.* The bacterium *Salmonella typhimurium* in cattle, and a related species in poultry, are easily transmitted in milk and in duck eggs, respectively, causing diarrhoea, severe colic and vomiting. In the industrialized countries any outbreak of salmonellosis is regarded as grave and must be notified to the Health Authority. Various species of the bacterium *Brucella*, which infect cattle, swine, sheep and goats in countries where the herds lack Government supervision, are transmitted in unpasteurized milk and cheese. Also, farm hands and slaughtermen can carry these organisms in their skin, leading to other avenues of transmission. Symptoms of brucellosis, which are slow to develop but very persistent, include undulant fever, physical weakness and loss of weight. Even the most effective treatment (with tetracycline) may take 6 weeks to cure this malady.

Mastitis in cows leads to transmission, through unpasteurized milk, of either *Streptococcus pyogenes* or *Staphylococcus aureus*, of which the first often causes sore throat, and even scarlet fever, whereas the latter can precipitate diarrhoea and vomiting.

Even countries that pride themselves on their hygiene in the raising and handling of food cannot avoid their farm animals becoming infested with worms; but the skills of the veterinarian, the slaughterman and the cook should see to it that these never have a chance to infect diners. Yet *Trichinella spiralis* infestations, which arise from eating undercooked pork, remain common in Europe, Canada and the USA. For treatment corticoids are administered during the agonizing migration of the worms from gut to the host's muscle; after which thiabendazole is given as an (only moderately effective) anthelmintic. Beef and pork tapeworm infestations can be rapidly and painlessly eliminated with either niclosamide or dichlorophen.

Infections from seafoods are common. Shellfish are the greatest offenders, probably because they are often eaten raw. Shellfish readily transmit the bacterium *Vibrio cholerae* that causes cholera*, also two kinds of virus, of which the first induces severe gastroenteritis whereas the other, more seriously, initiates a prolonged illness with hepatitis A. Scombroid poisoning arising from eating fish and characterized by headache and nausea seems to depend upon liberation of

---

* In the eighteenth century medical opinion held that cholera arose from 'lewdness', based on observations that it often followed consumption of oysters for their supposed aphrodisiac properties. Actually there is no such thing as a human aphrodisiac. The rich iodine content of shellfish could overcome the lassitude of undiagnosed myxoedema.

polyamines by bacteria. It comes from storing the catch without adequate refrigeration and affects particularly tuna and mackerel.

(b) *Toxicants*. Here we shall confine our attention to toxicants introduced *accidentally*. Seafoods that *naturally* contain substances poisonous to man were reviewed in Section 4.3 (p. 68).

Milk, provided by cows who get much kale or other cruciferous plants (p. 66) in their forage, is goitrogenic to man (Liener, 1980, p. 127). Cows who eat bracken fern rhizomes (p. 284) produce milk that is toxic and even carcinogenic (Evans, Jones and Mainwaring-Burton, 1972). Livestock which consume mouldy fodder absorb mycotoxins that remain after their death and usually survive cooking so that they are consumed by humans in meat, eggs and milk. Cattle can transmit aflatoxins in this way. Mycotoxic poisoning from animal foods is a fairly new subject but one that runs parallel to the older study of plant foods (pp. 266–268). Cows in the European Tyrol, if allowed to feed on the knee-high buttercups that are so plentiful in Spring, secrete toxic alkaloids in their milk.

Bees can collect from plants nectars that contain substances toxic to man when consumed in honey. Flowers of the shrub *Coriaria* (family Coriariaceae) in New Zealand have been found responsible for a honey made toxic by tutin (a bis-epoxy sesquiterpene) which, by its action on the CNS, causes excitement, convulsions and sometimes death (Connor, 1977). Mountain-laurel flowers in Western regions of the United States also yield a honey toxic to humans (NAS, 1973).

An epidemic of poisoning by methylmercuric chloride ($MeHg^+Cl^-$) began in 1953 among people who ate fish and shellfish harvested from Minamata Bay at the southernmost tip of Japan. The main symptoms were ataxia (difficulty in walking), loss of sensation of touch, pain, heat or cold, constriction of the visual field and even blinding. Nine hundred cases were officially recognized for compensation but 90 of these soon died. Some patients were greatly helped by physical re-education but no cure was discovered. The trouble was traced to a factory that made acetaldehyde by hydrating acetylene over mercuric sulfate catalyst. The much more poisonous methylmercuric salt, which arose as a minor byproduct in this process, was unknowingly discharged into the bay, dissolved in the wastewater. The incident received wide publicity, which makes it all the more surprising that another acetaldehyde plant, in Niigata on the West Coast of Japan's main island, caused a similar epidemic in 1965. Here 419 cases received official compensation and of these 18 died (Tsubaki and Irukayama, 1977). Sadly some children were born already injured by the methylmercuric cation (Takeuchi and Matsumoto, 1969). Other examples of mercury poisoning are reviewed on p. 272.

The high lipophilicity of methylmercuric salts ensures their concentration by simple forms of marine life. This happens because fat-soluble substances, provided that they are not subject to rapid biodegradation, can build up in what is known as the food chain. Another example of this concentration is furnished by DDT (*10.10*). Such substances easily become partitioned into the plasma membranes of marine bacteria which are eaten by plankton (mainly microscopically small crustaceans). This plankton (of which 1 g will have ingested, in its lifetime, about 10 g of microorganisms) forms the regular food of shrimps, mussels and very small fish, all of which are preyed upon by larger fish. Concentration occurs at each stage and further concentration takes place when birds or human beings consume the fish.

In one field study 0.005 ppm of a chlorinated insecticide found in marine bacteria led to a concentration of 0.06 ppm in the local plankton, 0.25 ppm in local clams, 1.5 ppm in the local fish, and 3.5–75 ppm in regional birds (Woodwell, 1967). Tin salts are similarly accumulated. Such sinister operations of the food chain are often and rightly quoted by environmental scientists. It is only fair to add though that most potential poisons are either easily biodegradable, or hydrophilic, or even have both of these desirable properties. Hence they are not accumulated in the food chain. In fact the more usual scavenging aspects of the food chain are very much to man's advantage.

(*c*) *Growth promoters*. By 1950 antibiotics were being manufactured from microorganisms on such a large scale that huge mounds of spent organisms were starting to accumulate. The mycelial mats from penicillin factories provide an example. These residues still contained antibiotics, but not in amounts economical to extract further. To dispose of these mounds they were offered for pig food. To everyone's surprise the pigs became much healthier, put on weight and fetched more in the market place. These animals, often kept in quite filthy conditions, benefitted greatly by losing their burden of pathogenic bacteria. It was then found that other farm animals responded well to similar feedings, and prize animals were actually fed pure antibiotics.

Many city dwellers think of the farm environment as cleaner and healthier than their own comparatively crowded suburbs. This is far from being the case because faecal matter is always blowing around on the farm, and in this dung-dust are many microorganisms pathogenic to man. Much more hepatitis A and poliomyelitis have always been contracted (per 10 000 population) in farming country than in town. This background, not of grave national consequence, became more alarming when it was realized that domestic livestock, if fed routinely on antibiotic residues, developed *transmissible multiple drug resistance* (TMDR) in their enterobacteria such as *E. coli*. The transmitted factors are small loops of DNA that consist of extrachromosomal genes. They are also known as plasmids or episomes, and one bacterial species can infect another, upon contact. Readily spread by eating with unwashed hands, they soon began to turn up in the enteric bacteria of human populations, even those that had never been exposed to an antibiotic (Smith, 1969). Thus many patients who might otherwise have benefitted from the penicillins, tetracyclines, and aminoglycoside antibiotics such as gentamicin, have been put at a disadvantage (Moorhouse, 1969;

Feingold, 1970). In spite of all reasonable precautions, such multiple drug-resistant infections sometimes spread in hospitals–examples of nosocomial epidemics (p. 116).

In spite of some conflicts of interest, governments are struggling to introduce legislation that would limit the antibiotic dosing of farm animals to types of drugs not used in human medicine. This is not proving easy.

(*d*) *Anabolics for livestock.* About 30 years ago, farmers began to use sex hormones on their livestock to induce them to put on more lean meat as opposed to fat before slaughter. This practice seemed to accord with the advice of Health Authorities that citizens should lower their intake of animal fats. Soon the use of diethylstilbestrol was banned because in 1971 an increased incidence was reported of vaginal and cervical adenocarcinoma in women whose mothers had been medicated with this drug (*12.1*) during the first trimester of pregnancy. The more expensive naturally-occurring hormones, estradiol (*12.2*), progesterone and testosterone continued to be used. Most of these excess amounts disappear by the time the meat is marketed and governments were at first content to carry out tests to verify this (223 000 tests annually in West Germany). However the European Economic Community banned this use of hormones as from January 1st, 1986. That leaves only the 'non-sexual' anabolics such as trembolone and zeranol, listed as 'under examination' in the 27th Report of the Joint FAO/WHO Expert Committee on Food Additives. For further reading on anabolics in livestock see Coulston and Korte, 1976.

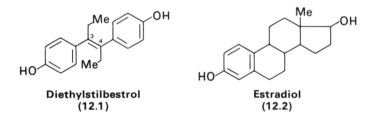

Diethylstilbestrol
(12.1)

Estradiol
(12.2)

Plant farming

The many microorganisms that infect plants seldom survive in human beings. However toxic *products* from fungi have often caused severe illness, even death. These products, and the residues left after insecticide sprayings, are the two main contaminants of plant foods in the field.

(*a*) *Toxicants from fungi.* Of all cereals, rye is the most subject to attack by ergot, which is the compact, horny sclerotium of the fungus *Claviceps purpurea*. Looking at an infected field one clearly sees how the rye grains have been replaced by the hard, black mass of the fungus. In Europe during the Middle Ages much ergot-tainted rye had to be eaten when the periodical famines occurred. Surprisingly an epidemic of ergot poisoning broke out in France as late as 1951. Truly, constant vigilance is the price of survival!

The most conspicuous feature of ergotism in man is a rapid vasoconstriction followed by gangrene of the extremities which turn black and sometimes drop off without any bleeding occurring. The symptoms are accompanied by a feeling of intense burning, which gave the name 'St Anthony's Fire' to the disease. Two other characteristics of ergotism are (a) the strong, catecholamine-like excitation of the central nervous system and (b) reinforcement of the contractions of the gravid uterus, up to the point of precipitating an abortion (Barger, 1931).

The ergot alkaloids are derivatives of lysergic acid (*12.3*). Their many pharmacological effects derive from some molecular resemblance to epinephrine (*8.1b*), dopamine (*7.33a*) or serotonin. The fragment (*12.4*) is regarded as playing a major part in the various effects. Two of the alkaloids have medical uses. Ergometrine (ergonovine) which is a simple derivative of (*12.3*), is employed in obstetrics to control post-partum bleeding. Ergotamine which has a more complex chemical structure and was first isolated in 1920, is used to alleviate an attack of migraine. It is a powerful vasocontrictor and being the constituent of ergot responsible for the typical gangrene, must be used only in small doses.

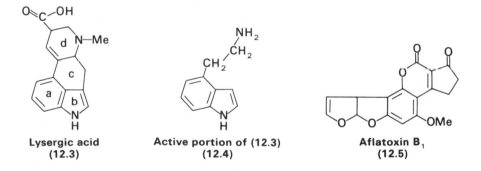

Lysergic acid
(12.3)

Active portion of (12.3)
(12.4)

Aflatoxin B₁
(12.5)

Aleukia is poisoning from eating millet and other grains that have become mouldy through delayed harvesting. Species of *Fusarium* are responsible and the toxin is a tricothecene (Joffe, 1978). Epidemics of aleukia occurred in the Soviet Union towards the close of the Second World War. Of the many thousands of people affected by bone-marrow damage about 60% died.

The aflatoxins are a family of oxygen heterocycles that are secreted by some strains of *Aspergillus flavus* and *parasiticus* which thrive on many kinds of food plants under hot, moist conditions. Peanuts (earthnuts; *Arachis hypogoea*) are particularly likely to be infected. Although they then show visible damage there is no change in taste and the toxin is not destroyed by heating. Aflatoxin B₁ (*12.5*), which is the most frequently encountered member of the family, is one of the most potent of the known carcinogens in experimental animals (rodents, birds, fish). Rats when fed a diet containing 15 ppb aflatoxin B_1 (1 part in 7×10^7) develop a hepatitis that is often followed by cancer of the liver. Field studies of inhabitants in Uganda, Kenya and Thailand showed close correlation between liver cancer and eating aflatoxin-contaminated food (Rodricks, Hesseltine and Mehlman, 1977; Liener, 1980, p. 345).

Other fungal toxins that sometimes are found in cereal grains are *Aspergillus* toxins (e.g. ochratoxin and sterigmatocystin), *Penicillium* toxins (e.g. luteoskyrin and patulin) and the *Fusarium* toxin zearalenone. The harmless practice of eating mouldy cheeses and the romance of the discovery of penicillin seem to have lowered the public's guard against the dangers that mould-infested foods present. It would be well to stay alert to what an adverse season, or the supplanting of a harmless by a pathogenic mutant, can do to an otherwise safe and nutritious crop.

(*b*) *Insecticide residues*. The persistence of the chlorinated insecticides after harvesting aroused much anxiety in the early 1960s*. As a consequence biodegradable insecticides were designed to replace them. This excellent result was promoted and is being steadily maintained by each country's principal Health Authority, and depends a great deal on its careful monitoring of the foods offered in wholesale and retail markets. Other factors important in securing this happy outcome were (a) the United Nation's Food and Agricultural Organization (FAO) policy of 'Integrated Pest Management' (IPM) (p. 248) which drew up a list of the most selective and biodegradable insecticides coupled with advice on sparing the pesticide through cooperating with climatic conditions; (b) the discovery and marketing by manufacturers of a range of safe organophosphate and carbamate insecticides designed to furnish whatever persistence-times a particular crop, grown in a particular area, may require before disintegrating harmlessly and (c) the discovery of new pyrethrins, harmless to mammals that could (unlike the traditional pyrethrins) resist destruction by sunlight.

The present position is mirrored in a recent report of the British Government's *Working Party on Pesticide Residues*, who concluded that over a five year period pesticide residues steadily declined and are now virtually absent (UK Steering Group on Food Surveillance, 1986).

(*c*) *Plant mutagens*. So far, no mutagen detected in food has been correlated with mutagenesis *in humans* although further studies may reveal an example. Typical mutagens occasionally found in food are aflatoxin B_1 (*12.5*) and nitrosamines (p. 90). Antimutagens have also been found, e.g. turnip and cabbage decrease the mutagenicity of the pyrolysis products of tryptophan and vitamins A, C and

---

* This refers to the chlorinated insecticides being used at that time, namely DDT (*10.10*) and the cyclodienes such as dieldrin, aldrin, chlordane, endrin and heptachlor, which are now banned in many countries. For the clinical neurobiology of the organochlorine insecticides see Taylor and Calabrese (1979). However, at no time did these pesticides contribute significantly to the risk of cancer in human beings (NRC, 1982).

E are credited with ability to inactivate mutagens. A large body of evidence shows that irradiation of food does not make it mutagenic (Anderson and Purchase, 1983).

12.2 Contaminants introduced during processing, marketing or meal-making

Food additives (dealt with as beneficial components of our daily diet, in Section 5.2) remain a prime subject of public disquiet. Yet it is beyond reasonable doubt that we enjoy a safer food supply than ever before in human history. The main toxic hazard in what we eat arises from microbiological contamination. The possible presence of heavy metals and the migration of organic substances from packaging need watching, as does possible adulteration by petty criminals.

Bacterial toxins

Whereas toxic fungi rather than toxic bacteria may threaten us in the growing plant, bacteria rather than fungi offer the principal threat once food processing begins. This is illustrated by the flesh of the coconut which, in Indonesia, is exposed to a friendly fungus to make the banqueting delicacy known as 'bongkrek'. However when the ever-present bacterium *Pseudomonas cocovenans* outgrows the mould, two poisons are accumulated – bongkrekic acid and toxoflavin. The first of these, a C_{28} aliphatic acid, blocks ATP translocase in the mitochondria and many people have died as a result (Henderson and Lardy, 1970).

In industrialized countries one of the commonest causes of food poisoning arises from *Staphylococcus aureus*, but only from those strains that produce the enterotoxin, a protein of MW about 30 000. It is usually transferred to the food by the infected hands of a preparer. As little as 1 μg of the toxin brings on vomiting, severe abdominal cramps and copious diarrhoea, but the patient recovers in two days and death from this cause is rare. The toxin is not destroyed by boiling in water for an hour. The foods most frequently affected are chicken (cold, or hot roasted), baked beans, cream- (or mock-cream-) filled pastries, and custard (a kind of egg sauce, much eaten in England).

Less common but far more serious is botulism which arises from the presence in food of the anaerobic bacterium *Clostridium botulinum*. The toxin is a heat-labile protein of MW 128 000. Many consider it to be the most poisonous substance known; 1 μg is thought to be a lethal dose for human beings but laboratory animals show symptoms at 10^{-6} μg/kg. After a little preliminary vomiting, death occurs by suffocation brought on by paralysis of the diaphragm. The actual site of action is at ACh-dependent synapses of the peripheral nervous system. Botulism is not a common disease; outbreaks mostly follow consumption of a consignment of canned seafood, such as tuna, where every can in a faulty batch is likely to be infected. The second commonest source of infection seems to be home-preserved peas and beans, insufficiently heat-processed.

Bacillus cereus is a Gram-positive rod, common in soil. It mainly troubles the diner who is served rice that had been boiled on the previous day and then set aside in a warm place. Of the two known toxins, the commoner one rapidly causes vomiting, whereas the other evokes a more leisurely diarrhoea with abdominal cramps.

Typhoid, paratyphoid fevers and cholera, can be contracted in restaurants if a carrier (who may be symptomless) is working in the kitchen. Brucellosis (p. 263) sometimes affects diners for the same reason. The infections mentioned in this paragraph are uncommon in temperate climates. For more on food poisoning derived from bacteria see Petersdorf, *et al.* (1983).

Heavy metals

Gross contamination of food by toxic metals such as lead, mercury and copper was commonplace until the various nations, influenced by Britain's pioneering *Sale of Food and Drugs Act* of 1875, introduced similar legislation. However the widespread presence of arsenic could not be controlled until nearer the end of that century when methods for measuring it finally became available. Whereas most organic chemical contaminants are rapidly metabolized and eliminated, mercury, lead, arsenic and cadmium become accumulated by the body and exert their toxic effects to an ever increasing extent by combining with substances vitally important for the body's daily metabolism.

(*a*) *Lead.* The heavy metal that is currently attracting most attention is lead. It has always, because of its wide distribution, been present in dust and soil. Mining and industrial practices now add to this burden, and more still comes from automobile exhausts because of the use of tetraethyl lead in fuel (used to prevent 'knocking' during combustion). The United States, which pioneered the virtual elimination of lead from motor fuel, recorded a marked decrease in the lead content of its citizens' blood measured after the first ten years (Annest, *et al.*, 1983). Most other countries have yet to decrease lead in their motor fuel. The EEC requires that new model motor cars, if their engine capacity exceeds 2 litres, must run on unleaded fuel from October 1988; the same will apply to *all* new model cars from October 1989. Unleaded fuel is already widely available in Austria, Switzerland and West Germany.

One peculiarity of high civilizations is that they consume their food and drink mainly from lead-glazed plates and cups. In the eighteenth century Europe broke away from the traditional tin and salt glazes when, country after country, they discovered how to apply the thicker, smoother, rich-looking lead glazes to achieve a result formerly available only in imports brought thousands of miles from China. Acidic foods such as pickles and fruits including the tomato continually extract traces of this lead. From this source and from the solder used to form the tinned-iron cans in which so much processed food is sold, the inhabitants of industrialized countries consume from 0.1 to 2.0 mg of lead daily. In addition, children, who are so much more vulnerable than adults to lead poisoning, receive more lead from the dust of their playgrounds and by swallowing chips of paint, and also the sweet-tasting water that rain produces as it flows over paint containing lead carbonate or red lead.

The lead that issues from motor-car exhausts as a fine dust is in the form of halides. When this is inhaled it is (oddly enough) not absorbed through the lungs but climbs up the airways in a film until it is swallowed. The traditional use of lead in ointments, which decreased about the middle of this century, did not raise the blood level of lead. Potentially more dangerous sources of lead intake are from childrens' lead toys and the paint of their wooden and metallic toys, also from soft (but not hard) water conveyed in lead pipes, wine stored in lead cisterns, dust from artist's pigments and fumes from the burning of painted wood. Until recently a severe industrial hazard was presented to printers setting type in hot metal (an alloy of lead, antimony, bismuth and tin) – a method of typesetting now being rapidly taken over by computerized photographic and electrostatic processes. Lead smelters and those workers who manufacture electric storage batteries remain at high risk.

It is thought that lead is absorbed from the small intestine by the calcium channel. It then appears in the erythrocytes and the liver as well as in the tubular epithelium of the kidney. Gradually it is transferred from these sites to hair, teeth and bones; about 95% becomes harmlessly stored in the latter. The half life of lead in the blood is about a month but in the bones it is about a quarter of a century. Lead is continually lost from the body mainly through the urine. Very little lead reaches the adult brain but infants are much more vulnerable.

Chronic poisoning in adults usually begins with the symptoms of constipation and loss of appetite but finally produces a colic that is paroxysmal and excruciating. Chronic poisoning in children involves the central nervous system. The first symptoms are usually vertigo and irritability, proceeding to delirium, vomiting, and convulsions. The mortality rate hovers around 25% if treated and 65% if untreated. In infants, exposure to lead produces a progressive mental deterioration after the first 18 months of life. This shows as loss of motor skills and retarded development of speech and there is often some hyperkinetic behaviour. These symptoms are not as was once thought confined to children in the crowded inner-city areas for lead tends to be present to the same extent in the dust of all playgrounds.

In addition to the above symptoms, exposure to above average concentrations of lead interferes with the biosynthesis of haem at several enzyme levels and this leads to hypochromic microcytic anaemia in humans of all ages.

Chronic lead poisoning is best treated by chelation therapy, initially with calcium edetate and mercaprol, given together intramuscularly, and then followed by oral penicillamine during the next several weeks. Because oral chelation therapy promotes absorption of lead from the gut, treatment must take place in a low lead environment.

The Joint FAO/WHO Expert Committee on Food Additives recommends 0.05 mg/kg body weight of lead as the maximum weekly intake for adults. This should be compared with 0.005 for mercury, 0.007 for cadmium, and 0.014 for arsenic (all mg/kg, weekly). By agreement between the UK Government and paint manufacturers lead will completely disappear from consumer paints by mid 1987. However playground equipment still exists with coats of paint received 30 or more years ago containing up to 20% lead. The US Congress passed a Lead-Based Paint Poisoning Prevention Act in 1971.

For more on lead poisoning in humans, young and old, see Lansdowne and Yule, 1986; Klaassen (1985) and also (for children) Boeckx (1986).

(b) *Mercury*. Formerly the most prescribed of all drugs, mercury and its derivatives have been replaced, largely since 1950, by less dangerous remedies. On the other hand concentrations of mercury in the environment have risen in proportion to the combustion of fossil fuels (which contain traces of mercury) and through the increased use of mercury in industry and agriculture. We have already had occasion to mention a former use of mercurials to quieten infants (p. 60), the current abuse of mercurial cosmetics (p. 259) and the often fatal eating of fish accidentally poisoned by methylmercuric salts (p. 264). Many other people have been poisoned by eating seeds, intended for sowing and not for human consumption, that had been preserved with a methylmercuric salt as protection from fungal attack. Such disasters have occurred in the latter half of this century in Ghana, Guatemala and Pakistan. The worst of these catastrophes followed importation by the Iraqi Government of wheat and barley protected in this way and distributed with proper warning for Spring planting in 1972. However the hungry farmers ate most of it as bread – an act that resulted in 6530 of them being hospitalized and about 500 dying (Bakir, *et al.*, 1980).

When inhaled, the vapour of elemental mercury enters the lung and readily crosses semipermeable membranes which uni- and bi-valent mercury salts cannot do. Chronic exposure to traces of mercury vapour shows up as tremor and gingivitis (sore gums); also there are evident psychological symptoms such as irritability, confusion and insomnia. Transferred to a mercury-free atmosphere the subjects usually make a complete recovery.

Inorganic mercuric salts are mainly adsorbed onto the intestinal mucosa although a proportion gains access to the blood, from where it concentrates in the kidney. Acute poisoning leads to violent intestinal pain, blocking of the kidney tubules and death. Chronic mercuric poisoning is more insidious – the glomerulus of the kidney is attacked, and other symptoms resemble those caused by elemental mercury. Treatment of mercury poisoning is by chelation therapy, usually with intramuscular dimercaprol followed eventually by a course of oral penicillamine. Poisoning by the methylmercuric ion (p. 264) is more severe and harder to remedy. For more on mercury poisoning and its treatment see Klaassen (1985).

(c) *Arsenic.* Used enthusiastically in medicine for at least two millenia, the employment of arsenic today is confined to advanced cases of trypanosomiasis where the brain has become infected. In no way does this virtual rejection of arsenic undervalue Ehrlich's epoch-making discovery, in 1910, of arsphenamine – the first effective remedy for syphilis, a hitherto incurable disease. This was the first drug able to eliminate an infection caused by a bacterium and, what is more, arsphenamine was the first remedy of any kind whose union with a receptor could be chemically specified. It is the nature of advances in science that they light the way for still more valuable advances, and the decline of arsenotherapy serves to illustrate this principle.

Today the impact of arsenic on health comes from its wide distribution in nature, particularly in edible fish and in drinking water. The smelting of ores, the traditional spraying of grapevines and fruit trees against fungi, its use as a rodenticide, in poison baits against the domestic ant and as a dressing for ectoparasites on sheep, although all declining uses, continue to distribute this element in its most poisonous forms namely as the trioxide (As_2O_3) and sodium arsenite. The frequent presence of arsenate in phosphate fertilizer, though small also plays a part in distributing this unwanted element. The average daily human intake of arsenic is only about 0.3 mg but those who rely heavily on fish for food get much more. After absorption from the intestine arsenic is stored mainly in the liver, kidney, heart and lung. It also is deposited in bone, teeth, hair and nails. Arsenic crosses the placental barrier and can damage the foetus.

The mild oedema brought on by low, regular doses of potassium arsenite (Fowler's Solution), evidenced as a gain in weight and fullness in the face accompanied by a pleasant-looking 'milk and roses' complexion, were formerly taken as proof of 'tonic' properties while this insidious drug was causing gastrointestinal, renal, hepatic, myocardial and neurological damage! Chronic arsenical poisoning is often not realized until muscular weakness and pain set in followed by skin pigmentation and gross oedema. The garlic-like odour of arsine (AsH_3) is noted in breath and sweat. If exposure is continued, evidence of kidney and liver damage cannot be ignored and eventually peripheral neuritis leads to paralysis of the legs. Chronic arsenical poisoning can be successfully treated with oral penicillamine.

Acute arsenical poisoning, as instanced on p. 217, produces excruciating abdominal pain, severe vomiting and diarrhoea followed often by coma and death and all symptoms are accompanied by the telltale odour of arsine. For more on arsenical poisoning and its treatment see Klaassen (1985). For the widespread, centuries-long use of arsenic as a 'tonic' in mediaeval China see Needham (1954).

(d) *Cadmium.* The average daily intake of cadmium in food is about 50 μg in the industrialized countries but larger than this if the diet is rich in mammalian kidney or liver, or in shellfish. From time to time iron cooking vessels, whose enamel owes its cheerful orange colour to cadmium sulfide, become officially banned on the grounds that if the glaze were faulty and if something acidic were cooked in it some cadmium could be ingested. The half life of cadmium in the human body is about 20 years; it is trapped by metallothionein, a cysteine-rich protein in kidney and liver that has a high affinity for cadmium and zinc (Goering and Klaassen, 1984). Hence most people do not seem to be at risk from cadmium poisoning but metal refiners react to cadmium fumes with dyspnoea (breathing difficulty), and grossly cadmium-contaminated food injures the kidney. Quite untypical (presumably because of concurrent calcium deficiency) was the incident at Fuchu in Japan which took place shortly after the Second World War. Cadmium, washed into the rice fields by effluent from a local lead and zinc processing plant, poisoned the rice crop. Those who ate the rice, and received about 2 mg a day of Cd^{2+} in it, suffered agonizing myalgic pains. For more on the toxicology of cadmium see Friberg, *et al.* (1974).

(*e*) *Antimony*. Citrus juices liberate antimony from enamelled jugs and buckets. Citizens who undertook to cater for large gatherings such as weddings or church bazaars often unwittingly produced mass vomiting in this way. However from about 1930 as plastic ware replaced enamel this hazard disappeared in proportion.

(*f*) *Aluminium*. Manufacturers of enamel saucepans directed much adverse propaganda against aluminium which began to capture their market early in the present century. Imposing and authoritative sounding names were mustered to convince a trusting public that cooking in aluminium would cause cancer. Slowly but surely the public decided in favour of aluminium. More recently anti-aluminium propaganda has been revived but with as little supporting evidence as before. One recalls another propaganda exercise from the first decade of this century when the manufacturers of leather shoes warned us that walking in the newly-introduced rubber-soled shoes would bring on blindness. Do we see through the thrust and parry of trade warfare as well today as we did in the early 1900s?

(*g*) *Iron*. The essentially poisonous nature of iron, and how ingeniously the human body limits its uptake, were discussed on p. 54. This protection is wanting in the disease haemochromatosis where excessive intestinal absorption of iron leads to lassitude, abdominal pain and greying of the skin, followed by diabetes and (if untreated) death from liver or heart conditions. A small proportion of white people inherit this condition but the greatest sufferers are the black Bantu people of South Africa who seem to acquire it by brewing ethanolic beverages in iron vessels.

Contamination by organic chemicals

The increased proportion of wives who daily left home to work, and an insistent demand by all people for more leisure, combined in the second half of this century to produce a demand for more packaging of foods. This demand proceeded hand in hand with growth of the plastics industry. The principal danger presented by food packaging materials is that they may be too permeable, or else difficult to seal, so that they may admit air, microorganisms, pests, or whatever they were designed to keep out. A secondary danger could be *migration* of unpolymerized monomer or of plasticizers from the wrapping into the food. Migration also occurs from the wax of waxed paper, the lacquer of lacquered cans, the solder of unlacquered cans and some inorganic ions from glass. In spite of these possibilities, little injury to human beings by such migrations has been reported, whereas many people have been made ill from bacterial infection of unwrapped foods.

Cut lunches are often packed, domestically, in a cling wrap (cling film) which usually consists of polyvinylchloride containing, as plasticizer, either di(2-ethylhexyl) phthalate or di(2-ethylhexyl) adipate. A little of these plasticizers can migrate into fatty foods such as cheese or ham. Polyethylene film which requires no plasticizer can be used instead but it is difficult to adapt to wrapping by machine.

Apart from film, bags and pods, food is often marketed in plastic jars and bottles and, even when marketed in glass vessels, these often have plastic closures. In its 28th Report (1984) the FAO/WHO Expert Committee on Food Additives provisionally allowed small amounts of unreacted monomer and of plasticizers, diffusing into foods from plastic in their containers. Of propellants they accepted nitrous oxide as completely without risk and dichlorodifluoromethane to a limit of 0.15 mg/kg (19th Report, 1975).

Residual solvents in food are still under review, but there is a complete ban on the use of benzene, chloroform and 1,2-dichloroethane (FAO/WHO 27th Report, 1983). The largely abandoned practice of decaffeinating coffee beans with trichloroethylene left about 0.5% of this solvent behind (Brandenberger and Bader, 1967). Although this practice seems to have done no harm extraction of soya beans with the same solvent (now discontinued) produced S-(dichlorovinyl)-L-cysteine, which produced aplastic anaemia in cattle (McKinney, et al., 1959).

For more on possible contamination from packaging see Katan (1985); for discussions on which toxicological problems in food processing are real and which imaginary see Gibson and Walker (1985).

Fumigants

These are used to control pests infesting bulk foods (e.g. weevils in wheat silos). Flour millers take similar precautions against the flour moth whose cobwebs block his sieves. Methyl bromide (bromomethane) is typical of these fumigants. While a small proportion of what is used in fumigation may combine with food protein there is no evidence of harm to consumers (Winteringham, 1955).

Adulteration

The conscienceless adulteration of foods that, in the industrialized countries, was rife until late in the nineteenth century (p. 81) has been replaced by honest merchandizing. For this very desirable change we can thank well-conceived legislation backed by regular and well-informed inspections. The sensitivity and diversity of modern analytical methods makes detection almost certain and punishment inescapable. All the more surprising that in 1985 several of Austria's wholesalers of the lower qualities of local wines chose to sweeten them with diethyleneglycol $(HO \cdot CH_2CH_2 \cdot O \cdot CH_2CH_2 \cdot OH)$ – a substance that had killed 105 people, mainly children, when it was used as a vehicle for sulfanilamide in 1937 (Calvery and Klumpp, 1939). The Austrian wine pollution was halted before anyone died of kidney necrosis but the wine-marketing industry suffered another scandal in 1986. A group of Italian wine merchants added inexpensive methanol to low-ethanolic wines to reduce the density, a property that governs the wholesale price. As little as 4 ml of methanol can cause permanent blindness (Ritchie, 1985), and up to 14% v/v of this poison was found in these wines. More than 30 consumers died and many more became permanently blinded.

Follow-up

Comparatively rare as food adulteration has been in recent years, try to collect further examples (e.g. of cooking oils in developing countries) and discuss their impact on the consumer.

13

Some foreign substances with consequences for public policy

The two subjects to be discussed in this Chapter are of importance both scientifically and socially. A great deal of scientific knowledge is available to help with the problems that these topics raise, and more is constantly being sought and acquired. However, in these subjects, Government decisions often have to be made urgently and in areas where the scientific evidence is as yet inadequate. Often too they lead to policy judgements made on grounds not of 'What is true?' but 'What is expedient?'. When briefed to give evidence the scientist needs to be careful to distinguish between established facts and such value judgments. What a searing dichotomy that can present! The scientist has professionally to uphold a rigid discipline of thinking based on facts found by well-established methods and capable of being verified by other scientists all over the world. Yet he is also, as a citizen, a participant in human society with all its competing wants and values.

Different social groups of course have different policies. For example some want 'No smoking in public' whereas others claim a right to smoke where they choose. A Government may respond to such pressures by expressing humanitarian concern and seek to improve the nation's health. It can aim to educate, influence by propaganda or discourage by taxation, an unhealthy activity. It may go further and declare the activity illegal, risking public resistance and even breakdown of public order as happened in the USA with ethanol. (Prohibition of the sale and consumption of ethanolic beverages was introduced in the USA in 1919, by the 18th Amendment to the Constitution, and repealed by another Amendment in 1933.)

While these are choices for Government as it seeks to harmonize the hopes and ideals within the community, its Treasury has other guiding principles: if smoking is reduced there will be a saving in health costs realized slowly over the years, but a counteracting and rapid drop in income from tobacco taxes which must be recouped, either by raising the general level of taxation or by heavily taxing other items of public consumption, even foods. The political consequence of such a compensation must be highly dissuasive to those who tread the corridors of power! Moreover several Governments have long ago constituted themselves as the sole tobacco merchants in their respective countries so that too-enthusiastic reforms would lose them revenue in excess of mere taxes. Nor are Governments always consistent, for several of them discourage smoking by public propaganda while paying subsidies to their tobacco growers!

13.1 Carcinogens

Cancer is a noun of assembly to describe about 200 different diseases, all of them characterized by unrestrained cell division. In this changed condition previously normal human cells grow faster and without restraint. That is what is meant by malignancy. All cancers are malignant. A carcinoma is a cancer situated in the boundary of an organ and is derived from epithelial cells. It is the commonest form of cancer and occurs with increased frequency in ageing populations. A sarcoma is a cancer in connective tissue (e.g. muscle, tendon, cartilage, bone) and is more frequent in younger populations. Several neoplasms (new growths) with names ending in 'oma' (e.g. lipoma, granuloma) are not cancers. As sanctified by usage the word carcinogenic now describes any agent that elicits a cancer and not just one that elicits a carcinoma.

The nature of cancer

In speed of growth cancer cells apparently do not outdo that of our intestinal cells which become sloughed off at a tremendous rate and have to be renewed urgently. The difference lies in the loss of that control exercised by normal cells when they have accomplished a task set by the whole organism. In short the cancer cell grows without regard to the needs of the complete organism. The enhanced rate of multiplication in the cancer cell is accomplished by an enhanced rate of mitosis, so that the nucleus completes the four phases of its mitotic cycle (also called the cell cycle) much faster.

When we watch a tissue becoming progressively more malignant we see cells, ones that were visually indistinguishable from those of the organ in which the tumour is growing, gradually losing the differentiation that made them recognizable as belonging to that tissue, and with it are lost the functional properties characteristic of that organ. This dedifferentiation seems to be secondary to a profound biochemical change in which the affected cell switches from respiration to fermentation, as first noted by Otto Warburg (1927). Such a change is not in itself pathological. A runner's muscles will switch from the aerobic to the anaerobic mode when he is yielding up his last quantum of strength to establish an athletic record. What is different is that the athlete's muscular biochemistry quickly reverts to its normal respiratory pattern. So far we do not know what makes the cancer cell turn anaerobic. To his dying day Albert Szent-Györgyi (Nobel Prize laureate in Medicine, 1937) held that regulation of this process is most likely effected by very simple, rapidly-diffusing molecules; but the evidence remains inconclusive (Szent-Györgyi, 1975).

What we are really sure of is that the malignant cell, unlike its healthy parent, no longer responds to messages from other cells – messages that would restrain its multiplication in the interest of coordination and harmony in the whole organism. It seems as though the whole process of evolution has been turned backwards in a great devolution from metazoan life which is rich in instructions for shared growth-information and mutual adhesion. That is to say the cancer cell has reverted to a protozoan life with complete independence for each cell.

What can we learn from the protozoa? Most of them are unicellular animals but a few form colonies and these may give some clues as how to initiate a more sociable lifestyle in human cancer cells. It is instructive to consider the family of protozoa known as the Volvocales. These green flagellates have some members like *Chlamydomonas* which are always unicellular; in contrast to the closely related species *Volvox* which exists only in spherical colonies (Coleman, 1979). Unfortunately the chemical basis for this difference has remained elusive but another protozoal family, the Acrasiales (familiarly but incorrectly called 'slime moulds') seems to be furnishing good clues. The most studied member is *Dictyostelium discoideum* which is about 10 μm in diameter. This animal multiplies unicellularly until all the surrounding nutritive material has been consumed. It then emits a chemical signal which draws about 1000 similar amoeboid cells together to form a multicellular structure which, when nourishment is more plentiful, releases many spores each of which grows into a unicellular creature like the first. This chemical messenger is 3',5'-cyclic adenosine monophosphate (cAMP) (*13.1*), a substance much employed by the human body as a 'second messenger' (Sutherland, 1970). Other species of *Dictyostelium* seem to use peptides as messengers but these have not been so well studied (for more on *Dictyostelium* see Mato and Konijn, 1979).

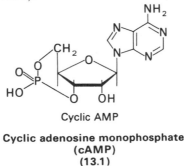

Cyclic AMP

Cyclic adenosine monophosphate
(cAMP)
(13.1)

In the mammalian situation cAMP is always generated intracellularly because it cannot diffuse through the plasma membrane. In experimental work this disadvantage is overcome by using the di-butyryl ($C_3H_7 \cdot CO-$) derivative, which was designed to be more liposoluble and hence more permeable (p. 119). It was hoped too that a non-specific esterase (such enzymes abound in mammals) would remove the two acyl groups intracellularly. With the help of this reagent a relevant experiment was carried out on what are called 'transformed cells'. These are not malignant but they share several properties with malignant cells. For example they are partly dedifferentiated, they multiply faster and they have diminished self-cohesion. The ones used here were fibroblasts, isolated from the ovaries of a Chinese hamster. When dibutyryl-cAMP was added to their culture medium all signs of 'transformation' rapidly disappeared and they reverted to being normal fibroblasts (Puck, 1977). This result suggests that the network of microfibrils and microtubules which relays information from the plasma membrane to the nucleus (Buckley and Porter, 1967) is cAMP-dependent. However how to use such information to help cancer patients remains to be discovered.

Prevalence of cancer, past and present

Cancer is not as is sometimes supposed a disease peculiar to our present times for it was well known in classical antiquity, as is recorded in many surviving writings of Claudius Galen, eminent physician of the second century AD. That cancer seems to be widespread today (one in four citizens of the United States contract it and one in five die from it) may reflect improved diagnostic methods. It is also relevant that we live longer than our ancestors did, so that many slowly-developing cancers have the time to become evident. Industrialized countries rejoice in a high level of accountability. The USA annually reports the number of deaths from cancer, not only State by State but also County by County. Looking at these we can observe small trends of difference between city and rural life or between industrial and pastoral areas; also we may note regions where the concentration of a recognized carcinogenic occupation (such as the wood-working or leather industries) confers a typical cancer on a proportion of its practitioners. However no areas free from cancer emerge and no general correlations are indicated (Blot, *et al.*, 1977).

Cancer may in general be advancing on a broad front but there are also cases where a large malignant growth has undergone spontaneous recovery. Well authenticated, though few in number, these instances suggest the presence of a self-repairing mechanism in our bodies. Although gross manifestations of it are rare there are indications that it is proceeding all the time on a very small scale. That is to say, it may be quite normal for our cells to become precancerous and then be normalized quickly by self-repair, as in the response of normal skin to ultraviolet light (Hanawalt, *et al.* 1979).

Cancer is common in developing countries although the major types differ from those encountered in industrialized countries. For example cancers induced by the Epstein-Barr virus (p. 283) are often noted in developing lands. These tend to be highly disfiguring and usually result in death. One such cancer is Hodgkin's lymphoma which causes large tumours of the head and neck; it is most frequently seen in northern and eastern Africa. Another example is nasopharyngeal cancer, very common in southern China and among Chinese populations of south east Asia; this attacks tissues at the back of the nose and spreads to lymph nodes in the neck (Epstein and Achong, 1979).

In spite of the seeming universality of cancer we know of a few communities that are apparently free from it. They are ones that have preserved a very individual way of living, seemingly unchanged through the millenia. An example is the Hunza community, who live in Kashmir on the mountainous borders of China and Afghanistan at a height of about 3000 m. A noted physician and nutritionist who lived among them reported that these farming people were free from cancer and lived long, healthy lives (McCarrison, 1922). The Eskimos, with whom the arctic explorer Stefansson often resided, were reported by him to be free from cancer except for those whose way of life had been modified by close contact with other races (Stefansson, 1960). What have these two communities in common? The Hunzas are lacto-vegetarian, the Eskimos live almost exclusively on flesh. The Hunzas, living in a mountain pass, have long been exposed to foreigners whereas the Eskimos have enjoyed isolation. Balancing these differences are some similarities: both peoples value freshness and variety in their food, both suckle their young for 2–3 years, both lead a hard life with evident enjoyment. The most important clues though may lie elsewhere.

Genetic and environmental factors in carcinogenesis

The fact that not all humans exposed to an established carcinogenic influence (such as traditional wood or leather work) go on to develop cancer, indicates the reality of a genetic contribution. That there is also an environmental contribution is shown in people who change their circumstances by migration or by simply embracing a cultural change without leaving their country. Such people are apt to incur a change in the type of cancer to which they are subject (reviewed by Kmet, 1970).

About twenty kinds of cancer (or precancerous states) are known to be strongly inherited but these are fairly rare types, constituting together only about 2% of all cancer cases (Creasey, 1981; Petersdorf, et al., 1983). One example is retinoblastoma, an eye tumour with an incidence of 1 in 20 000 live births. There is a 95% probability that a child who carries the defective gene will develop this form of cancer. Again almost every person who inherits the genetic defect for polyposis (1 in 8 000 live births) develops cancer of the colon.

Turning from conditions such as these, where the hereditary component is strong and measurable, we encounter the commoner category where a cancerous tendency can be seen 'to run in the family'. Thus daughters of women who develop breast cancer have a roughly fourfold greater chance of acquiring this condition than women without such a family history. In Australia it is evident

282   Consequences for public policy

how people of Scottish or Irish inheritance suffer from an extraordinarily high incidence of basal cell cancers which develop, one after another, on exposed parts of the body under the propitious influence of a sunny climate. Fortunately this is one of the most treatable forms of cancer. Genetic factors can also act protectively as with black people who are excluded from contracting melanoma. For more on genetic predisposition to cancer see Knudson (1977) who has contributed so much to this aspect.

It is currently thought that about 80% of all cases of cancer have a mainly environmental origin. It is an impressive fact that when populations migrate their pattern of cancer susceptibility changes after a time lag from that of their country of origin to one similar to that of their country of adoption. For example the Japanese people who migrated to the United States developed few of the stomach cancers that were so characteristic of the country they had left. Instead they developed cancer of the breast and colon, which were rare in Japan (Haenzel and Kurihara, 1968). However a similar alteration in cancer patterns is now developing in Japan where the diet is changing to include less fish but more quadruped meat and fat. Coincident with this change mortality from breast cancer began to increase sharply (Hirayama, 1978).

Such changes are easiest to follow when the migrating population has an individual pattern of malignancy. An example is carcinoma of the mouth which is one of the commonest cancers in India and Sri Lanka but rare elsewhere. Conversely cancer of the colon, the commonest malignancy of non-smoking Caucasian males, is rarely found in Africans or Asians. Again primary hepatoma is uncommon among Caucasians but frequently encountered in Africans and Southern Chinese. We have already mentioned the striking regional distribution of Hodgkin's lymphoma and nasopharyngeal cancer but the latter at least has a demonstrable genetic component.

Environmental influences in causing cancer were divided by Hueper (1948, 1961) into radiation, heat, the atmosphere, diet and foreign chemicals. The last two, which are closely related to the subject of this book, will be dealt with more fully on pp. 293–300. We have already encountered radiation in the form of strong sunlight and from radionuclides (p. 226). Concerning heat a small but constant percentage of burn scars turn to epidermal carcinomas (Treves and Pack, 1930). Clay pipes used for tobacco smoking burn the lip in the habitually-grasped position where it often becomes cancerous. Similarly the *kairo* box, of metal foil containing hot coals, worn in rural Japan close to the abdomen for winter comfort, often elicits a cancer. So does 'reverse smoking', as practised in Sardinia, Venezuela and parts of Africa, in which the burning end of the cigar is the one held in the mouth (Doll, 1977).

The carcinogenic potential of a dirty atmosphere was revealed more than 200 years ago when Percival Pott correlated scrotal cancer with exposure to coal soot (p. 69). Today we are more concerned about hidden dangers in industrial effluents and automobile exhaust, and we control them by legislation (p. 245).

The hazards of consuming atmospheric contaminants in our drinking water were reviewed by Harris, Page and Reiches, 1977.

(a) *Viruses as carcinogens.* To Hueper's environmental influences we must now add infection by certain viruses, although scientific opinion was slow to realize the importance of this factor in human beings. These viruses may not cause cancer directly but there is no longer any doubt that they are essential steps in triggering at least five types of cancer (Burkitt's and Hodgkin's lymphoma; also nasopharyngeal, cervical and primary hepatic carcinomas).

One turning point in appreciating the influence of viruses in evoking human cancer was a statistical finding (Martin, 1967). This showed that the highest incidence of cancer of the uterine cervix occurred in women who had the largest number of sexual partners. Such a correlation suggested an infection and a papillomavirus (normally resident in a genital wart in the male partner) was found to be the culprit. The other turning point was the demonstration that two human cancers common in Africa and Asia (Hodgkin's lymphoma and nasopharyngeal carcinoma) are associated with infection by the Epstein-Barr virus, a DNA herpes virus (Epstein and Achong, 1979).

Hopes are now entertained that virus-associated cancers can be fought with vaccines. Indeed a vaccine is already used to protect poultry against cancer conferred by a herpes virus that used to kill millions of these birds in the 1950s. Another attack is being made by chemotherapy. On the mountain slopes of East Africa and New Guinea, Burkitt's lymphoma attacks children between four and eight years of age; it is manifested as a tumour of the jaw and is rapidly fatal. However if treated early with methotrexate (*9.11*) or cyclophosphamide (*7.42*), a cure can be rapidly achieved (Bertino and Johns, 1967).

(b) *The social environment in carcinogenesis.* The list of environmental factors responsible for cancer can usefully be extended by considering social influences. Concerning cervical cancer in women, while many cases may have been acquired accidentally it is evident that most of the 800 000 cases reported annually arise in the more permissive strata of society (unknown in nuns, common in prostitutes) (Doll, 1977). Another example of a social influence is the rarity of breast cancer in women who have their first child before the age of 18. Such early primiparity is encouraged more in some countries than in others, and within each country there is likely to be some social or educational group that defers childbirth. Cigarette smoking, a common cause of lung cancer, is very much subject to social influences.

The carcinogenicity of foods and other foreign substances

We have already reviewed what the National Research Council, in their 1982 report, considered the most carcinogenic components of meals eaten in the USA (see p. 42, which should be re-read at this point). Their findings and recommendations were based on a retrospective survey. Note their conclusion that no food additive or pesticide residue seemed to be making any appreciable contribution to the risk of cancer in the American population.

When we look around our world more widely we come across areas where, from tradition or from necessity, carcinogenic foods are regularly consumed. For example in the Transkei region of South Africa, the people eat a good deal of sorghum, of which the high content of tannin predisposes to cancer of the oesophagus (see also p. 292).

Aflatoxin B$_1$ (12.5) is found in nuts and grains which through storage under hot, moist conditions have attracted toxic strains of the fungus *Aspergillus flavus*. Because it is one of the most potent known carcinogens, it has been studied more than any other fungal carcinogen, and hence has provided most of the quantitative data linking spoiled foods with cancer (see further p. 267).

We have already referred to the winning of starch from the seeds of cycads in tropical lands. This ancient family of gymnosperms generates the toxic and carcinogenic glycoside, cycasin. However those races that depend on the Cycadaceae for food have long known how to free it from the carcinogenic principle (see further p. 11).

The seeds of the palm *Areca catechu*, when mixed with lime (to liberate the alkaloids) and the leaves of a climbing pepper, have been chewed for many centuries by inhabitants of the East Indies as a mild stimulant of the central nervous system and the gastrointestinal tract. This practice often leads to oral cancer (Arjungi, 1976).

Safrole, a flavouring agent widely distributed in plants, is carcinogenic in rodents and hence has been withdrawn from its former use in flavouring soft drinks in Europe and the USA (p. 84).

The young fronds (often called fiddlesticks) of the bracken fern *Pteridium aquilinum*, eaten in parts of Canada, the USA, New Zealand and Japan, have often been spoken of as carcinogenic. This thought flowed from knowledge that the rhizome evokes cancer in cattle, whose milk is carcinogenic in mice (Evans, Jones and Mainwaring-Burton, 1972). However, the fronds are thought to be safe human food (Hirono, 1973; Grasso, 1983).

The highly controversial N-nitrosamines, mostly found in processed fish and meats, often result naturally from the nitrosation of amines present in foods (see, further, p. 90).

Many hundreds of chemicals are known to induce malignant tumours when administered experimentally to rodents. The news media have repeatedly drawn attention to the fact that some of these are (or were formerly) used as food additives or are possible food contaminants, or are introduced, through human activity, into the air that we must breathe. Actually, very few substances are known *for certain* to be carcinogenic in man, but it is only right that we should constantly be on guard against others. On pp. 287–293 we shall review how such tests are made, on p. 293–300 we shall discuss the results of these tests, and we shall look at the administrative problems on p. 300–304. However, first of all we should review what is known of the formation and development of a cancer.

The process of carcinogenesis

While, as we have seen, many factors are known to favour development of an established cancer, it is much harder to pinpoint the event that first sets malignancy in motion. Much of the difficulty in detecting the underlying process lies in the large number of precipitating circumstances which have been catalogued. Arcos, Argus and Wolf (1968) begin their three volume work on the chemical induction of cancer with this observation: 'It is possible that under certain conditions, in some species and towards some tissue, practically every agent may prove to be carcinogenic to some degree'. They instance the production of sarcomas in rats by seemingly inert materials such as glass, ivory, transparent cellulose foil, metal foils and concentrated solutions of glucose or sodium chloride. More recently we have learnt that bladder cancer in rats can be provoked by feeding such common nutrients as L-leucine, L-isoleucine and L-valine, provided that a known tumour initiator (in this case: N-butyl-N-4-hydroxybutylnitrosamine) is fed at the same time (Nishio and Fukushima, 1986). Hueper (1961a) suggested that the carcinogenic action of the glass and foils arose from their causing a local anoxia which imposed the switch to anaerobic metabolism, correlated with malignancy by Warburg (1927).

From the confusing wealth of data one helpful principle has emerged very clearly: chemical carcinogenesis is a multi-stage process. The first example of this was demonstrated by Berenblum (1941). He showed that after application of a *promotor* (itself non-carcinogenic), mice rapidly developed cancer when a normally non-carcinogenic dose of the hydrocarbon benzo[a]pyrene (*7.31*) was painted on their skin. He called the benzopyrene an *initiator*, and for a promotor he used croton oil, of which the active principles are esters of phorbol (*13.2*) – a tetracyclic polyhydroxy compound. One of the most successful of these promotors is TPA, which is the 12-O-tetradecanoyl 13-acetate derivative of (*13.2*).

Several well-known dyestuff intermediates of former times, such as 2-naphthylamine, benzidine and 4-acetamidobiphenyl (*13.3*) become initiators

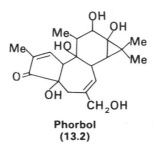

Phorbol
(13.2)

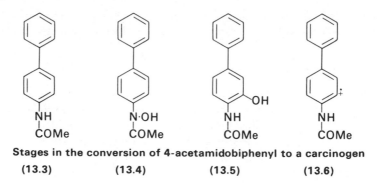

Stages in the conversion of 4-acetamidobiphenyl to a carcinogen

(13.3)   (13.4)   (13.5)   (13.6)

only when the human body's cytochrome-dependent oxygenases (in the endoplasmic reticulum, p. 30) have chemically altered them to electrophilic substances, which are the true carcinogens. Therefore we should call these intermediates *pro-carcinogens* (or proximate carcinogens). Thus 4-acetamidobiphenyl (*13.3*) is N-hydroxylated to (*13.4*); the hydroxy-group then migrates to the *ortho* position (as in *13.5*), then is removed, leaving (traces of) the positively charged carbocation radical (*13.6*) (Miller, Miller and Hartmann, 1961; Miller and Miller, 1981). Such electrophiles react covalently with one of the electron-rich (nucleophilic) centres in DNA, thus providing the initial carcinogenic step. Nevertheless if normal excision-repair is operating in the nucleus (Friedberg, 1985), the DNA should revert to its normal state, except when a promotor (also called a co-carcinogen) is present to develop these dormant cancer cells.

It is characteristic of the specificity of multistage processes that, in the original Berenblum project, no cancer resulted if the promotor and the initiator were applied to different sites of the skin. Also no result was obtained if the initiator was applied before the promotor, using the same site (Berenblum, 1941, 1974).

Another type of multi-stage process starts with 'transformed cells' (p. 279) which can be produced from normal cells by the action of viruses, vegetable lectins or some simple chemicals such as acetamide, benzyl chloride, methyl iodide or succinic anhydride. Hamster embryo cells in cell culture are often used for this procedure which was first effected by Sachs (1965); many examples are listed by Searle (1984). Transformation is heritable, i.e. it is transmitted to progeny. Some transformed cells seem to be spontaneously malignant but most of them require activation by a true carcinogen.

In yet another multi-stage carcinogenic model, dimethyl sulfate is used to change healthy cells into an 'immortal strain', namely one that can be cultured indefinitely – a characteristic more of malignant than of normal cells, which seem to have an inbuilt mortality. Yet, other than having acquired this unlimited lifespan for their progeny, these treated cells retain all the properties of normal cells and (quite unlike transformed cells) they have a normal growth rate and they remain differentiated. Yet they can be converted to malignant cells in a single step when incubated with an oncogene (Newbold and Overell, 1983).

An oncogene may be defined as a sequence in a viral DNA that closely resembles a sequence in the host's genome. It has been suggested that cancer may arise through the viral sequence replacing the host's sequence, or else that a chemical factor may transform the host's sequence into the viral sequence (Todaro and Huebner, 1972). An example of the minimal character of difference between oncogenic and normal sequences is illustrated by the induction of a bladder cancer following a change in a single nucleotide, one that specified a single amino acid: valine was substituted for glycine in the twelfth residue from the amino-terminal of one of the host's proteins (Tabin, *et al.*, 1982).

From initiation of the cancerous process in the human body to its florid clinical manifestation takes many years, seemingly about three years for a leukaemia but 10–20 years for a solid cancer (i.e. a tumour).

Among the *anticancer influences* in the human body must be counted selenium (p. 55) and the glutathione-S-transferases, of which there are at least six (Mantle, *et al.*, 1987). Unfortunately a considerable proportion of the human population seem to lack the genes to produce some of these enzymes.

The interferons seem to exert a modest degree of cancer control in the human body. They are glycoproteins with about 160 amino acid residues and are formed in three kinds of human cells after invasion by a virus (lymphocytes, leucocytes and fibroblasts). They are usually classed as lymphokines (biologically-active agents produced by lymphocytes). Interleukin II, a similar polypeptide, encourages growth of cytotoxic T-cells which attack cancer cells. Both types of lymphokine are being made industrially by the hybridoma technique for experimental work. So far, the results in the Cancer clinic have not been striking.

Tumours possess antigens against which the body's immune system could operate. Individual observations have been recorded of monocytes, T-cells and macrophages recognizing and then killing cells. This suggests that, in health, an immune surveillance system may be eliminating cancer cells at an early stage (Smith and Landy, 1970). Evidence is also accumulating that major histocompatibility antigens play an important role in host defences against both the development and the spread of malignant growths (Festenstein and Garrido, 1986). Consonant with this thinking is the increased frequency of cancer in patients undergoing immunosuppressive treatment during organ-grafting.

Many have hoped to establish immunity-based treatments for clinical cancers. Unfortunately, tumours have several ways of protecting themselves from immunological attack. Moreover stimulation of the immune system in a tumour-bearing experimental animal has often stimulated the tumour to grow! Clearly the immunology of cancer is complex and far from being understood. Any form of cancer treatment depending on an immune technique must be approached with extreme care.

Tests for carcinogenicity

Relatively quick, simple and inexpensive tests are in regular use for finding whether a substance is mutagenic or not. Such information can provide a useful warning because most carcinogens are mutagens although mutagens are not necessarily carcinogens. Hence when a positive result is obtained in a mutagenic test it becomes necessary to test the substance in an animal such as a rodent, although this procedure is both long and expensive. At the end of that test one will know if the substance is a carcinogen for the selected species, rat or mouse. Happily not all rodent carcinogens are active in man for two reasons: (a) when, as is often the case, the true carcinogen arises by hepatic metabolism – the metabolic pathways of man are known often to differ from those of rodents, which themselves display important differences, and (b) human cells vigorously excise and repair damaged DNA whereas rodent cells are sluggish (Regan and Setlow, 1973; Lieberman, *et al.*, 1971; Klimek, 1966; Ben-Ishai and Peleg, 1975).

Epidemiological studies usually take the form of studying a group of workers who have been exposed to the suspected substance for, say, the last 20 years. This is called a retrospective study. For a newly employed chemical a prospective study must be initiated, although it is hard to keep track of the workers who change their employment. Even when it is agreed that only epidemiological studies can settle the question at issue, two imperfections remain. First if the number of exposed workers is small no clear-cut answer may emerge unless the substance is potent. Second even if the number of participants is adequate a feeble carcinogen may not be detected if it leads to forms of cancer that are common in the unexposed community; however if it leads to an unusual type of cancer it will certainly be recognized.

In epidemiological work accepted statistical methods must be used, for one is not looking just for cases of cancer but for an *excess* over what a well-matched group produces. In such work a small difference, one way or the other, may not fall outside the 95% confidence limits of the test, or whatever other statistical safeguard against random variability has been agreed upon. Possibly because of this limitation no direct study has shown that city air produces more cancer in humans than country air does. Epidemiological studies perform better in the workplace where concentrations tend to be higher (Cartwright, 1984).

(a) *Tests using laboratory animals.* The animals most often used in testing for carcinogenicity are the rat and the mouse because they are the least expensive to maintain and can conveniently be observed over a whole lifetime. Rats live in reasonable health for about three years and mice for about two. It is not practicable to test throughout a lifetime because of the increased natural incidence of cancers in ageing rodents. Thus rats usually show a dramatic increase in the number of natural tumours after 27 months and it is seldom possible to detect chemically-induced tumours against this background. Adequate controls (untreated animals) have to be maintained throughout every test, and this essential provision adds expense to the routine. Rats, though a little more expensive to maintain than mice, seem to use metabolic transformations more akin to those of man.

To achieve valid statistical significance a group size of 50 animals is desirable. Separate experiments at three different dose levels, conducted simultaneously, will usefully add to the information obtained. The pros and cons of testing at high dose levels such as would never be encountered in man, are discussed by Grasso (1979). The most common form of dosing is oral, but for special purposes injection, inhalation, or skin-painting have been used. According to Lehninger (1982), to test one chemical thoroughly for carcinogenicity in rodents costs about $100 000. Apart from rats and mice, hamsters (and occasionally rabbits) are sometimes used, but guinea pigs are considered to be too insensitive. Dogs and monkeys have been employed for special purposes but the high cost of upkeep and long lifespan are against them.

One serious shortcoming of testing on experimental animals is that a substance that produced tumours in only 5% of the animals would be judged a weak carcinogen, one that the investigator was lucky to be able to detect. Yet, if this substance produced 5% of tumours in a human population, it would be regarded as a major health hazard (Arcos, Argus and Wolf, 1968, vol. 1, p. 343). Even so low an incidence of a cancer as 0.01% would represent 20 000 people in a population of 200 million. To detect this low incidence experimentally would require at least 30 000 animals according to Klaassen (1985).

(b) *Tests on isolated cells.* Much of the time required for completion of an animal test is spent in waiting for a tumour to become evident. Hence since about 1970 it has become customary to start with some short-term tests that use uniform populations of single cells in which any genetic change can rapidly be detected under the microscope. Adoption of these methods presumes that a carcinogenic substance will damage the genes directly and this is what usually occurs. However there are also agents, named epigenetic, that elicit cancer indirectly. Here we shall deal first with tests for the more numerous genotoxic agents, and come to the epigenetic agents later.

No single short-term test is capable of detecting all the substances found to be carcinogenic in rodents, so that it is prudent to use two, or even more, of such tests, which may run concurrently. For these tests one employs either mammalian or bacterial (occasionally fungal) cells. The test may be selected to give any of the following endpoints: damage to DNA, aberrations in the chromosomes or simply mutagenesis.

DNA damage can be produced by strand breakage, base destruction or change in cross-linking; these injuries, plus any attempts at DNA repair, can be measured by autoradiography. Such tests are usually conducted on freshly isolated, non-dividing rat liver cells, which have the advantage of containing the metabolizing enzymes that are frequently required to convert a pro-carcinogen to a carcinogen (Williams, 1980).

Tests for chromosomal aberrations conducted on rat hepatocytes or on human lymphocytes, over the last several years, have given excellent correlations with carcinogenicity. However these tests usually need the attention of an expert cytogeneticist who has the time for karyotype analysis. This objection does not apply to observation of any rapid increase of sister chromatid exchange. A special benefit of this test is that it can be conducted in human lymphocytes in an exposed population (Sandberg, 1982).

Single cell tests can also be devised for a particular mammalian tissue although the results may apply only to that tissue. Some Japanese researchers recently worked out a rapid (4 weeks) assay, using rat bladder cells in culture, to detect possible bladder carcinogens. Confirmation of their results on entire rats took 60 weeks (Nishio and Fukushima, 1986).

Many mutagenic tests are conducted as a first step in screening chemical substances for possible carcinogenicity.

A mutation may be defined as a permanent change in the genetic material of a cell, a change that is transmitted to successive generations. Mutations may be advantageous or disadvantageous. Advantageous mutations make important contributions to evolutionary adaptation whereas the majority of mutational events are lethal or deleterious. Mutagens and carcinogens both impose a change on a cell that its progeny inherits. Carcinogens were long thought to produce cancer through inducing a mutation. However mutation is a unique type of event and, while carcinogenic processes may proceed in parallel with mutation, they appear to be different and more complex.

Often in mammals and other eukaryotes the effect of a mutation is seen only after a few generations because so many mutations are recessive and are manifested only when two individuals with mutations on the same point of the DNA molecule happen to cross-breed. This type of difficulty seldom arises with prokaryotes who make little use of sexual reproduction, but usually divide vegetatively, by binary fission. This behaviour has brought about a preference for bacteria as cells for use in tests for mutagens.

A much-used procedure of this kind is the reverse mutation test devised by Bruce Ames and his colleagues in the University of California (Ames, Sims and Grover, 1972; Ames, 1979). This test is sensitive, rapid, inexpensive and can be carried out by supervised technicians. It uses a strain of the common bacterium *Salmonella typhimurium* that has a mutational defect in the gene that normally orders synthesis of the enzyme phosphoribosyladenosine triphosphate. This enzyme is essential for histidine synthesis and hence the bacterium cannot grow in a histidine-deficient medium unless a reverse mutation is induced. Because many chemicals become carcinogens only after activation by the enzymes of the liver's endoplasmic reticulum (p. 130), a suspension of rat microsomes (known as S9) is often added to a second series of Ames tests, run in parallel.

The Ames test is carried out in this way. A thin layer of nutritive agar (histidine-free), containing about 1000 million of the test organisms, is poured into a Petri dish. When the pour has set a small disc of filter paper, impregnated with the test chemical, is placed in the centre of the plate which is then incubated at 37°C for 2 days. If the chemical is a mutagen it will make many new kinds of mutants of which a few will be of such a nature that they reverse the original mutation and permit synthesis of histidine, as signalled by the prolific growth of the organism. The amount of back-mutation is used to compare the mutagenicity of different substances through the construction of dose-response curves. These are usually linear, suggesting that there is no threshold for mutagenesis.

Special strains of *Salmonella typhimurium* are available for these tests. All strains are selected to lack the lipopolysaccharide capsule which this organism frequently sports, but which is inimical to free-diffusion of the test substance. Some available strains are especially responsive to base-pair substitutions whereas others detect frame shifts (deletions or additions of base pairs). The sensitivity of the specialized strains can be enhanced by genetically deleting their excision–repair mechanism.

How well does the Ames test behave as an indicator of carcinogenicity? When about 300 substances, each one definitely established as a carcinogen in rodents, were submitted to this test (with and without liver microsomal modification); only 90% proved to be mutagenic. For example the following eight substances were Ames-negative, although fully carcinogenic in rats or mice: acrylonitrile, benzene, *o*-toluidine, safrole (*5.7b*), diethyl hexylphthalate, diethylstilbestrol (*12.1*), phenobarbital (*7.26*), and hexamethylphosphoramide. However not even the long and expensive rodent test is final where human beings are concerned for we tend to be less susceptible (p. 288). Of these eight substances only benzene is known to be carcinogenic in humans. True, diethylstilbestrol can exert carcinogenic properties if used during pregnancy (which is no longer practised) but it is firmly established for treatment of post-menopausal cancer of the breast. Phenobarbital, introduced in 1912 by Hauptmann for the treatment of epilepsy and still widely used for that purpose, has given no evidence of carcinogenicity during that long period.

It is evident that the Ames test on its own cannot detect all substances carcinogenic to rodents. Conversely many Ames-positive substances are known that produce no tumour in rodents (e.g. benzoin and caprolactam – which is a monomer for making nylon). Indeed many long and (apparently) safely used substances from everyday life are Ames-positive, including many natural essences and flavourings, well-established cosmetics, food preservatives and sweeteners. It is disturbing too that two common constituents of human cells, cysteine and glutathione, give a positive Ames test because these substances are known to play a part in preventing cancer (Glatt, Protić-Sabljić and Oesch, 1983). Again 'dioxin' (TCDD) (*10.8*), whose often violent activity seems to be of a mutagenic character, at least in susceptible mice (p. 223), is not mutagenic in the Ames test.

Although the thought is much nurtured by the news media, we can no longer logically suppose that every mutagen is a potential carcinogen. The biological effect which the Ames test is monitoring (ability to effect a frameshift) is not the kind of biological effect that cancer cells exhibit (independence of growth and acceleration of the cell cycle). A quantitative lack of correspondence between carcinogenicity and mutagenicity is frequently reported (e.g. Coombs, Dixon and Kissonerghis, 1976). Special attention should be paid to the aniline-mustard series, in which carcinogenicity (among the members) goes up as the mutagenicity comes down and *vice versa* (*13.7–13.8*). Fifteen members of this series were examined in a collaborative programme between the Mutagenesis Screening Section of the Frederick Cancer Research Center (Maryland) and two Californian Schools. These members were graded for mutagenicity by the Ames test (with and without prior incubation with the S9 microsomal fraction of liver) and for carcinogenicity by a count of the increase in lung tumours in a strain of mice prone to this malignancy in mature life but tested here only for the first six months. It was found that the 4-phenoxy derivative (*13.7*) ranked as the highest for mutagenicity and lowest for carcinogenicity whereas the reverse was found for the 3,5-diureido analogue (*13.8*) (Leo, *et al.*, 1981).

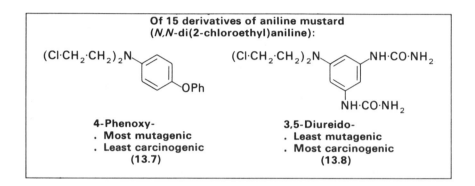

All these irregularities serve to remind us that the Ames test can provide only an initial sorting in any attempt to find if a substance is carcinogenic. The high degree of agreement found between mutagenicity and carcinogenicity in rodents, coupled with its speed and cheapness, makes the Ames test a good beginning to what can only be a long programme of investigation. Help in choosing a short-term test to complement the Ames test is offered by Weisburger and Williams (1984) and by Ashby, *et al.* (1985). The Ashby-edited report (from the International Programme on Chemical Safety's collaborative study on *in vitro* assays) was published jointly by the World Health Organization, the International Labour Organization and the United Nations Environmental Programme.

There are many tests available, but quite a few give differing results when different collaborating laboratories examine a submitted specimen. One of the best of these tests, although it requires special skills not widely available, is the Styles cell-transformation test (Purchase, *et al.*, 1976). This test depends on the observation that most mammalian cells will not grow in semi-solid agar. However if a substance that can elicit cell transformation (p. 279) is supplied growth (as single cells) occurs freely. This test, which can use human liver cells or hamster kidney cells, was positive for the (no longer used) dye butter yellow but negative for 2-naphthylamine, whereas the Ames test returned exactly the opposite verdict. Both substances are known mammalian carcinogens.

This leads to a discussion of epigenetic substances which are those which promote malignancy without showing any damaging effect on chromosomes. They do not react directly with genes but produce a biological change favourable to later genetic damage. This change may be a tissue injury, a hormonal imbalance, an immunological disturbance or simply promotional activity (in the Berenblum sense, p. 285) on cells that have been independently affected by a genotoxic agent. Although epigenetic substances are returned as negative by an Ames test they become positive if a dose of a genotoxic agent is added at the same time. Several classes of epigenetic materials are distinguished (Weisburger and Williams, 1984). Some (azathioprene and 6-mercaptopurine) are immunosuppressors; others (estradiol, diethylstilbestrol) are hormones; others (phorbol esters, tryptophane metabolites, bile acids) are promotors; others (asbestos, foils of metals or cellulose) are insoluble; a fifth class contains some of the cytotoxic agents used in treating cancer (chlorambucil, cyclophosphamide and melphelan) and a sixth class is formed by several chlorinated hydrocarbons including some of the earlier discovered insecticides such as dieldrin, aldrin and heptachlor, also the polychlorinated biphenyls (p. 252) and 'dioxin' (p. 223).

Quite apart from all these tests for carcinogenicity many chemicals are constantly under test for teratogenesis (birth defects), perinatal and postnatal toxicity and effects on fertility. Congenital malformations can be induced by exposing a mother to teratogens (e.g. thalidomide) in early pregnancy, but there is no evidence of increased incidence of birth defects in progeny of women or men exposed to atomic radiation (Miller, 1968) nor of men in long-term treatment for cancer with cytotoxic agents (Brown, 1985).

What is carcinogenic for man?

The most astonishing thing about carcinogens is how very few substances are known *for certain* to cause cancer in man. This situation has two origins: (a) the great difficulty in obtaining definite human figures and (b) the relatively efficient human repair system (p. 288) as a result of which there can be fewer figures to obtain than, say, with rodents. The most reliable pronouncements about what is carcinogenic in man are usually considered to be those of the International Agency for Research on Cancer (IARC), situated at Lyon in France, which, as the relevant arm of the World Health Organization, is steadily occupied with sifting the evidence. Up to 1982 they had examined 585 substances suspected of evoking cancer in human beings. Of these only 147 were found carcinogenic in experimental animals and of these 147 substances only 44 presented any evidence that they might cause cancer in man*.

In making this survey important evidence was obtained by analysing the health records of factory workers. For example those engaged in manufacturing benzidine (4,4′-diaminobiphenyl) which is a dyestuff intermediate, had 25% extra incidence of bladder cancer after 15 years' exposure and 75% excess after 20 years. The manufacture of benzidine is now illegal in many industrialized countries whereas others (such as Yugoslavia, Korea and Taiwan) still make it and convert it to dyes for which there is no satisfactory equivalent, such as Direct Black 38 (IARC, 1982). These dyes are often imported by benzidine-banning countries, an apparent example of NIMBY (p. 228). However this is not all plain sailing. Black dyes need to be applied to fabrics in very high concentrations, often 10% w/w of the fabric. Dyers exposed to both the dust and splashes (and even eventual wearers of the garments) constantly absorb minute amounts of these dyes which are quantitatively reduced to benzidine in the body. Hence attempts are currently being made to exclude the use of these dyes (Anon., 1985e).

In another example of IARC's work it was established that those exposed to 100 ppm of benzene in the air of their factory, for a working lifetime, sustained 14–17% excess deaths from leukaemia. The use of benzene as a solvent (e.g. for rubber) is now widely banned. However benzene remains an essential building block in the synthesis of many indispensable drugs and other highly useful substances. Hence its manufacture and use is tolerated but only under carefully monitored conditions.

The 1982 IARC list of substances carcinogenic in man which has, in spite of continuing investigations, received no addition since that time goes as follows:

1. *Inorganic materials*: arsenic, asbestos (principally blue asbestos), cadmium, chromates, haematite (one of the mineral forms of ferric oxide);
2. *Organic intermediates*: 2-naphthylamine, 4-aminobiphenyl, benzene, benzidine, and vinyl chloride (through its metabolite, chloroethylene oxide);
3. *Drugs used in the treatment of cancer*: chlorambucil, cyclophosphamide, melphelan, and diethylstilbestrol; and chlormethine when used with vincristine, procarbazine and prednisone in the so-called MOPP regime; also the immunosuppressant drug, azathioprene;
4. *Cancer-inducing occupations*: woodwork, particularly furniture manufacture, making and repairing shoes, manufacturing rubber, the refinement of nickel (apparently from nickel carbonyl), the manufacture of benzaldehyde by chlorinating toluene (but other methods are harmless), and any trade that brings the worker into contact with soot, tar or crude oils (IARC, 1982).

Members of the public are similarly at risk if they smoke cigarettes, chew

---

* IARC regularly prints an invitation to anyone who is aware of data that may alter current evaluations of carcinogenic risk to humans to get in touch with the Unit of Carcinogen Identification and Evaluation, Division of Environmental Carcinogenesis, International Agency for Research on Cancer, 69372 Lyon Cedex 08, France.

tobacco or take snuff (IARC, 1985), or eat food contaminated with aflatoxin (p. 267). Soldiers are at risk of contracting cancer from mustard gas in areas where it is in use (p. 218). Those being treated with the anticancer drugs listed above under 3. are at minimal risk because timing and dosage are carefully controlled, but these substances have to be handled carefully in manufacture and when being dispensed in hospital pharmacies.

No evidence could be found to place the following items on the IARC carcinogenic list, although each one has been subjected to adverse publicity in the news media: caffeine, saccharin, sodium and calcium cyclamates and formaldehyde (IARC, 1982). In each case an animal model acquired cancer but at an inappropriately high dose or because of a metabolic pathway completely different from the human one. It is interesting to compare this list with one issued in 1974 by the US Occupational Safety and Health Administration (OSHA) which restricted the hours and concentrations of exposure of factory and laboratory workers to the following 14 animal carcinogens: 2-acetamidofluorene, 4-aminobiphenyl, 4-nitrobiphenyl, 3,3'-dichlorobenzidine, benzidine, 1- and 2-naphthylamines, 4-dimethylaminoazobenzene, methyl chloromethyl ether, bis(chloromethyl)ether, N-nitrosodimethylamine, 4,4'-methylene-bis(2-chloroaniline), β-propiolactone and ethylenimine. OSHA added that it knew of about 2000 substances which at least one test had indicated to be 'suspect carcinogens' out of the 50 000 or more chemicals currently used in industry (about 1000 more are brought into use every year). OHSA stated its intention to add to its 1974 list, at intervals.

This section will conclude with references to the carcinogenic status of several substances that have been subjects of public debate within living memory.

(a) *Caffeine.* Caffeine has been accused of eliciting cancer in the pancreas, kidney and lower urinary tract but there is no evidence that caffeine is related to development of cancer in man (Rall, 1985; Armstrong, 1976; Jick and Dinan, 1981) nor is it mutagenic in mammals (Rall, 1985). See Section 5.3 for lack of mutagenicity.

(b) *Saccharin.* The reputed carcinogenic properties of this artificial sweetener were dealt with on p. 87. It remains only to add that 6000 diabetics, identified by the British Diabetic Association, who had a high daily intake of saccharin over many years, showed no increased incidence of cancer of the bladder, which is the organ affected in rats given unrealistically high doses of saccharin (Armstrong, *et al.*, 1976).

(c) *Butter yellow.* Butter yellow (synthetic 4-dimethylaminoazobenzene) ceased to be used for colouring margarine after Kinosita (1937) showed that it was a powerful hepatic carcinogen in the rat. However it was not carcinogenic in any other experimental animal and seems to have done no harm to man. The current position is that some countries do not need their margarine to be coloured because they feed little hay to their cows and hence are used to pale butter whereas farmers in yellow-butter countries exert lobbying to prevent margarine being coloured (an effort more successful in some countries than in others), while yellow-margarine countries generally use natural carotene.

(*d*) *Tannins.* Tannins are a class of astringent-tasting substances of diverse chemical composition that occur widely in foods, including nuts and the caffeinaceous beverages. The International Agency for Research on Cancer's working party on tannins could find no data suggestive of a carcinogenic effect in man (IARC, 1976). Injection of tannic acid into rats produces liver cancer but primary hepatoma is most uncommon in industrialized countries where so much caffeine-rich beverages are drunk. The high incidence of small intestine carcinoma in New Zealand sheep may be correlated with the high tannin content of their forage (Ferguson, *et al.*, 1985).

(*e*) *Oestrogenic hormones – the pill.* Before discussing artificial oestrogens it is necessary to emphasize the strong carcinogenic effect of the principal female hormone estradiol (*12.2*). To the layman it is highly disturbing to learn of the many injurious substances that the human body manufacturers, from simple chemicals like hydrochloric and hypochlorous acids, carbon monoxide and hydrogen cyanide, to large molecules like the proteases and other hydrolytic enzymes in lysosomes which, by digesting some restraining cells, enable the body to grow. All of these potent substances act in the interests of our health, provided that they are secreted in the right place at the right time, and in the right microdoses. These limitations apply also to estradiol.

After menopause most women experience a whole battery of highly unpleasant symptoms which medication with an oestrogen relieves. However this treatment brings an increased risk of endometrial carcinoma which varies from 5- to 15-fold, depending on the dose and the duration of treatment (Murad and Haynes, 1985). About two out of three cases of breast cancer are estradiol-dependent; often the main source of this hormone is the tumour itself! Such cases improve when an anti-oestrogen such as tamoxifen (*13.9*) is administered. Paradoxically a smaller proportion of breast cancers are not oestrogen-dependent and actually regress when oestrogens are given.

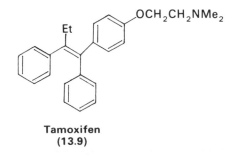

Tamoxifen
(13.9)

Because estradiol is inactive when given by mouth prolonged oestrogen treatment requires the orally-active diethylstilbestrol (*12.1*) or ethinylestradiol. Since 1971, there have been reports of a small increase (0.01–0.1%) in vaginal and cervical adenocarcinoma in the daughters of women who had been given one of these oestrogens during the first trimester of pregnancy. It has been agreed that patients should not be given any form of oestrogen during pregnancy, particularly during the first trimester – a time when the foetal reproductive tract is developing (Murad and Haynes, 1985).

Turning now to oral contraceptives; provisional studies, published in 1983, suggested that their use by those under 25 increased risk of breast and endometrial carcinomas. Fortunately this has turned out not to be the case generally. The Cancer and Steroid Hormones study (CASH) of the Centers for Disease Control, Atlanta, Georgia examined 4700 cases of breast cancer and as many controls. It found no association between this form of cancer and use of the Pill (Stadel, 1985). The 1985 study of the Royal College of General Practitioners on 23 000 oral contraceptive users showed a slight rise in cervical cancer. The study recommended that women taking the Pill regularly should have an annual smear test to detect any change in the cervix of the womb before malignancy sets in. The same study showed that a woman who takes the Pill regularly has a lessened risk of acquiring endometrial and ovarian cancers.

(*f*) *Formaldehyde.* A four year study by the National Cancer Institute of 26 561 workers in the 10 sites that had the longest history of making or using formaldehyde (pathologists, embalmers) reported an 'overwhelming negative' for carcinogenesis (Anon., 1986a). (See also p. 246 and the book by Turoski (1985)).

(*g*) *Hair dyes.* The familiar two-bottle type consists of *p*-phenylenediamine (or a derivative) which is oxidized on the hair with hydrogen peroxide together with *m*-aminophenol, resorcinol or *m*-phenylenediamine (or a derivative). These choices offer a wide range of shades. Following the US National Cancer Institute's 1979 report that 4-methoxy-*m*-phenylenediamine was carcinogenic in laboratory animals, this coupler was dropped by the industry. A range of tones can still be offered which are generally regarded as safe. Lead acetate and henna leaves (principal constituent 2-hydroxy-1,4-naphthoquinone) are also used as toning accessories by the public. Data gathered from 120 557 married registered nurses (all female) in the USA showed no evidence of a carcinogenic risk during the 20 or more years that followed first regular use of hair dyes (Hennekens, 1979).

(*h*) *Vinyl chloride.* Vinyl chloride (*13.10*) is a colourless gas and the raw material for making polyvinylchloride (PVC) which is one of the most used of all plastics. The polymer is sold as clear foil (food wrap), bottles, buckets, bins, raincoats, floor tiles and the soles of sports shoes, to mention only a few of its uses. Hence it was disconcerting when the Italian scientist, C. Maltoni reported in the early

1970s that a tumour was present in some of those who worked with vinyl chloride (Maltoni, 1977; Haley, 1975). Although only a minute proportion of the work-force was affected, the tumour was of such an unusual nature (angiosarcoma of the liver) that it could be attributed only to the vinyl chloride. This discovery led to a survey of 10 173 people in 37 USA plants who had either worked at making vinyl chloride or polymerizing it. The results showed that workers with even a high exposure to vinyl chloride did not tend to die earlier than the control population, nor were they more likely to die of cancer. However such cancers as they did contract were more apt to be localized in the liver or brain than was the case in the controls (Rawls, 1980). Clearly, vinyl chloride causes a rare type of cancer to which only a small fraction of people are susceptible.

Legislation was promptly introduced in the USA to limit the concentration of vinyl chloride in factory air and emissions, to reject any PVC that had bubbles of unpolymerized gas and to ban its use as a propellant in pressure packs. Work with rodents indicated that the mixed function oxidases of the liver converted vinyl chloride to chloroethylene oxide (*13.11*), seemingly the true carcinogen.

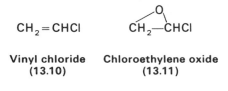

$$CH_2=CHCl \qquad CH_2\!-\!CHCl$$

Vinyl chloride   **Chloroethylene oxide**
(13.10)   **(13.11)**

(*i*) *Tobacco.* Tobacco was brought to Europe from the West Indies at the end of the fifteenth century; in the next century the smoking of this herb spread as far as European trading reached. The active principle, nicotine, was isolated by Posselt and Reimann in 1828, but smokers still preferred the leaves. About 3800 compounds are generated when tobacco is burnt. Some 50 of these elicit cancer in experimental animals. The components which contribute most to the injurious effects of smoking are nicotine, carbon monoxide and tar (a mixture of polycyclic hydrocarbons). Associated with these in harmfulness are hydrogen cyanide, acrolein, phenols and nitric oxide. Whereas the cardiovascular disease attribut-able to smoking seems mainly to be caused by the nicotine and carbon monoxide, the neoplastic diseases are related to the tar. The principal neoplastic disease is cancer of the lung, but cancers of the bladder, tongue, larynx, oesophagus and pancreas also occur.

Cancer of the lung (small-cell bronchial carcinoma) accounts for half of all male deaths from malignant disease and occurs most often between the ages of 50 and 75 although these age figures are becoming lower as manufacturers switch their advertising to appeal to school children, in order to compensate for decreasing sales to adult males. Cigarette smoking is responsible for most cases and the risk is proportional directly to the amount smoked and the content of tar. The average period of survival, after diagnosis, is usually less than a year.

Fortunately cessation of smoking gradually reduces the risk so that after 15 years of abstinence the ex-smoker's risk is no more than that of a non-smoker. Cigar and pipe smokers are much less subject to cancer than are cigarette smokers. An estimated 120 000 lung cancer deaths due to smoking occur annually in the USA. For further reading see American Cancer Society (1987); Petersdorf, *et al.* (1983, p. 1302); Surgeon General of the USA (1979, 1981).

Tobacco chewing is found in communities in every continent of the world. It produces much cancer of the tongue thanks to a series of *N*-nitroso compounds such as *N*-nitroso*nor*nicotine (*13.12*). These compounds are present in the tobacco but in cigarette smoking they mainly escape in the sidestream whereas in chewing tobacco they can be reinforced by any nitrite present in the saliva (p. 90). For further reading on this practice and on snuff taking see the International Agency for Research on Cancer's monograph (IARC, 1985). For more on the formation and toxicity of nitrosamines see p. 91.

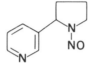

N-Nitroso*nor*nicotine
(13.12)

(*j*) *Asbestos.* In addition to the lung injury (pneumoconiosis) produced by inhaling asbestos dust (pp. 229–230) this fibrous mineral can also produce a rare but fatal type of cancer known as mesothelioma. This tumour becomes evident only after a latent period of 10 to 40 years. It affects only a very small proportion of those who work with asbestos (suggestive of a genetic predisposition) and seems to present no danger to the general population. The US National Cancer Institute estimates that about 970 new cases of epithelioma occur yearly in the USA. In cities, asbestos in the outdoor air arises from remodelling or demolition of buildings and from car brakes. The US National Research Council puts the risk of a person contracting mesothelioma, if exposed for a lifetime to 1 fibre in each 2.5 l of inhaled air, as approximately 9 persons in a million. This figure escalated from 9 to 64 for a cigarette smoker but death would be from small cell lung cancer (NRC, 1984). At the present time many countries are removing any *exposed* asbestos insulation from schools, libraries and offices. For further reading see Zurer (1985).

(*k*) *Food and drink.* The very significant role that heavy eating and over-moderate drinking play in the genesis of cancer was discussed on p. 42, which should be re-read at this stage. It is specially noteworthy that a reduced intake of ethanol is recommended by the (US) National Cancer Institute (1979), the (US)

National Research Council (NRC, 1982) and the American Cancer Society (1982). For further reading see Finley and Schwass (1985). For the possible perils of roasting, toasting and frying see pp. 69–73).

(*l*) *Some unusual correlations.* That there should be 'cancer families' (p. 281) is understandable on genetic grounds. Stranger though is the concept of 'cancer houses'! Houses have been found in Poland from which cases of leukaemia have long been reported. They were found to be damper than control houses, hence carcinogenic fungi were searched for and located (Alexandrowicz and Smyk, 1975). Similar cancer houses have been reported from Texas (Wray and O'Steen, 1975).

Another important factor in the occurrence of carcinogenic mycotoxins is the weather, determining as it does the conditions for growth, for insect attack, and for the initial storage of a crop. In 1977, an early drought in the Southeast of the USA led to an intense attack by the European corn borer on the maize crop. The borer provided transport for *Aspergillus flavus* to develop. This raised the level of aflatoxin B_1 to above the statutory interstate maximum of 20 ppb, for almost the entire crop.

Carcinogens and the community

Almost everyone who lives in a country that has an ageing population has known the grief of seeing relatives or close friends suffer, and even die, from some form of cancer. The high hopes that all cancers could soon be eliminated, much as bacterial diseases were mastered by chemotherapy, prompted massive public support for research funds. If some dissatisfaction is now starting to appear, it could be that the man in the street had expected better prevention, or more cures, to have come out of the intense research efforts of the last thirty years. There is so far only hesitant public enthusiasm for the current and well founded advice that environmental factors (including wholesome food, good drink, enjoyable smoking and plenty of strong sunlight) are potent contributing factors. For the public 'cancer' and 'the good life' are by definition 'poles apart'. How is it that they are not better informed?

The turmoil of the current cancer debate is distributed between several groups of people. First there are the medical scientists whose patient, often frustrating, labours aim to discover important facts relevant to the cancer problem. The discoveries and knowledge of these scientists are freely available, whether by publications or by solicited consultations, to the governmental regulating authorities. The latter, which constitutes our second group, also amass extra information from the many excellent scientists whom they employ. These governmental health authorities also keep informed of what a third group – the manufacturers – are doing in the drug and food industries, and elsewhere where effluents and emissions could lower the quality of air or water. The Government also issues information to the news media and, through special publications, to the public – our fourth and fifth groups, respectively.

The news media, some of them conscientiously informative others callously sensationalist, are often influenced by pressure groups who plead their special causes, often with missionary zeal. One group delights in arousing strong feelings about our daily bread which they claim has become carcinogenic through pesticide contamination and 'chemicals' heedlessly added. Even more powerful advocates are the producers of, for example, special foods, cigarettes or ethanolic beverages, who spare no cost to recommend their product, healthy or otherwise. Slimmers and consumers' unions compete in this advice-giving. Exposed to all of these often contradictory opinions the average person is becoming bewildered. What he/she really needs is a ready source of disinterested information attractively presented.

When called upon to advise the Government on a carcinogenic issue, the scientist becomes conscious of certain limitations when what the Government needs to know so urgently has not yet been discovered. Nor can the scientist even hazard a guess as to when the desired discovery will be made, so delicate is the balance between reason and chance in this field of research. The Government's task, whether in its parliamentary or its administrative sectors, is also a difficult one because it involves those areas of judgment and decision-making where the potential hazards have to be weighed against the likely benefits, whether economic or elector-satisfying. Only too often regulatory decisions have to be made in the absence of sufficient knowledge.

As an example of this dilemma let us compare the different approaches of typical industrialized countries to the question of whether there is a concentration for each carcinogen below which exposed workers will not be harmed. Britain has replied in the affirmative. In 1978 the British Health and Safety Executive proposed a method for determining 'a practical threshold of neoplastic exposure'. However this policy has its own checks and balances and Britain has been foremost in completely banning chemicals whose carcinogenic effects have broken through such reasonable precautions as a completely enclosed plant operated by remote control and a carefully monitored and ventilated workplace (benzidine and 2-naphthylamine received such a ban).

In Germany scientific committees of the Health Ministry believe that there is no safe threshold for a carcinogen. However checks and balances also operate here and their Federal Labour Ministry regularly sets exposure standards for carcinogens, guided by what is economically and technically possible. The French state that they 'combine strict medical monitoring with reporting and personal hygiene requirements'. The United States prefers to introduce early legislation that is open to revision through discussion in the Law Courts. Too strict standards for carcinogens as recommended initially by the Regulatory Agencies have often been watered down after such hearings. Curiously, despite these differences in approach by the different countries the end results are much the same (Brickman, Jasanoff and Ilgen, 1985).

Is there a threshold dose for each carcinogen?

The notion that there may be no threshold sprung from some experiments made by Druckrey and Küpfmüller (1948, 1949). They found the relationship:

$$d \cdot t^n = k$$

where d is the daily dose of a carcinogen (in mg/day), t is the latent period before a tumour becomes palpable, n is a small positive integer and k is a constant. The value of n is obtained from the slope of a linear plot of log d against log t. For the hepatomas produced by butter yellow (4-dimethylaminoazobenzene) in rats, the value of n was 1, and t turned out to be 350 days when the dose was 3 mg/day but 34 days when 30 mg/day was given. The total dose $d \cdot t$ remained a constant with one exception: doses below 1 mg/day gave a lower value of $d \cdot t$. This and related work suggested that chronic administration of very small doses may be more carcinogenic than larger doses given over a shorter period of time.

From these results it has even been suggested that as little as one molecule of a carcinogen could produce cancer in man provided that he lived long enough. However exposure of humans to small amounts of chemical carcinogens is considered relatively safe by many responsible scientists because of (a) the excellent DNA repair system (p. 288) and (b) the detoxification system whose processes of degradation and elimination should not be overtaxed by small doses. Nevertheless the US Government has legislated for 'zero levels' of carcinogens (although this is scarcely possible) whereas Britain regards complete prohibition as a last resort and hence legislates for those low levels of exposure that are considered to be safe. Hence in Britain a substance need not be labelled carcinogenic unless it has been shown to cause human cancer, whereas in the USA positive results from laboratory animals lead to official classification as a carcinogen.

Cancer can also arise from too little of a chemical

The notion that no dose of a carcinogen can be so low that it is no longer capable of eliciting cancer is challenged when we recall cases that are not caused by the presence of a substance but by its absence! A deficiency of *vitamin A* for instance enhances susceptibility to lung cancer in man (Bjelke, 1975). Also treatment with this substance is enough to change pre-cancerous cells to normal cells in experimental animals (Hill and Grubbs, 1982).

Deficiency of *selenium* in the human diet increases the incidence of cancers of the colon, lung, bladder, breast and pancreas, according to surveys in selenium-poor areas of the United States, New Zealand and Venezuela (Schrauzer and White, 1978). For further reading see Milner (1985).

It seems that oesophageal cancer, an untreatable disease, is often associated with a deficiency of *zinc* in the diet (Finley and Schwass, 1985, pp. 164–67). It seems likely, though not yet substantiated, that a substance whose deficiency is associated with cancer normally functions as part of a detoxification system.

The so called 'Delaney Amendment'

This is actually only a clause in the 1958 Food Additive Amendment to the Federal Food, Drug, and Cosmetic Act of 1938 [Title 21 USC 348(c)(3)(A)]. Its relevance to this part of our narrative is that it assumes that there is no safe human dose for a (laboratory) animal carcinogen. Specifically it prohibits the use in foodstuffs of any substance that has been shown to produce cancer in any experimental animal *at any dose*. This clause is still valid in US law, but its application to saccharin was bitterly fought and eventually suspended in view of the exemplary record of this sweetening agent in humans (pp. 82, 295).

Should a useful drug be rejected because of adverse laboratory data?

The decision whether to use such a drug rests on balancing the benefits against the risk of its causing human cancer. An interesting light is thrown on this problem by the antitubercular drug isoniazid. During the late 1950s and early 1960s the US Public Health Service conducted studies on the efficacy of isoniazid in preventing tuberculosis. A total of 25 033 household contacts of known tuberculous patients and 27 924 patients in mental institutions received, at random, either isoniazid or a placebo in a double-blind test (defined on p. xxx). The incidence of tuberculosis was substantially lower in the treated patients. Surveillance was maintained and death certificates reviewed. After the first ten years no difference in death rate from cancer appeared between the treated and the control groups (Ferebee, 1970). After 15 years this result remained unchanged (Goldman, Ingelfinger and Friedman, 1977). However in the meantime it was found that isoniazid is Ames positive and that a dose of 0.5–5.0 mg per mouse daily, produced a 50% increase in pulmonary adenomas. Had the laboratory results come first the drug may never have been used in treating tuberculosis where it continues to occupy a dominant position.

The last-named authors went on to discuss metronidazole (6.7) which was found to behave like isoniazid in laboratory tests in *Salmonella* and *mice*, but only after it had been used for the treatment of human trichomonal vaginitis for many years with great success and no signs of cancer. For this drug though there were no epidemiological data. Treatment requires only a single dose of 2 g and there is no other drug of comparable efficacy (Petersdorf, *et al.* 1983, p. 895).

Conclusion

A wide variety of factors, some of them genetic, hormonal or microbiological, others meteorological, physical (radiation) or chemical, can initiate a complex chain of events that may eventually produce a cancer. This book is concerned only with the chemical factors, whose action is often demonstrably indirect. When evaluating the cancer risk of a traditionally-used chemical, we should try to make a (retrospective)epidemiological analysis. As for new substances it is current practice to start with the Ames mutation test, using the appropriate strain of *Salmonella* both with and without addition of rat liver centrifugate (the S9 fraction). In addition a different type of single cell test needs to be run in parallel to locate some of the mammalian carcinogens that are Ames negative.

It must be kept in mind that the Ames test reports many more mutagens (for *Salmonella*) than can elicit cancer in rodent tests. In particular any molecule with a rigid framework (a single benzene ring often suffices) is likely to trigger the reverse mutation mechanism in this bacterium.

Hence *in vitro* assays must be seen as only indicative of a potential carcinogenicity in a chemical. Each positive result must be followed up *in vivo* to ascertain if this potential is expressed in mammals. A positive result in one mammal needs to be confirmed in a different species, particularly if the test substance is metabolized differently in the first species from what occurs in humans. Because tests on experimental animals are lengthy and expensive some agile decision-making may be required at this stage!

One can be left with a difficult problem when the test substance proves carcinogenic in two or more laboratory animals. However exceptional cases arise; for example no one would deny administration of a promising new drug to a terminally-ill patient. Perhaps we are too prompt to reject low-dose carcinogens when, in the United States alone, half a million human beings die prematurely each year from smoking cigarettes and 25 000 annual deaths are ordained by drivers who have drunk more ethanol than a driver should.

Follow-up

From your own observations, your reading and from discussions with family and friends, what attention do you think is being given to health and lifestyle as contributions to lowering the cancer death toll? Some items to check: eating healthier food, stopping smoking, cutting down on ethanolic drinks, taking more exercise, living at a less stressful pace.

Further reading

Introduction to the Cellular and Molecular Biology of Cancer, Franks and Teich, 1986;
Carcinogens in Industry and the Environment, Sontag, 1981;
Chemical Carcinogens, Searle, 1984, 2 vols;
Chemical Induction of Cancer, Arcus, Argos and Wolf, 1968–1985, 5 vols;
Origins of Human Cancer, Hiatt, Watson and Winsten, 1977, 3 vols;
Cancer, Creasey, 1981;
Carcinogenesis (periodical begun in 1980) IRL Press, Oxford, UK.

13.2 Mood enhancers and drug dependence

From the earliest times humans have sought to enhance their perceived feelings in periods of leisure or celebration. Whether the mood of the group centred on elation or depression, on excitement or tranquillity, there were rituals and customs on hand to enable the mood to be shared by the whole community. When occasion dictated, this goal was accomplished through singing, chanting, laughing or weeping which engendered release of the appropriate hormones or other body chemicals. From history and the work of anthropologists we have learnt how some communities, on special occasions, would enhance the gathering's mood by providing an appropriate foreign substance (like champagne at a wedding to cite a modern instance). Thus the non-medical use of drugs is as old as humanity itself. No doubt there existed individuals who deviated from accepted practices in the timing or quantity of what they chose to consume!

Unfortunately regular use of a mood enhancer can lead to dependence on it. This dependence may vary from a mild desire to repeat the experience even if inappropriately, to an irresistible compulsion that ignores all social and medical consequences. Progressive intensification of the drive to consume pushes the consumer more and more into solitary rather than group indulgence, and his dependence becomes further reinforced by the lack of conventional group restraints. When deprived of his regular intake the habitual drug consumer feels miserable and his mind is preoccupied with procuring the next supply.

Dependence on a drug is no matter for concern if the substance has a low toxicity. The worldwide dependence on tea, coffee and other caffeinaceous beverages can be seen as a civilizing influence, by promoting social cohesion, and affording agreeable hours of companionship at little, if any, cost to health. Such drinks abolish fatigue (though at the expense of creating it later), maintain wakefulness and create good cheer, all from the intake of 100–150 mg of caffeine in a cup of coffee. Yet drinking too many cups of it leads to tremor and insomnia and a still greater excess produces cardiac arrhythmia and delirium. Most pharmacologists classify caffeine as a typical drug of dependence, physically and psychologically, and the abrupt cessation of intake usually leads to an excruciating headache, experienced often on waking, after two days of abstinence (Shorofsky and Lamm, 1977).

The amazing thing about coffee is that most people stop drinking it when they have had enough! However the minority who abuse it, that is to say who consume it uncontrollably, have attracted much investigation (Gilbert, 1976; Greden, 1981). We are now in a position to review caffeine in its three Paracelsian aspects, as an accompaniment to food (p. 94), as a medicine (p. 165) and now as a poison. If only we could discover how the majority of caffeine enjoyers manage not to consume a damaging excess, we may begin to understand how it is that individuals, so well in control of their early encounters with ethanol or nicotine, become lured down seductive pathways until, swept off their feet, they find themselves uncontrollably entangled in a mesh of dependence.

In general compulsive non-medical use of drugs is detrimental to both the user and society. In common parlance, this way of life is called habituation or addiction – terms too vague to serve scientific use. Thus a person may be habituated to taking a daily vitamin pill and then run for the 7.30 a.m. train. He may implement these habits from Monday to Friday yet cast them aside in the weekend, his precious days of diminished routine. As for addiction, many people are addicted to eating chocolate or watching television. When such occasions offer, their extreme enjoyment is evident; but in between these occasions, life proceeds for them quite differently, yet pleasurably. It is quite otherwise with drug *dependence** which can be recognized by three signs (a) compulsive use, (b) overwhelming involvement with securing supplies and (c) tendency to relapse after withdrawal. Dependence inevitably has a strong psychological basis but most of the mood enhancing drugs confer physical dependence as well. That is to say some process in the normal physiology of the body is so greatly altered that discontinuance of the drug becomes agonizing.

Three decades ago M. H. Seevers, at the University of Michigan, showed that laboratory animals in appropriately furnished cages, quickly learnt to inject themselves with all the human drugs of dependence. Reinforcement (i.e. habituation intensified by rewarding repetition) frequently led rats and monkeys to become so preoccupied with self-injection that hunger, thirst, and the sex drive are neglected (Seevers and Deneau, 1963). Because these animals are clearly not psychopaths it has been argued that drug dependence in humans does not require a pre-existent psychopathic trait. Others point out that depressive illness, anxiety disorders, and antisocial acts are over-represented among alcoholics and those dependent on illegal drugs (Rounsaville, *et al.*, 1982). Yet no personality trait has been recognized that would identify all the various kinds of compulsive drug user. This should not surprise us because the three main mental states (retreat, over-participation, and wild fantasy) achievable through the three main types of mood enhancing drug must appeal to three very different types of people.

Tolerance. Tolerance is a phenomenon often associated with mood-enhancing drugs and has three aspects. Firstly there is metabolic tolerance of the kind elicited by many medicinal drugs; in short the body learns how to destroy the drug, mainly in the liver (pp. 25, 130) so that a higher dose must be taken to get the same effect. This adds to the expense of drug procurement and enhances the risk of poisoning other centres in the body. The second form of tolerance is behavioural, e.g. learning to exercise caution by making a strong mental effort (in reality this is exerted more fitfully than the attempter realizes). Thirdly some drugs evoke pharmacological tolerance, usually through the adaptation of selected cells in the nervous system. These tolerances do not develop in parallel. Many an alcoholic, wishing to obtain a formerly experienced effect on the central nervous system, achieves the effect by increasing the dose to a level which, unfortunately, damages his liver.

---

* Rather awkwardly the person who is dependent has to be called an addict because dependent is an older word with a different meaning (e.g. a wage-earner with a wife and children as dependents).

We should next look briefly at representatives of the different kinds of mood enhancers. Abuse of two that are legal, ethanol and nicotine, constitutes the most serious drug problem of industrialized societies. It is a problem that exists also in developing countries. Even tribal societies, at points where they make contact with more developed countries, find the effects of ethanol utterly dehumanizing.

Illicit drugs, deleterious though they can be, have a much smaller circle of users because (a) they are not subjected to prominent advertising like cigarettes and ethanolic drinks and (b) they are available only surreptitiously and inconveniently, and at an exhorbitant price. Many a victim of extreme dependence on an illicit drug is forced into a life of crime to obtain the money to sustain his drug needs. Such cases attract intense publicity, as do the pursuit and apprehension of the illegal suppliers. Yet health authorities in all the affected countries maintain that the total cost of illicit drug use, to families and to the community, falls far short of what smoking and excess drinking impose. One hears much argument about the wisdom of legalizing, or at least decriminalizing, the drugs that are currently illicit. Those in favour assert that a great social benefit would be the disapperance of the criminal network of procurement and supply. Those against argue that legal relaxation would bring about a vast increase in drug use through the various pleasures being as widely advertised, and as compellingly, as are cigarettes and alcoholic drinks. Governments aiming to limit consumption by taxation, would intensify the dilemma in which cigarettes and ethanolic beverages already hold them (p. 277).

For further reading, see Goldstein, Aronow and Kalman (1974); Crossland (1979); Jaffe (1985).

Ethanol

Ethanol exhibits all three aspects of the Paracelsian doctrine. Taken in small amounts, it can be metabolized as a food and often graces the meal table (pp. 25, 93). It also has medical uses (p. 163). In this Section we come to the third aspect – that of ethanol as a poison.

A great many people consume ethanolic drinks when in the company of friends, particularly on convivial occasions. Such social drinking, although completely forbidden by several religions (notably the Moslem, Mormon and Seventh Day Adventist faiths) has little adverse effect on physical health when practised in moderation, say within the range of 1–6 drinks* a day for a man, or 1 to 4 for a woman (based on average body weight).

Comfortably adapted to their habit such social drinkers are exposed to two hazards. Firstly they may be tempted from time to time to go on a spreee, social or solitary, and secondly they may become dependent on ethanol. Let us look at these two phenomena in that order:

---

* The familiar unit of 'one drink' usually means 10 g of ethanol. For the strengths of the various ethanolic beverages, in various countries see p. 26.

(a) *The spree.* This lasts for several hours during which time a great deal of ethanol (up to 500 g) is consumed with very little food to accompany it. Manifestations of gross ethanolic intoxication appear while the liver is trying hard to remove the ethanol but cannot exceed the inadequate hourly rate of about 100 mg per kg body weight. In fact the blood is unlikely to be clear of ethanol until two days later. Then, provided that the subject has not driven a car or become otherwise involved with the police, or developed the acute gastric erosion to which many are subject under these circumstances, he/she may be little the worse for the episode. Many people never repeat it, others do so infrequently and their health and nutrition remain sound. However if the spree is repeated each weekend, which some find a tempting pattern, there is risk of developing pancreatitis, a painful and often terminal condition (Davidson and Passmore, 1986).

A few words on the distribution and fate of ethanol may be helpful. It is rapidly absorbed, unchanged, from the stomach and gut, and it diffuses to all the organs and fluids of the body. About 90% of it is eliminated by slow oxidation to carbon dioxide and the rest is excreted in the urine, sweat and breath. The principal metabolizing enzyme is liver alcohol dehydrogenase (LAD) in the cell sap of the hepatocyte; the enzyme requires NAD (*3.5a*) as a cofactor. This oxidation to acetaldehyde proceeds under zero order kinetics at the slow rate of 10–25 mg per 100 ml of blood per hour. This reaction is the bottleneck of the oxidation because conversion of acetaldehyde to the acetyl residue (*3.9*) by mitochondrial aldehyde dehydrogenase is rapid, as are the incorporation of this residue into acetylcoenzyme-A and the final oxidation to carbon dioxide. One may ask why the performance of LAD is so feeble. Although human metabolism is much concerned with substances that have only two or three carbon atoms, ethanol is not among them. The normal function of LAD seems to be to protect us from the faintest trace of ethanol by dealing with the minute amounts absorbed from any stray yeasts in the gut. The presence of LAD in most mammals suggests that this scavenging had an evolutionary advantage (Hathway, 1984, pp. 164, 181). The ethanol-dependent person has an extra pathway for losing ethanol, for his continual exposure to it induces another oxidase in the endoplasmic reticulum (p. 130) of the liver.

We resume the narrative of the non-dependent imbiber by giving some attention to the effects on the central nervous system. Even in small doses ethanol impairs the judgment and inhibits the skills necessary to make fine movements. The prevailing euphoria usually prevents the subject noticing these losses. That is why ethanol is especially dangerous for the motorist even in small amounts. On the scale compiled by Miles, at the level of 30 mg/100 ml of blood (0.03%) there is mild euphoria, at 50 mg/100 ml a mild incoordination. At 100 mg/100 ml the subject finds it hard to walk, whereas at 200 mg/100 ml confusion and drowsiness sets in. At 300 mg/100 ml the subject is usually in a stupor and at 400 mg/100 ml is likely to be in deep anaesthesia, which may prove fatal (this scale does not apply to the dependent individual). All of these effects, including the initial rapid flow of ideas, garrulousness and even any aggressiveness are due to inhibition (never stimulation) of various parts of the brain.

(b) *Dependence.* To become dependent on ethanol, that is to become an alcoholic, is a much more serious matter than coping with the occasional spree. An alcoholic is defined as *someone who cannot stop drinking when there is every reason for him to do so.* In the range of 6–12 drinks a day for a man and 4–8 for a woman there is a high risk of incurring physical, mental and social problems. More than 12 drinks a day bring definite physical and mental damage coupled usually with severe social problems. Established alcoholics if they can afford it often consume a bottle of spirits every day. In addition to their faster than normal oxidation of ethanol (see above) alcoholics have usually developed some CNS tolerance so that they seldom show signs of severe intoxication. Yet they are far from sober for their reactions are capricious and their judgments far from trustworthy. Moreover in spite of their acquired tolerances there is no elevation of the lethal dose. For most alcoholics family life and personal relations deteriorate when those tracts of the brain that keep these links warm, human and harmonious become damaged. Many alcoholics remain astute enough to keep their employment in spite of the steady decline in competence.

Despite their ruddy, healthy appearance, alcoholics suffer badly from digestive and neurological illnesses. They tend to develop a chronic gastritis and hence have a poor appetite. This leads to malnutrition characterized by deficiency of folic acid, thiamine, nicotinic acid, pyridoxin, vitamin B_{12}, potassium, zinc and magnesium [see Russell (1980) for ethanol-induced loss of zinc leading to increased cancer liability]. The incidence of peptic ulcer is exceptionally high in alcoholics and many such patients vomit blood. Drinkers admitted to hospital following a period of prolonged drinking almost invariably show a (reversible) enlargement of the liver (alcoholic fatty hepatitis). About 8% of alcoholics go on from there to develop a permanent liver damage (cirrhosis) which results from an attempt by fibrous tissue to repair normal lobular tissue that has been eroded away. Pancreatitis occurring as an often fatal abdominal catastrophe is the next most frequent ailment. Many neurological symptoms also are evoked by the abuse of ethanol. Of these, coma is the most serious and is always treated as a medical emergency to forestall extinction of breathing. Haemodialysis can save such a threatened life.

(c) *Abstinence (withdrawal) symptoms.* These characterize the over-frequent spree drinker and (even more) the alcoholic whose way of life has impoverished him so that he can no longer afford to buy his daily supplies. Abstinence symptoms comprise the tremulous, the hallucinatory, the epileptiform and the delirious states (Victor and Adams, 1953, 1983). The tremors can be so violent that the patient cannot stand without help, nor can he speak clearly nor even feed himself. The tremors may subside within a few days but two weeks usually pass before the patient can sleep undisturbed. Nightmarish hallucinations occur in about one quarter of the tremulous patients. In one form the hallucinations are purely auditory; the voices come from a distance but are very clear and terrifying. Another type of withdrawal symptoms take the form of epileptiform seizures. The most serious of all withdrawal symptoms is the *delirium tremens*, characterized by profound confusion, delusions, agitation and hallucinations. In most cases it ends abruptly, about three days after it begins, but about 5% of these cases collapse and die.

Most withdrawal symptoms (but not delirium tremens) are accompanied by a drop in serum magnesium levels and a rise in arterial pH (an alkalosis) – two factors that evoke hyperexcitability of the CNS. The aim of treatment of withdrawal symptoms is to blunt agitation and ensure rest. This is best done by administering paraldehyde or a benzodiazepine sedative such as diazepam (Gessner, 1979).

Apart from their digestive and neurological symptoms, alcoholics are vulnerable to myopathy affecting both skeletal muscles and the heart. Mothers who drink much ethanol throughout pregnancy give birth to microencephalic children who often have other deformities. The early mortality is about 17% but the children who survive usually fail to grow normally and are mentally retarded (Clarren and Smith, 1978).

(*d*) *Treating alcoholism.* The only successful treatment for alcoholism requires total abstinence for life, in spite of some random claims to the contrary. If the patient has a will to recover, three things help: an understanding physician (who need not be a specialist), the use of disulfuram ('Antabuse') (which allows nauseating acetaldehyde to build up) and membership of Alcoholics Anonymous (AA) (Jaffe, 1985). Alcoholism seems to have a genetic factor in its makeup being 4–5 times more frequent in the offspring of alcoholic parents (Goodwin, 1976).

In recent times most of the industrialized countries have legislated to give alcoholism the status of a disease instead of (as formerly) a crime. Treatment however is expensive and relapses frequent, so that each country is finding its medical resources strained by this behavioural problem.

In 1970 the USA passed a law called the Comprehensive Alcohol Abuse and Alcoholism Prevention, Treatment and Rehabilitation Act and created the National Institute on Alcohol Abuse and Alcoholism (NIAAA). The latter was brought into being in order to devise and administer all Federal anti-alcoholic activities, also to serve as a centre for anti-alcoholic education. It aims to promote better understanding of the alcoholic's problems and to encourage the establishment of programmes to help alcoholic employees in industry.

In most of the United States a driver with a blood alcohol concentration of 0.10% or higher is prosecuted but the World Health Organization recommends a limit of 0.05% because research shows that driving skills start to become impaired at 0.04% for most people. Many European countries impose a penalty if the level is in excess of 0.08% and a stiffer one (usually confiscation of driver's licence) if it exceeds 0.15%.

(e) *Ethanol and cancer.* Government health departments in several countries have produced statistics that led them to advocate more moderation in drinking ethanol in order to lessen the risk of acquiring cancer (e.g. Swedish National Food Administration, 1981; Canadian Department of Health and Welfare, 1977; US Department of Agriculture, 1980). In their report 'Diet, Nutrition and Cancer', the US National Academy of Sciences draws attention to an excess of rectal cancer in heavy beer drinkers and notes that cigarette smoking acts in synergy with ethanol drinking to increase cases of cancer of the mouth and oesophagus (NAS, 1982). For a correlation of cancer with loss of zinc from the body see p. 302.

(f) *Developing countries.* Developing countries which are traditionally rather low consumers of ethanolic drinks are currently experiencing a sharp increase in the production and drinking of these beverages. With this trend has arisen an increase in ethanol-related social problems. Several of these countries are obtaining help from the World Health Organization to develop alcohol policies and programmes within the context of national health planning (Walsh and Grant, 1984). For further reading, see Victor and Adams, 1983; Jaffe, 1985.

Nicotine

Introductory observations on tobacco, leading to a discussion of its carcinogenic properties, have already been made (pp. 298–99). It remains to review other aspects of this warm climate crop. The adverse effects of smoking derive more strongly from cigarettes than from pipes or cigars because of the higher temperatures reached in cigarette smoking, the shorter pathway of the fumes into the body and the more widespread custom of deep inhalation.

That it is the nicotine (*8.24*) in tobacco which conveys most of the pleasure of smoking and confers dependence became evident when it was found that intravenous injection of nicotine abolishes (temporarily) the longing for tobacco experienced by heavy smokers deprived of their cigarettes. Similarly the use of nicotine-impregnated chewing gum (available on medical prescription) also reproduces these mood enhancing effects. Most of what is known of the pharmacological action of nicotine has to do with its action on the peripheral autonomic system, whereas its powerful effect on the central nervous system has proved more difficult to elucidate.

As absorbed by the average smoker, nicotine elicits an *alerting* pattern in electroencephalography. In contrast, the electromyography reveals muscular *relaxation*. Studies on laboratory animals indicate that nicotine stimulates the brain to release the catecholamines, particularly dopamine and norepinephrine.

Also, according to the dose, release of acetylcholine may be either inhibited or increased. Nicotine appears to facilitate recollection and reduce aggression (Jaffe and Jarvik, 1978). In the human body nicotine is metabolized to cotinine by replacement of two hydrogen atoms in the pyrrolidine ring by one oxygen atom. This product has few cardiovascular or subjective effects and because of its slow clearance ($t_{0.5}$ 19 h) is a better measure of overall intake than that of nicotine itself ($t_{0.5}$ about 2 h) (Benowitz, et al., 1983).

Upon taking up cigarette smoking the beginner soon learns to operate it in a biphasic manner as follows. To stimulate mental activity he smokes slowly; whereas to reduce nervous tension he makes large deep inhalations or takes several sharp puffs. The latter choice decreases cortical activity, apparently through decreasing acetylcholine output (Armitage, Hall and Morrison, 1968). These authors point out that the smoker has finger-tip control on how much nicotine he transfers instantly to his brain.

This skill as a titrator of nicotine is shown in another context, by the smoker's ready adjustment to the nicotine content of various cigarettes. When offered some with a higher or lower nicotine content than that he is used to, the smoker, after the first puff, adjusts his smoking pattern and the number of cigarettes smoked so as to reproduce his usual dosage of nicotine. The effect of the introduction of 'low nicotine and low tar' cigarettes has been unfortunate, for smokers smoke more of them and get more carbon monoxide than formerly but not any less nicotine or tar (Ebert, et al., 1983; Benowitz and Jacob, 1984).

(a) *Morbidity and mortality.* The smoking of tobacco continues to be described as the largest preventable cause of death in the industrialized countries. For smokers the mortality ratio is 1.7 compared to non-smokers. Cardiovascular disease, which is related to both the nicotine and the carbon monoxide intake, shows as coronary artery disease, cerebrovascular disease (including stroke) and peripheral vascular disease, all of which tend to terminate in premature death. Impairment of respiration is found in young adults after only a few years of smoking and often leads to chronic bronchitis or emphysema. Peptic ulcers are more prevalent in smokers, both male and female, than in non-smokers, and cause more deaths from perforation.

In women smoking leads to an increased incidence of abortions, and it significantly lowers the weight of the new-born as well as increasing the likelihood of their sudden death. Smokers sleep less well than non-smokers and on the whole are more subject to anxiety and depression. The social cost of cigarette smoking is illustrated by some recent figures: in 1984, 81% of the deaths caused by the use of drugs were attributable to tobacco, 16% to ethanol but only 1% to heroin and other opiates. For example about 340 000 US citizens die prematurely each year from smoking-related diseases; treatment costs the nation about $40 billion annually (stated in 1986 by the US Surgeon General, C. E. Koop).

(*b*) *Passive smoking*. Everywhere, indoor atmospheres contaminated by tobacco smoke are inhaled involuntarily by non-smokers. Most of this contamination arises from what is called sidestream smoke which the cigarette distils while smouldering anaerobically between puffs. This effluent is particularly strong in nitrosamines, 2-naphthylamine and 4-aminobiphenyl, all established as human carcinogens. Sir Richard Doll, doyen of medical statisticians, observed (when addressing the 14th International Union against Cancer in 1986) that there is an increased rate of cancer among the non-smoking wives of husbands who smoke in bed.

(*c*) *Cessation of smoking*. This is something that many victims find extraordinarily difficult. Steadily reducing the number of cigarettes smoked seldom works and immediate complete cessation is advised by the many community programmes available. Prospective epidemiological studies have shown that ten years after quitting, the death rate of those who had smoked more than 20 cigarettes a day decreased by about two thirds, while the death rate of those who had smoked less approximated to that of non-smokers. For further reading: see Jaffe, 1985; Holbrook, 1983.

Depressants of the central nervous system

The first central nervous system depressants (used as sedatives and hypnotics) were chloral hydrate (*13.13*) (introduced in 1869) and paraldehyde (*13.14*) (introduced in 1882). Oddly named though they now seem to be these two sturdy pioneers have an excellent safety record and seldom induced dependence. They are still used in hospitals particularly for treating abstinence symptoms arising from other CNS depressants. However, private patients greatly dislike these two drugs for their unpleasant taste and for their property of filling the breath with their vile odours. Were it otherwise they would most likely be as favoured items of abuse as most of the more recently discovered CNS depressants. Some clinicians consider those CNS depressants that have anti-anxiety properties as in a distinct class from those used as hypnotics but no such difference has been clearly established. On the other hand those that have, in addition, anti-epileptic properties do form a distinct category.

The first barbiturate (barbital) was introduced in 1903 and other members of this family followed. However in 1959 the benzodiazepines began to replace

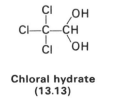

**Chloral hydrate
(13.13)**

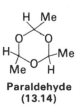

**Paraldehyde
(13.14)**

barbiturates on the grounds of a higher therapeutic index and less tendency to induce dependence. The steps by which a prescribed barbiturate such as pentobarbital (7.13), can so easily set a patient on the road to dependence are detailed on p. 133. The short-acting barbiturates such as amobarbital 'Amytal', pentobarbital ('Nembutal') and secobarbital ('Seconal'), after a long period of widespread use as hypnotics, have been largely replaced in medical practice by benzodiazepines such as diazepam (7.41), chlordiazepoxide, triazolam, temazepam and flurazepam.

The long-acting barbiturate phenobarbital (7.26) is still used in treating epilepsy and is not much abused. It is quite otherwise with the three short-acting barbiturates named above. These have two classes of abusers (a) those who began taking them for a time-limited illness but who are unable to surrender their use and (b) those who began taking them in large doses for mood enhancement, to achieve, in kindred company, a kind of excited, somnolent intoxication not unlike that produced by ethanol. The former are more likely to experience chronic intoxication characterized by sluggish movements, difficulty in thinking, slurring of speech, diminished comprehension and memory, faulty judgments and emotional instability. The latter are more subject to acute intoxication from overdosing during a spree. Both intoxications resemble those encountered with ethanol and are similarly treated. There is, as with ethanol, a third category of addict: the habitual daily user of large doses. Such a person becomes a hospital emergency when (a) he takes a dose in excess of that to which he has built up a tolerance or (b) he can no longer afford his daily dose.

Withdrawal symptoms from the abrupt cessation of chronically taking small doses of a barbiturate include headache, vomiting, rebound insomnia and, if the dose were larger, delusions, delirium and epileptiform fits. Treatment is carried out in hospital as for ethanol 'drying out'.

Many abusers of sedatives have come to prefer the more lipophilic benzodiazepines, particularly diazepam, over the short-acting barbiturates (Griffiths, Bigelow and Liebson, 1983). Other CNS depressants which attract mood enhancers are meprobamate (13.15) ('Miltown') and methaqualone (13.16) ('Quaalude').

Further reading Jaffe (1985); Victor and Adams (1983).

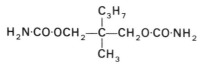

Meprobamate
(13.15)

Methaqualone
(13.16)

Opioids

The term 'opioids' refers to those drugs that have the pharmacological properties typical of morphine: powerfully analgesic, cough-relieving and constipating. Opium, the juice of the poppy *Papaver somniferum*, was already known in the third century BC and its most active principle, morphine *(8.11a)*, was isolated in Germany in 1804 (p. 103). Codeine, a monomethyl ether of morphine, has a similar but milder action and is also present in opium. Diamorphine (synonym: heroin) is the *O,O*-diacetyl derivative of morphine from which it is made in the laboratory. There are many entirely synthetic analgesics that act like morphine although they usually have much simpler molecular structure. These include methadone *(8.12)* and pethidine (meperidine) *(8.13)* both of which induce a morphine-like dependence; related analgesics such as pentazocine ('Talwin') and dextro-propoxyphene ('Darvon') exhibit less of this adverse effect.

(a) Acute poisoning. Acute poisoning by opioids arises from suicidal intent or from miscalculation of the dose when an addict switches from one street-bought product to another which by chance is less adulterated. The victim is usually brought to hospital in a comatose state and exhibits slowed respiration, bradycardia and a body cool to the touch. If untreated, death occurs from respiratory and circulatory failure.

(b) Chronic poisoning. Those who are chronically poisoned experience faintness, loss of apppetite, vomiting and constipation. Treatment of the severely intoxicated calls for artificial respiration, gastric lavage (if medication was oral) and injection of phenylephrine or other pressor amine. If the patient remains unresponsive a specific opioid antagonist is injected intravenously. When the patient eventually regains consciousness, the opioid abstinence syndrome usually appears, with its profuse sweating, weeping, running of the nose and severe abdominal pain, proceeding to extreme restlessness and the appearance of waves of gooseflesh, the skin resembling that of a plucked turkey.

Dupont (1979) estimated the number of opioid addicts in the USA (with its population of 250 million) to be about half a million – a figure that may be compared with the estimated 10 million alcoholics and problem drinkers (Liska, 1986). About 100 000 of these opioid addicts are receiving treatment (65% of them for heroin dependence) in special drug-abuse clinics of which several hundred are available throughout the USA. This treatment alone costs the nation about $10 billion each year.

Dependence as a consequence of medical treatment is uncommon. More usually one addict recruits another into opioid abuse, most often at the age of 17 or 18 (Hughes, *et al.*, 1972). Most addicts have to engage in criminal activities to support this expensive habit. The goal of the opioid abuser is the euphoria, described as a 'high'. The victim quickly discovers a need to increase the dose to obtain the original effect because of quickly developing tolerance. At this stage the drug has to be injected intravenously if that was not done before. Heroin, more lipophilic than morphine, enters the brain faster and produces transient excitement; however it is soon hydrolysed to morphine whose action is thus duplicated.

When increasing tolerance makes it too expensive to inject enough of an opioid to recapture the euphoria, the addict still has to inject a smaller dose to counteract the extremely painful abstinence symptoms described above. These symptoms reach their peak after 2–3 days, then decline gradually. Agonizing as this process is reported to be, death rarely occurs. These physical symptoms of withdrawal are accompanied by a psychological one of intense craving for the drug. Drug-seeking activities become substituted for any other aim and this powerful driving force leads to frequent relapse. Abstinence symptoms from codeine and *d*-propoxyphene, although morphine-like, are much milder. Babies born to mothers who have been using heroin prior to delivery exhibit withdrawal symptoms immediately upon delivery.

(*c*) *The molecular basis for opioid dependence.* The molecular basis for opioid dependence and withdrawal symptoms is still not clear. Levitzki (1986) presents evidence that the primary effect is inhibition of adenylate cyclase, the enzyme that produces cyclic adenosine monophosphate (cAMP) (*13.1*). By the usual rebound phenomenon this enzyme proliferates, which would explain the tolerance (the need to increase dose). After withdrawal of the opioid this overfunctioning enzyme inflicts distress on the patient. These reactions apparently take place on the receptors that exist in the brain, spinal cord and gut and which receive the body's natural opioid regulators, namely the enkephalins and endorphins, all of them polypeptides.

(*d*) *Treatment.* In Britain, State-registered chronic opioid users may obtain heroin for self-administration free of charge. The mortality rate of these patients varies from 2 to 6% a year (Stimson and Oppenheimer, 1982). Alternatively the patient may choose oral medication with methadone. In the United States most treatment for opioid dependence is by oral methadone. This drug is longer-acting than heroin and its withdrawal symptoms are less dramatic. This treatment is not a cure but a substitution of one form of dependence for another. The patient's gain is having a ready source of cost free opioid and freedom from the sorry business of intravenous injections. The patient's loss, if he prefers the insane excitement of a heroin injection, is the steadiness of the euphoria that methadone produces. The State's gain is that many of the methadone-treated patients return to stable employment, also the avoidance of sharing hypodermic needles spreads less infectious disease.

Alternative treatments are available by the use of opioid antagonists such as naltrexone or cyclazocine. The well-known anti-hypotensive drug clonidine (*13.17*) is another effective extinguisher of physical dependence (Charney, *et al.*, 1982). Regrettably only a small proportion of highly motivated patients wish to

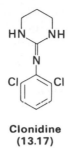

Clonidine
(13.17)

lose their opioid dependence. Apart from these drug treatments all patients require psychological help in readjustment to living and working in the community.

(e) *The legal regulation of opioids.* Before refrigeration became as widespread as it is today, much 'tainted' (bacterially contaminated) food was eaten and dysentery often resulted. Opium, in various forms, was the standard treatment: it soothed the spasm and stopped the diarrhoea. Whether it was wise to *imprison* toxic germs in the gut was pondered by few. Until about 1940, and in spite of the gathering net of legislation, many preparations of opium and morphine were freely on public sale in pharmacies. For their dysentery most people took drops of chlorodyne, which was an ethanolic solution of morphine, cannabis (!), chloroform, licorice, treacle and peppermint. In time, the cannabis was omitted but not the morphine. Similarly, oncoming fevers were aborted with Dover's Powder (opium, ipecacuanha and lactose). Colds and influenza were treated with paregoric (also called Compound Tincture of Camphor to prettify its opioid nature) which contained opium, camphor, aniseed and benzoic acid. Gee's Linctus, highly esteemed for subduing a severe cough, contained all of these ingredients plus 'the honey of squill.'

The beginning of regulation may be dated from the international conference (1911), held in The Hague, which was called to discuss the uncontrolled abuse of opium throughout the world. The participating nations agreed to introduce restrictive legislation but deliberations were delayed by outbreak of the First World War (1914–1918). One of the earliest countries to act was the USA which introduced what became known as the *Harrison Narcotic Act* (1914), designed to register and tax all who distributed opium, coca leaf and their products. This Act only slowly became the basis for Federal prosecution of smugglers, peddlers and addicts. A parallel may be seen in the US legislation against the manufacture and consumption of ethanol, introduced (as 'Prohibition') in 1919 but repealed in 1933. However legislation against opioids and other 'narcotics'* was intensified

---

* In scientific usage a narcotic is a down-regulator of cell metabolism, acting through the nervous system. As adopted by the Law (and thence the public) the word has lost its defined meaning and has become synonymous with 'illegal drug'.

stepwise. In 1924 US Federal Law banned heroin, even from being prescribed by a registered medical practitioner. Then in 1970 the Comprehensive Drug Abuse Prevention and Control Act (usually briefly called the 'Controlled Substances Act') was introduced to list and control five Schedules of drugs assigned in accordance to their perceived degree of promoting dependence. The drugs in Schedule 1 were never to be used, even in medical practice; inclusion in lower Schedules brought increasing degrees of freedom in prescribing.

In Britain the 1968 Drug Addiction Act was introduced to limit issue of heroin and cocaine to named physicians working in designated treatment centres.

For further reading on opiates, see Victor and Adams, 1983; Jaffe, 1985.

Stimulants of the central nervous system

In the foregoing we reviewed three types of mood enhancing agents that are fundamentally depressants, even though they can provide transient excitement by depressing a control centre. The true stimulants, which we should now consider, act quite differently, namely by releasing a cerebral neurotransmitter, dopamine (*7.33a*). (Caffeine, a stimulant which acts by blocking the adenosine receptor in the brain, was discussed on p. 305.) Whereas the CNS depressants evoke a lethargic (if fitfully animated) mood, the CNS stimulants provide an alert one, and the individual seems to be purposefully engaged, even if untypically overactive. The often repetitive prattling of the former is replaced by the clear consecutive speech of the latter, the bonhomie by cool detachment.

Pharmacologists were surprised to find that two such chemically different substances as amphetamine (*7.24*) and cocaine (*8.16*) should elicit similar actions. Cocaine is extracted from the shrub *Erythroxolon coca* which grows in the Peruvian Andes. It was introduced into medical practice in 1884 as the first local anaesthetic, but was replaced by simplified molecules in which the tendency to produce dependence was reduced more than tenfold. Amphetamine 'Benzedrine' was synthesized as a structural analogue of epinephrine (*8.1b*) and marketed in 1932 as a nasal decongestant; it lacks local anaesthetic properties. Users of amphetamine inhalers soon noticed some mental stimulation; students adopted the inhalers as an aid to concentration. Some truck drivers replaced their comparatively harmless caffeine tablets by amphetamine ones, as an aid to keeping awake during their long and tedious journeys.

(*a*) *Amphetamine (7.24)*. This was first used as the racemate but was later made available as the *d*-stereoisomer (dextramphetamine) which carries most of the pharmacological activity. The *N*-methyl derivative, methamphetamine, has essentially similar properties. The anorectic (appetite-diminishing) effect of amphetamine led to its being prescribed for obesity but as this use often led the hapless patient into dependence it has been replaced by fenfluramine (*8.15*) or phenylpropanolamine. In most countries the use of the amphetamines is illegal except for the treatment of narcolepsy, a rare disease. However they are available in most industrialized countries as a result of illegal synthesis. The users receive a strong impression of an increased mental and physical drive and competence, whereas onlookers see only excitability, irritability and restlessness.

Those who use amphetamines intravenously experience euphoria that is particularly powerful at the moment of injection; they also acquire mental alertness and an illusion of increased physical strength. These people feel little need for either food or sleep, thus incurring physiological debts that must be repaid later.

(*b*) *Cocaine.* Cocaine is usually insufflated up the nostrils as a snuff which may consist of a salt alone, or mixed with sodium bicarbonate to liberate the base for an intenser effect. The ensuing euphoria lasts only a few minutes and leads to repetitions at half-hourly intervals. Cocaine is also available as a paste, for smoking, and is sometimes injected intravenously to obtain a more vivid euphoria, though one of brief duration. When patients accustomed to the intravenous use of cocaine (16 mg) were given *d*-amphetamine (10 mg) similarly, they were unable to tell one from the other, so similar are the pharmacological properties (Fischman and Schuster, 1982). Severe dependence, with psychological, physical, and vocational impairment is seen among those who inhale cocaine regularly, and death from respiratory depression and cardiovascular collapse is not uncommon. In general the acute and chronic symptoms of cocaine abuse and dependence closely follow those described above for amphetamines. As the street price of cocaine is usually higher than that of amphetamines the hospitals receive more amphetamine-distressed patients. In Peru, where popular mythology supposes that cocaine could do no harm, the smoking of it is currently producing psychiatric problems, criminal activities and indifference to employment opportunity (Jerí, 1980).

(*c*) *Toxicity.* Adverse effects from CNS sympathetic stimulants, whether amphetamine or cocaine, strike erratically. They can be mild for the beginner and severe for the inveterate user, or the other way around. Acute toxicity in the newly-recruited takes the form of dizziness, irritability, confusion and hallucinations, accompanied by tremor, sweating and cardiac arrhythmia. Death is usually preceded by convulsions and shock. Hospital treatment is with chlorpromazine, to which diazepam is added if the convulsions continue. Continued use of amphetamine produces tolerance. Hence doses have to be increased, both in size and frequency, to reproduce the old effect. At this stage psychiatric symptoms often step in. The subject complains of sensations like insects running under his skin and is apt to pick at his face. Other futile and repetitious movements may follow. He grows suspicious and complains of 'being watched'.

Although small doses of amphetamines do not necessarily lead to dependence, by the time the subject has become dependent he is not easily dissuaded by these toxic symptoms, but tends to inject the drug every two to three hours right around the clock, stopping only when he has become too disorganized to perform the next injection. A deep sleep finally overtakes the emaciated body followed by several days of utter physical exhaustion. Progressive social deterioration occurs and friends who offer good advice are often attacked physically during the paranoid delusional episodes. Hospitalization consists of treatment with dopamine antagonists (e.g. haloperidol); acidification of the urine helps to excrete the load of amphetamine (Angrist, *et al.*, 1974). The psychotic episodes clear up in about three weeks. If the discharged patient resumes use of amphetamines, permanent brain damage often develops, characterized by microvascular injury in areas rich in dopaminergic neurons, particularly the caudate nucleus (Ellinwood, 1979). The patient is then apt to adopt freakish postures and be easily startled.

(*d*) *Abstinence symptoms.* Sudden withdrawal of amphetamines or of cocaine precipitates unpleasant physical symptoms. Four to eight hours after a single nasal 'snort' of cocaine (96 mg) subjects reported tiredness and loss of energy. After chronic administration of either drug, abrupt withdrawal is followed by craving, and profound physical and mental exhaustion. These symptoms, although highly unpleasant, are not so catastrophic as those that follow withdrawal of opioids but it is surprising that earlier workers overlooked them.

(*e*) *Combinations of drugs.* Those who dislike some of the side-effects of CNS stimulants tend to take these drugs with ethanol, barbiturates or even opiates. These combinations are apt to produce anxiety and severe depression, the mixed pharmacological origins of which can frustrate hospital treatment.

For further reading on CNS stimulatns, see Mendelson and Mello, 1983; Jaffe, 1985.

Cannabis

Hemp (*Cannabis sativa*) has a psychoactive principle known as Δ^9-tetrahydrocannabin-1-ol (THC) (*13.18*), described as Δ^1 in an earlier numbering. This highly lipophilic substance, whose highest concentration is in the flowering tops, has long been known as a distracting agent for painful medical conditions but its use in industrialized countries had faded away by the 1930s. Yet a couple of decades later a fashion for smoking it arose in these countries, particularly among the young. Known for this purpose as marihuana, hashish or pot, it produces striking effects on the central nervous system. The concentration of THC in marihuana may vary from 0.5 to 10%, the higher concentrations often being obtained by adding an extract from normally discarded parts of the plant.

Within 7–15 min from the beginning of smoking a marihuana cigarette (a 'joint'), the subject's plasma concentration of THC reaches its peak, yet neither physiological nor mental effects reach their maxima for 20–30 min (Perez-Reyes, *et al.*, 1982). Because of this delay marihuana smokers cannot titrate their puffing

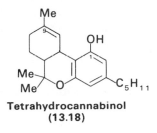

Tetrahydrocannabinol
(13.18)

frequency to obtain the desired level of euphoria whereas tobacco smokers habitually do so. What is at the root of this delay? Does the drug have to penetrate to a particular compartment first (see p. 119 for definition of compartments)? Or does a more active metabolite have first to be formed? The answer is not yet known. True, THC is quickly converted to a metabolite, which is the 11-hydroxy derivative (the new hydroxy group replaces a hydrogen in the 9-methyl group). This metabolite has all the effects of THC but is formed too quickly to explain the puzzling delay.

The subjective effects of smoking marihuana, which last for two or three hours, consist of euphoria and a feeling of relaxation – not unlike what is experienced with ethanol. If alone the subject feels sleepy, whereas in the presence of company there may be laughter but less social involvement than occurs with ethanol. Instead there is a tendency to confuse past, present and future ('temporal dislocation') and the subject often feels that he is outside the self, strange and unreal. Irrelevant ideas and words diversify the sparse conversations.

While under the influence of the drug short term memory is diminished and difficulty is experienced in carrying out those tasks that require attention and quick response to information. For that reason cannabis users are dangerous in motor traffic or when flying planes. This danger persists for 4–8 hours after smoking one or two such cigarettes. Unfortunately this impairment persists long after the pleasant subjective effect of the cigarette has terminated and the smoker is back on the road. The well-known impairment in road-sense produced by ethanol is additive to that induced by marihuana. The connexion with impaired driving is discussed by Reeve (1979) and with automobile fatalities by Sterling-Smith (1976).

(*a*) *Toxicity and tolerance.* Although acute toxic effects are mild in people who see themselves as 'recreational users', namely those who smoke one or two cigarettes once or twice a week, marihuana does precipitate severe emotional disorder in those who bring to it a naturally unstable mind. All users tend to have bloodshot eyes and a racing pulse while smoking but tolerance to the tachycardia develops with time. Because effective marihuana smoking demands deep inhalation and prolonged retention of the smoke, bronchial irritation is a common complaint.

The psychological effects of chronic use resemble those seen with ethanol. The job, family and hobbies progressively lose their interest and more time is devoted to procuring and using the drug. High doses produce hallucinations and paranoid feelings of persecution. The depersonalization and temporal disintegration are accentuated as euphoria yields to panic. Such extreme symptoms affect only a small percentage of marihuana smokers but, because of the prevalence of cannabis use, such psychiatric emergencies are regularly admitted to hospitals.

There is some evidence that links the smoking of marihuana by pregnant women with impairment of foetal development. The many youths of 12 and upwards who smoke marihuana tend to have retarded spermatogenesis and a prolonged period of *Sturm und Drang*, an extension of emotional adolescent behaviour for parents and teachers to endure.

(*b*) *Withdrawal symptoms.* Withdrawal symptoms in cannabis users are comparatively mild. They include tremor, sweating, nausea, irritability and loss of appetite and sleep. Severer and more protracted abstinence symptoms are associated with chronic use of high-potency marihuana. Much that is known is still vague, and even contradictory, about the long-term effects of marihuana use. Studies are continuing.

Many attempts have been made to revive the use of cannabis in legitimate medicine and many analogues of THC have been tried as well. The two most promising fields of use were (a) lowering intra-ocular tension in glaucoma and (b) overcoming nausea in the treatment of cancer with cytotoxic drugs. However nothing more effective than existing remedies was found and most patients disliked those subjective symptoms that marihuana enthusiasts so highly treasure.

Further Reading

Agurell, Dewey and Willette, 1984; Mendelson and Mello, 1983; Jaffe, 1985. Every year the National Institute on Drug Abuse issues the review '*Marijuana and Health*', directed to Congress and printed by the US Government Printing Office, Washington, DC.

Miscellaneous

Psychedelic substances are characterized by their capacity to change perception and feeling in a way that is otherwise experienced only in dreams. The subject has a heightened awareness of what he sees and feels but a diminished control over this input. It is as if one half of the self is passively reviewing what the other half is receiving. Everything perceived in this way is judged by the subject to be of extraordinary interest. A sense of union with mankind, or even with the whole universe, is often experienced.

Most of the psychedelic drugs are either indolealkylamines such as psilocin, dimethyltryptamine (*13.19*) and LSD, or they are phenylalkylamines such as mescaline (*13.20*). It is noteworthy that tryptamine, a natural bodily constituent, has mild properties of this kind, but the omnipresence of monoamine oxidase usually keeps them in abeyance. The peyote cactus (*Lophophora williamsii*) has an active principle, mescaline; the sacred mushroom (*Psilocybe mexicana*) owes its activity to psilocin [the 4-hydroxy-derivative of (*13.19*)] and psilocybin (the phosphate ester of psilocin). Both of these plants were in use in Mexican religious ceremonies at the time of the Spanish conquest.

In 1943 the Swiss chemist Albert Hofmann accidentally discovered lysergic acid diethylamide (LSD) while working on the chemistry of ergot alkaloids (p. 267) to which LSD is chemically related. Later a cult developed for experiencing the so-called mind-expanding properties of psychedelic substances, based largely on the writings of the English novelist, Aldous Huxley (1894–1963). The general results were so dire that by 1970 these drugs came under the same bans as heroin. By that time the medical profession realized that LSD did not, as had been hoped, give information on the workings of the human mind, healthy or insane. LSD and related psychedelic substances act as antagonists on presynaptic receptors for 5-hydroxytryptamine – a neurotransmitter in the midbrain. Chlorpromazine (*7.20*) and haloperidol can be used to block the hallucinogenic effects of LSD and mescaline.

When an average·dose, say $70\mu g$, of LSD is taken orally, sensations of vertigo and weakness precede the euphoria. After about 2 h, visual (but seldom auditory) illusions set in. These have a highly varied character but any human content tends to be mechanized, e.g. a scene where hundreds of people, each one consisting of a triangle of brightly coloured paper, swarm in and out of church. Boundaries between the senses are blurred and time passes slowly. The mood shifts between elation and fear, the latter often giving way to panic. Although the half life of the drug in man is only 3 h, the mental effects do not begin to clear for about 12 h. The experience seems not to have much long-term effect on the subject provided that he does not do something foolish while under the influence such as to fall, as many have, from a tall building, completely unaware of the danger.

LSD is more than 100 times as potent as psilocin and longer acting too. Mescaline acts for about the same length of time as LSD but is about 4000 times less potent. Dimethyltryptamine is only short-acting and is not effective orally. Intravenous tryptamine reproduces many of the effects of LSD but very weakly. LSD is not a drug of dependence and 'acid trips' tend to be separated from one another by many months. The few chronic users tend to complain of impaired memory and they appear strangely passive. The principal adverse effect of psychedelic substances is the 'bad trip', a panic that can last for 24 h. Another unpleasant after-effect is the 'flashback' – a recurrence of the mental effects of the drug without any more of it having been taken (these may recur for several years).

(*a*) *Phencyclidine*. Phencyclidine (*13.21*) is 1-(1-phenylcyclohexyl)piperidine. This substance has legitimate use in wild-game management to stun large

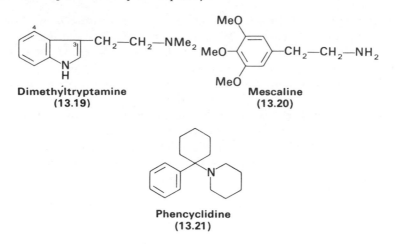

Dimethyltryptamine
(13.19)

Mescaline
(13.20)

Phencyclidine
(13.21)

animals temporarily. In the 1970s children began to steal it from circuses and more was sold illegally on the streets as 'angel dust'. Phencyclidine stimulates parts of the central nervous system while inhibiting other parts. It is hard to think of any other drug that induces so wide a range of subjective effects. An oral dose of 5 mg produces a wild elevation of mood and feelings of detachment from reality. This is accompanied by disorganization of thinking and a distorted perception of the body's image. Along with these effects the subjects report anxiety and disorientation as their most unpleasant feelings. Physical signs include excitement, restlessness, impaired motor coordination, stupor and vomiting. A dose of 10 mg can cause convulsions and grotesque posturing, followed sometimes by a prolonged coma. Although the subjective effects of phencyclidine reach a peak in 4–6 h, the half life in the body is about 3 days. Chronic users have impairment of speech, memory and thinking – effects that may last for a year after withdrawal, or there may be a long-lasting psychotic state. Many deaths have been reported, some arising from sheer toxicity, others from violent behaviour. There is no specific antidote for phencyclidine. Because hospitalized cases tend to exhibit violence towards the staff, Jaffe (1985, p. 567) recommends that four or five strong attendants should be retained nearby.

(b) *Anaesthetics and solvents.* There is hardly a substance with an action on the nervous system that has not been found to enhance mood. For at least half a century before they began to be used as general anaesthetics, both ether and nitrous oxide ('laughing gas') were inhaled for fun at carnivals and 'ether frolics' were a feature of social life in Europe and the United States. In 1841 a young American physician named Crawford Long noted that participants at an ether frolic suffered no pain when they became badly injured through their uninhibited horseplay. It took only five more years for William Morton to establish ether as the world's first general anaesthetic (Crossland, 1970).

In the nineteenth century efforts to reduce alcoholism in Ireland by means of adding ether to ethanolic drink led to the use of ether becoming so favoured that it became necessary to discontinue it. With this background of adult behaviour in mind the current trend of children to inhale solvents ('glue sniffing') seems less surprising (see also p. 258). The psychedelic effect of nutmeg and the deadening mental grip of absinth were referred to on p. 84.

(c) *Testing*. Drug taking has long ceased to be seen as a private indulgence – a matter for the individual alone. There are consequences for relationships within the family, and larger social groups too. Moreover there are the community losses such as the loss of production and the cost of remedial treatment. These are proving formidable. How far dare a modern State go in regulating its citizens' conduct? That will vary from country to country. At the present time even the most freedom-loving nations are reacting against the widespread use of drugs of dependence among their citizens. In addition to the drain on the economy there have been many incidents where human life has been endangered through the use of drugs by individuals responsible for public safety. Some governments are seeing this as an emergency situation.

As one expression of this concern, the United States in 1986 introduced a $900 million programme against the drug abuse that is estimated to cost that country about $60 000 million each year. A significant fraction of the programme is directed to medically testing Civil Servants to ensure, under pain of dismissal, that they do not use illegal drugs, either at work or during their leisure. The larger private enterprises seem willing to support this new order, whereas the American Civil Liberties Union has called it a flagrant violation of the US Constitution.

This is not the place for any debate on that issue but we can look briefly at the means available for testing. Much expertise is available from the US Navy which runs five laboratories to test sailors' urine for barbiturates, opiates, amphetamines, cocaine, marihuana and phencyclidine. (The absence of ethanol from this list must be an oversight?) The method of detection is a series of radioimmunoassays (RIAs) one for each substance; positive results are confirmed by gas chromatography followed by mass spectrography (GCMS). The cost works out at about $13 a test. The Navy launched this programme after a fatal accident on the aircraft carrier Nimitz in 1981. In 1985 this programme led to the discharge of about 30 officers and 6000 enlisted men.

Another type of urine test, considered equally sensitive and reliable, is the EMIT or enzyme-multiplied immunoassay test. Thin layer chromatography is also suitable but requires more skill to operate reliably. Some of the substances are estimated not as such but as their principal metabolite. For cocaine the major metabolite is benzoylecgonine, namely the acid of which cocaine is the methyl ester. The major metabolite of tetrahydrocannabinol (*13.18*) is a substance that has the 9-methyl group of THC changed into a carboxylic acid group. This acid can be found in the urine for about a month after a frequent user of marihuana has stopped smoking it. It is not hard to see how evidence of a discarded lifestyle could tell against an individual unless consideration and understanding inform the final judgment.

For further information on testing programmes for drug abuse see Hanson (1968).

Follow-up

In the context of Section 13.2, gather a small panel of concerned citizens from among your circle of friends to discuss how the scientist's contribution can best fit into this many-facetted social issue. A saying of La Rochefoucauld (1613–1680) may be a useful opener for discussion: 'When we do not find peace within ourselves, it is futile to seek it elsewhere' (Premier Supplément des Maximes, viii).

Appendix I: Lipid/water partition coefficients

A partition coefficient (P) is a measure of the way a substance is distributed, at equilibrium, between two immiscible phases. The lipid/water partition coefficients, much used in drug studies, usually employ octanol for the non-aqueous phase. These coefficients form a record of lipophilicity – the higher the figure the more lipophilic the substance. The relevance of lipophilicity is that it governs the rate of diffusion of a substance through semipermeable membranes, particularly biological membranes of the most frequently encountered 'Type 1' (Section 7.1).

Partition coefficients can conveniently be measured in a 250 ml glass-stoppered centrifuge tube. This is charged with (a) the weighed solute and (b) such proportions of the two solvents as previous runs on analogous solutes may suggest. The tube is usually inverted about 100 times in 5 min, although equilibrium should occur within 2 min. The mixture is then centrifuged, after which either phase can be analysed (e.g. by ultraviolet spectrography) for its content of solute (Leo, Hansch and Elkins, 1971).

Many values for partition coefficients have been collected and discussed by Leo, Hansch and Elkins (1971). An approximate value of P can quickly be calculated by the addition of fragmental constants taken from a Table, but there are some pitfalls (Rekker, 1977).

Table 8.1 listed the partition coefficients of some commonly used hypnotics and general anaesthetics. The partition coefficients of some other types of drugs are listed in Table A1.

Table A1: Partition coefficients (between octanol and water) of some commonly used drugs

Substance (and formula number)	log P
Tetracycline (*9.1*)	−1.47
Adenosine (cf. *3.6*)	−1.10
Sulfadiazine (*8.40*)	−0.13
Sulfanilamide (*6.5*)	−0.83
Caffeine (*5.17*)	−0.07
Sulfamethizole	0.54
Morphine (*8.11a*)	0.76
Ephedrine (*7.22*)	0.93
Prednisolone	1.42
Atropine (*8.27*)	1.79
Benzylpenicillin (*9.31*)	1.83*
Procaine (*8.19*)	1.87
Phenytoin (*8.9*)	2.47
Erythromycin	2.48
Diazepam (*7.41*)	2.82
Progesterone	3.87
Imipramine (*8.18*)	4.62
Chlorpromazine (*7.20*)	5.16

*Corrected for ionization but as this is a strong acid (pK_a 2.8), the effective log P is in the *minus* region. (Leo, Hansch and Elkins, 1971).

Appendix II: On searching the literature

The reader with unanswered queries may find it handy to consult one or more of the following books (for publisher and year see References).

Nutrition: The 8th edition of *Human Nutrition and Dietetics* by Davidson and Passmore.

Biochemistry: The 2nd edition of Stryer's *Biochemistry*. For further detail see Lehninger's *Principles of Biochemistry*.

Medicine: Davidson's *Principles and Practice of Medicine* (14th edition) by Macleod. For a more detailed text see *Harrison's Principles of Internal Medicine* (10th edition) by Petersdorf *et al.*

Drugs: It is best to use the generic name rather than one of the proprietary names. The authentic list of generic names is the World Health Organization's *International Nonproprietary Names (INN)* (6th cumulative list plus annual supplements). Both generic and proprietary names are used in *Martindale's Extra Pharmacopoeia* (28th edition) (Reynolds, 1982) which gives also the full chemical name but no structural formula. Martindale thoroughly covers the uses and side effects (with references to recent literature), also doses. For structural formulae see *The Merck Index* (10th edition). Further chemical information is available in a multivolume work: *Heilbron's Dictionary of Organic Compounds* (5th edition, with supplementary volumes). Heilbron lists the chemical structure (including absolute configuration), also chemical and spectrographic properties of an immense number of organic compounds. For the generic and proprietary names of agrochemicals see the British Crop Protection Council's 'Pesticide Manual'.

A full description of the pharmacological properties of all the most used drugs is available in *Goodman and Gilman's Pharmacological Basis of Therapeutics* (7th edition) by Gilman *et al.* This massive work has full physiological details of the modes of action; many structural formulae are included and doses too. *Burger's Medicinal Chemistry* (4th edition in 3 volumes) places the emphasis on chemistry but the effect on the action brought about by exchanging substituents is given prominence. The 7th edition of *Selective Toxicity*, by Albert, outlines the physical and chemical basis of therapy as seen from the viewpoint of structure-action relations as modified by selectivity.

Quantitative data can be obtained from reference books, for example *Substituent Constants for Correlation Analysis in Chemistry and Biology*, by Hansch and Leo. A selection of ionization constants and full details for determining them is in Albert and Serjeant's book *The Determination of Ionization Constants*. The *Registry of Toxic Effects of Chemical Substances* (RTECS) is published annually by the US National Institute for Occupational Safety and Health, Ohio. A computerized version that contains data on more than 40 000 compounds is available via the TOXLINE system of the US National Library of Medicine and the Chemical Information Service (CIS) sponsored jointly by the National Institutes for Health and the Environmental Protection Agency, Washington, DC. Within CIS there exists a database called CESARS (Chemical Evaluation Search and Retrieval System) which includes physical and chemical properties, toxicity, carcinogenicity and environmental fate. Also within CIS is the SANSS (Structure and Nomenclature Search System) for selecting a cohort (sub-population) of substances with a desired structural feature in common. A more exhaustive search for cognate structures can be carried out with the *CAS Online System* where more than 600 000 substances are searchable through *Chemical Abstracts*. One may also insert the CAS number into the US National Institute of Health's MEDLARS system (available without charge in many countries) and retrieve relevant literature references.

Toxicology: See the range of books recommended on p. 237, also the databases recommended above.

References

Abeles, R. and Maycock, A. (1976) *Accounts Chem. Res.* **9,** 313

Accum, F. (1820) *A Treatise on Adulterations of Food and Culinary Poisons, and Methods of Detecting Them* (2nd edn) Longman, Hurst, Rees, Orme and Brown, London

Addis, P. B., Csallany, A. S. and Kindom, S. E. (1983) in Finley and Schwass (1983) p. 85

Agurell, S., Dewey, W. L. and Willette, R. E. (1984) *The Cannabinoids: Chemical, Pharmacologic, and Therapeutic Aspects*, Academic Press, New York

Ahlquist, R. (1948) *Amer. J. Physiol.* **153,** 586

Aksoy, M., Erdem, S. and Dincol, G. (1974) *Blood,* **44,** 837

Alarie, Y. (1985) *Ann. Rev. Pharmacol. Toxicol.* **25,** 325

Albert, A. (1944) *Med. J. Austral.* **1,** 245

Albert, A. (1958) *Nature, (Lond.)* **182,** 421

Albert, A. (1976) *Adv. Heterocycl. Chem.* **20,** 117 (a review)

Albert, A. (1985) *Selective Toxicity* (7th edn) Chapman and Hall, London and New York

Albert, A. and Brown, D. J. (1954) *J. Chem. Soc.* p. 2060

Albert, A., Gibson, M. I. and Rubbo, S. D. (1953) *Brit. J. Exper. Pathol.* **34,** 119

Albert, A., Goldacre, R. J. and Phillips, J. N. (1948) *J. Chem. Soc.* p. 2240

Albert, A., Rubbo, S. D. and Burvill, M. I. (1949) *Brit. J. Exper. Pathol.* **30,** 159

Albert, A., Rubbo, S. D. and Goldacre, R. J. (1941) *Nature, (Lond.)* **147,** 332

Albert, A., Rubbo, S. D., Goldacre, R. J. and Balfour, B. (1947) *Brit. J. Exper. Pathol.* **28,** 69

Albert, A., Rubbo, S. D., Goldacre, R. J., Davey, M. and Stone, J. (1945) *Brit. J. Exper. Pathol.* **26,** 160

Albert, A. and Serjeant, E. P. (1984) *The Determination of Ionization Constants*, Chapman and Hall, London and New York

Alexandrowicz, J. and Smyk, B. (1975) *Rpts Biol. Med.* **31,** 715

Alhadeff, L., Gualtieri, T. and Lipton, M. (1984) *Nutrit. Rev.* **42,** 33

Allen, J. R. and Norback, D. H. (1977) in Hiatt, *et al.* (1977) p. 173

Alleyne, G. A. O., Hay, R. W., Picou, D. I., Stanfield, J. P. and Whitehead, R. G. (1977) *Protein Energy Malnutrition*, Arnold, London

Alving, C., Steck, E., Chapman, W., Waits, V., Hendricks, L. *et al.* (1978) *Proc. Natl Acad. Sci. USA,* **75,** 2959

Amdur, M. O. (1985) in Klaassen, Amdur and Doull (1985)

American Academy of Pediatrics, Committee on Nutrition (1972) *Pediatrics,* **49,** 456

American Academy of Pediatrics, Committee on Nutrition (1974) *Pediatrics,* **53,** 115

American Academy of Pediatrics, Committee on Nutrition (1981) *Pediatrics,* **68,** 501

American Cancer Society (1982) *Nutrition and Cancer: Cause and Prevention*, ACS, New York

American Cancer Society (1987) *Cancer Facts and Figures,* ACS, New York (gratis)

Americal Chemical Society (1985) Division of Environmental Chemistry's Symposium on Dioxins in the Environment, *Chem. Eng. News,* **63** (May 27), 41

American Dietetic Association (1978) *Vitamin-Mineral Safety, Toxicity and Misuse*, ADA, Chicago
Ames, B. N. (1979) *Science*, **204**, 587
Ames, B. N., Sims, P. and Grover, P. (1972) *Science*, **176**, 47
Anderson, D. and Purchase, I. F. H. (1983) in Conning and Landsdown (1983)
Anderson, T. W. (1977) *Acta Vitaminol. Enzymol., Milano*, **31**, 43
Angrist, B., Sathananthan, G., Wilk, S. and Gershon, S. (1974) *J. Psychiatr. Res.* **11**, 13
Annest, J. L., Pirkle, J. L., Makue, D., Neese, J. W., Bayse, D. D. *et al.* (1983) *New Engl. J. Med.* **308**, 1373
Anon. (1977) Editorial *Morbidity and Mortality Weekly Reports*, **26**, 383, Centers for Disease Control, Atlanta, Georgia
Anon. (1977a) *Med. Lett. Drugs Ther.* **19**, 17
Anon. (1978) *New York Times*, Nov 21; *Time*, **112** (Dec 4), 10
Anon. (1978a) *Chem. Eng. News*, **56** (Aug 7), 6
Anon. (1979) Editorial *Lancet*, **ii**, 617
Anon. (1985) *Chem. Indust., (Lond.)* p. 770
Anon. (1985a) *Chem. Eng. News*, **63** (Sept 16), 28
Anon. (1985b) *Chem. Eng. News*, **63** (Aug 19), 6
Anon. (1985c) *Chem. Indust., (Lond.)* p. 314
Anon. (1985d) *Chem. Eng. News*, **63** (May 20), 6
Anon. (1985e) *Chem. Eng. News*, **63** (March 4), 8
Anon. (1986) *Nature, (Lond.)* **321**, pp. 457, 459
Anon. (1986a) *Chem. Eng. News*, **64** (March 10), 6
Anon. (1986b) *Chem. Eng. News*, **64** (July 21), 15
Arcos, J. C., Argus, M. F. and Wolf, G. (1968) *Chemical Induction of Cancer*, Academic Press, New York
Ariëns, E. J., Simonis, A. M. and Offermeier, J. (1976) *Introduction to General Toxicology*, Academic Press, New York.
Arjungi, K. N. (1976) *Arzneimittel-Forsch*, **26**, 951
Armitage, A. K., Hall, G. H. and Morrison, C. F. (1968) *Nature, (Lond.)* **217**, 331
Armstrong, B. (1976) *Brit. J. Cancer*, **33**, 127
Armstrong, B., Lea, A. J., Adelstein, A. M., Donovan, J. W., White, G. C. *et al.* (1976) *Brit. J. Prevent. Social Med.* **30**, 151
Artman, N. R. and Smith, D. E. (1972) *J. Amer. Oil Chemists' Soc.* **49**, 318
Asbury, C. H. (1985) *Orphan Drugs: Medical vs. Market Value*, Heath and Co, Lexington, MA
Ashby, J., de Serres, F. J., Draper, M., Ishidate, M., Margolin, B. *et al.* (1985) *Evaluation of Short-term Tests for Carcinogens*. Elsevier, Amsterdam
Aub, J. C., Evans, R. D., Hempelmann, L. H. and Martland, H. S. (1952) *Medicine*, **31**, 221
Australia, Commonwealth Department of Health (1985) *Fluoridation of Water*, Australian Government Publishing Service, Canberra
Australia, National Health and Medical Research Council (1984) *Dietary Allowances for Use in Australia*, Australian Government Publishing Service, Canberra
Australian Heritage Commission (1980) *Nomination of the Willandra Lakes Region for Inclusion in the World Heritage List*, AHC, Canberra
Australian Senate Standing Committee on Science and the Environment (1982) *Pesticides and the Health of Australian Vietnam Veterans*; First Report, Australian Government Publishing Service, Canberra
Australian Veterans Health Studies (1984) *The Mortality Report* (3 vols), Australian Government Publishing Service, Canberra
Avery, C. B. (1972) *Italian Renaissance Encyclopedia*, Appleton-Century-Crofts, New York

Awad, S., Downie, J. and Kiruluta, H. (1979) *Canad. J. Surg.* **22,** 515

Awramik, S. M., Schopf, J. W. and Walter, M. R. (1983) *Precambrian Res.* **20,** 357

Baekland, F., Lundwall, L. K. and Kissen, B. (1975) in *Research Advances in Alchohol and Drug Problems,* (vol. 2) (ed. Y. Israel) Wiley, New York, p. 247

Baker, B. R. and Shapiro, H. S. (1966) *J. Pharm. Sci.* **55,** 308

Bakir, F., Rustin, H., Tikriti, S., Al-Damluju, S. F. and Shihristani, H. (1980) *Postgrad. Med. J.* **56,** 1

Balaban, A., Chiriac, A., Motoc, J. and Simon, Z. (1980) *Steric Fit in Quantitative Structure-Action Relations,* Springer-Verlag, Berlin

Balentine, J. D. (1982) *Pathology of Oxygen Toxicity,* Academic Press, New York

Ballard, B. E. (1980) in *Remington's Pharmaceutical Sciences* (16th edn) Mack Publishing Co., Easton, Pennsylvania

Ballard, B. E. and Nelson, E. (1962) *J. Pharm. Sci.* **51,** 915

Barger, G. (1931) *Ergot and Ergotism,* Gurney and Jackson, Edinburgh

Barger, G. and Dale, H. H. (1910) *J. Physiol. (Lond.)* **41,** 19

Barlow, R. B. (1980) *Quantitative Aspects of Chemical Pharmacology,* Croom Helm, London

Barnard, C. (1980) *Good Life, Good Death: A Doctor's Case for Euthanasia and Suicide,* Prentice Hall, Eaglewood Cliffs, NJ

Baselt, R. C. (1982) *Disposition of Toxic Drugs and Chemicals in Man* (2nd edn) Biomedical Publications, Davis, CA

Basu, T. K. and Stiles, F. A. (1985) *Food and Drugs, Interactions, Toxicology and Safety,* Croom Helm, Beckenham, UK

Baumhoff, M. A. (1963) *Ecological Determinants of Aboriginal California Populations,* University of California Publications in American Archeology No. 49, University of California, Davis, CA

Bedau, H. A. (1982) *The Death Penalty in America* (3rd edn) Oxford University Press, Oxford

Bell, E. A. (1973) in NAS (1973) p. 153

Bell, P. and Roblin, R. O. (1942) *J. Amer. Chem. Soc.,* **64,** 2905

Bend, J. R., Serabjit-Singh, C. J. and Philpot, R. M. (1985) *Ann. Rev. Pharmacol. Toxicol.* **25,** 97

Ben-Ishai, R. and Peleg, L. (1975) in *Molecular Mechanisms for Repair of DNA, B* (eds P. C. Hanawalt and R. B. Setlow) Plenum, New York, p. 607

Benovic, J. L., Shorr, R. G. L., Caron, M. G. and Lefkowitz; R. J. (1984) *Biochemistry,* **23,** 4510

Benowitz, N. L. and Jacob, P. (1984) *Clin. Pharmacol. Ther.* **35,** 499

Benowitz, N. L., Kuyt, F., Jacob, P., Jones, R. T. and Osman, A.-L. (1983) *Clin. Pharmacol. Ther.* **34,** 604

Berenblum, I. (1941) *Cancer Res.* **1,** pp. 44, 807

Berenblum, I. (1974) in *The Physiopathology of Cancer* (ed. W. Homburger (3rd edn) Karger, Basel, p. 393

Bert, P. (1878) *La Pression Barométrique. Recherches de Physiologie Expérimentale,* Masson et cie, Paris (reprinted in English translation by the Undersea Medical Society, Bethesda, Maryland (1978))

Bertino, J. and Johns, D. (1967) *Ann. Rev. Med.* **18,** 27

Bikle, D. D. (1983) *Annals Intern. Med.* **98,** 1013

Bird, A. and Marshall, A. (1967) *Biochem. Pharmacol.* **16,** 2275

Bistrian, B. R. (1978) *J. Amer. Med. Assoc.* **240,** 2299

Bjelke, E. (1975) *Int. J. Cancer,* **15,** 561

Blackman, G. (1946) *Agriculture,* **53,** 16

Blaney, J., Jorgensen, E., Connolly, M., Ferrin, T., Langridge, R. *et al.* (1982) *J. Med. Chem.* **25,** 785

Blaschko, H. (1952) *Pharmacol. Rev.* **4,** 415

Block, R. J. and Mitchell, H. H. (1946) *Nutrition Abstr. Rev.* **16,** 249

Blot, W. J., Mason, T. J., Hoover, R. and Fraumeni, J. F. (1977) in Hiatt (1977) p. 21

Boeckx, R. L. (1986) *Analyt. Chem.* **58,** 275A

Bois, P. (1963) *Brit. J. Exper. Path.* **44,** 151

Bolin, J. T., Filman, D. J., Matthews, D. A., Hamlin, R. and Kraut, J. (1982) *J. Biol. Chem.* **257,** 13650

Boobis, A. R., Caldwell, J., De Matteis, F. and Elcombe, C. R. (eds) (1985) *Microsomes and Drug Oxidations*, Taylor and Francis, London

Boxer, G. E. and Rickards, J. C. (1952) *Arch. Biochem. Biophys.* **38,** 287

Boyd, E. M. (1973) *Toxicity of Pure Foods*, CRC Press, Ohio

Braithwaite, J. (1984) *Corporate Crime in the Pharmaceutical Industry*, Routledge and Kegan Paul, London

Brandenberger, H. and Bader, H. (1967) *Helv. Chim. Acta*, **50,** 463

Brantom, P. G., Gaunt, I. F. and Grasso, P. (1973) *Food Cosmet. Toxicol.* **11,** 735

Brickman, R., Jasanoff, S. and Ilgen, T. (1985) *Controlling Chemicals: The Politics of Regulation in Europe & the United States*, University Press, Cornell, NY

British Crop Protection Council (1983) *The Pesticide Manual* (ed. C. R. Worthing) BCPC, Croydon, England

British Medical Association (1986) *Report of the Board of Science's Working Party on Alternative Therapy*, BMA, London

Brobeck, J. R. (1960) in *Handbook of Physiology*, 2 (eds J. Field, H. W. Magoun, and V. E. Hall) American Physiological Society, Washington, DC, p. 1197

Brodie, B. B. (1956) *J. Pharm. Pharmacol.* **8,** 1

Brodie, B. B. (1964) *The Pharmacologist*, Washington, **6,** 12

Brodie, B. B. and Axelrod, J. (1949) *J. Pharmacol.* **97,** 58

Brodie, B. B., Gillette, J. R. and Ackerman, H. (1971) *Concepts in Biochemical Pharmacology*, Parts 1 and 2 (for Part 3 see Gillette and Mitchell, 1975) Springer-Verlag, Berlin

Brodie, B. B. and Hogben, C. (1957) *J. Pharm. Pharmacol.* **9,** 345

Brody, J. A. (1984) *US Public Health Report*, **99,** Government Printing Office, Washington, DC, p. 468

Brody, J. A. (1985) *Nature, (Lond.)* **315,** 463

Brown, D. (1980) in *The New Grove Dictionary of Music and Musicians* (ed. S. Sadie) **18,** 627, Macmillan, London

Brown, G. M. (1962) *J. Biol. Chem.* **237,** 536

Brown, M. S. and Goldstein, J. L. (1985) in Gilman, *et al.* (1985) p. 834

Brown, M. S., Kovanen, P. T. and Goldstein, J. L. (1981) *Science,* **212,** 628

Brown, N. A. (1985) *Nature, (Lond.)* **316,** 110

Brown, S. S. and Savory, J. (eds) (1983) *Clinical Toxicology and Clinical Chemistry of Metals*, Academic Press, London

Browning, C. (1929) in *A System of Bacteriology in Relation to Medicine*, HMSO, London

Bruce-Chwatt, L. J. (1985) *Drugs Under Exper. Clin. Research,* **11,** 899

Bruck, S. (ed.) (1983) *Controlled Drug Design*, CRC Press, Boca Raton, Florida

Bryan, L. (1982) *Bacterial Resistance and Susceptibility*, University Press, Cambridge

Buckley, I. and Porter, K. (1967) *Protoplasma*, **64,** 349

Bundgaard, H. (1985) *Design of Prodrugs*, Elsevier, Amsterdam

Burchall, J. and Hitchings, G. H. (1965) *Molec. Pharmacol.* **1,** 126

Burckhardt, J. (1929) The Civilization of the Renaissance in Italy (15th edn) (tr. S. Middlemore) Harrap, London

'Burger's Medicinal Chemistry' (4th edn, 3 vols) (1981, see Wolff (1981))

Burkitt, D. P. and Trowell, H. C. (1975) *Refined Carbohydrate Foods and Disease. Some Implications of Dietary Fibre*, Academic Press, London

Burnet, J. (1911) *The Phaedo of Plato*, Oxford University Press, Oxford

Burnstock, G. and Costa, M. (1975) *Adrenergic Neurons*, Chapman and Hall, London and New York

Cade, J. (1949) *Med. J. Austral.* **2,** 349

Caldwell, J. and Paulson, G. D. (eds) (1984) *Foreign Compound Metabolism,* Taylor and Francis, London

Calloway, D. H. (1971) *Environ. Biol. Med.* **1,** 175

Calvery, H. O. and Klumpp, T. G. (1939) *Sth. Med. J., USA,* **32,** 1105

Came, P. and Caliguiri, L. (cds) (1982) *Chemotherapy of Viral Infections,* Springer-Verlag, Berlin

Campbell, R. K. (1982) *Am. Pharm., N.S.* **22,** 78

Canadian Department of National Health and Welfare (Bureau of Nutritional Sciences) (1977) *Recommendations for Prevention Programs in Relation to Nutrition and Cardiovascular Disease,* CDHW, Ottawa

Carmichael, W. W. and Mahmood, N. A. (1984) in Ragelis (1984)

Carr, D. J. and Carr, S. G. M. (eds) (1981) *People and Plants,* Academic Press, New York

Carson, J. F. and Wong, F. F. (1961) *J. Food Agric. Chem.* **9,** 140

Cartwright, R. A. (1984) in Searle (1984), **1,** 1

Casley-Smith, J. R. (1958) *Aust. J. Exper. Biol. Med. Sci.* **36,** 23; **37,** 451

Cattabeni, F., Cavallaro, A. and Galli, G. (1978) *Dioxin – Toxicological and Chemical Aspects,* Wiley, New York

Cattell, W., Chamberlain, D., Fry, I., McSherry, M., Broughton, C. *et al.* (1971) *Brit. Med. J.* **1,** 377

Chacko, G., Villegas, G., Barnola, F., Villegas, R. and Goldman, D. (1976) *Biochim. Biophys. Acta,* **443,** 19

Chambron, J., Daune, M. and Sadron, C. (1966) *Biochim. Biophys. Acta,* **123,** 306

Chance, B. and Boveris, A. (1978) *Lung Biology in Health and Disease,* **8,** 185

Changeux, J.-P. (1969) *Proc. Nobel Symp.* **11,** 235

Changeux, J.-P., Devillers-Thiery, A. and Chemouilli, P. (1984) *Science,* **225,** 1335

Charney, D. S., Riordan, C. E., Kleber, H. D., Murburg, M., Braverman, P. *et al.* (1982) *Arch. Gen. Psychiatry,* **39,** 1327

Chinn, H. I. (1979) *A Review of the Adverse Effects of Intakes of Vitamin D,* Report by Life Sciences Research Office to the Food and Drugs Agency, FDA, Washington, DC

Chittenden, R. H. (1909) *The Nutrition of Man,* Heinemann, London

Chowaniec, J. and Hicks, R. M. (1979) *Brit. J. Cancer,* **39,** 355

Clark, A. J. (1926) *J. Physiol. (Lond.)* **61,** 530

Clark, A. J. (1933) *The Mode of Action of Drugs on Cells,* Edward Arnold, London

Clarren, S. K. and Smith, D. W. (1978) *New Engl. J. Med.* **298,** 1062

Clayson, D. B. (1981) in Reeves (1981) p. 155

Cochrane, A. L. and Moore, F. A. (1980) *Brit. J. Indust. Med.* **37,** 226

Colebrook, L. and Kenny, M. (1936) *Lancet,* **i,** 1279

Coleman, A. W. (1979) in *Biochemistry and Physiology of Protozoa,* **1** (2nd edn) (ed. S. H. Hutner) Academic Press, New York, p. 307

Coleman, E. C., Ho. C.-T., and Chang, S. S. (1981) *J. Agric. Food Chem.* **29,** 42

Conn, E. E. (1973) in NAS (1973) p. 299

Connell, D. W. (1964) *Austral. J. Chem.* **17,** 130

Conning, D. M. and Lansdown, A. B. G. (1983) *Toxic Hazards in Food,* Croom Helm, Beckenham, UK

Connor, H. E. (1977) *The Poisonous Plants of New Zealand* (2nd edn) Government Printer, Wellington, NZ

Cook, J., Hewitt, C. and Hieger, I. (1933) *J. Chem. Soc.* p. 396

Coombs, M. M., Dixon, C. and Kissonerghis, A.-M. (1976) *Cancer Res.* **36,** 4525

Cope, J. D. (1985) *Pharmaceutical J.* **234,** 712

Coronary Drug Project Research Group (1975) *J. Amer. Med. Assoc.* **231,** 360

Costzias, G., Van Woert, M. and Schiffer, L. (1967) *New Engl. J. Med.* **276,** 374

Coulston, F. and Korte, F. (1976) *Environmental Quality and Safety,* Suppl. 5, Thieme Verlag, Stuttgart

Coulston, F. and Pocchiari, F. (eds) (1983) *Accidental Exposure to Dioxins,* Academic Press, New York

Creagan, E. T., Moertel, C. C., O'Fallon, J. R., Schutt, A. J., O'Connell, M. J. *et al.* (1979) *New Engl. J. Med.* **301,** 687

Creasey, W. A. (1981) *Cancer: An Introduction,* Oxford University Press, New York

Crosby, N. T., Foreman, J. K., Palframan, J. F. and Sayer, R. (1972) *Nature, (Lond.)* **238,** 342

Crossland, J. (1979) (ed.) *'Lewis's Pharmacology',* Livingstone, Edinburgh

Crum Brown, A. and Fraser, T. R. (1869) *Trans. Roy. Soc. Edinburgh,* **25,** 151

Cucinell, S. A., Coney, A. H., Sansur, M. and Burns, J. (1965) *Clin. Pharmacol. Therap.* **6,** 420

Curley, A. (1971) *Lancet,* **ii,** 296

Cushny, A. R. (1926) *Biological Relations of Optically Isomeric Substances,* Ballière, Tindall and Cox, London

Dagani, R. (1981) *Chem. Eng. News,* **59** (June 29), 18

Dahl, L. K. (1972) *Amer. J. Clin. Nutrit.* **25,** 231

Daly, J., Brons, R. and Snyder, S. (1981) *Life Sciences,* **28,** 2083

Daniel, G. (ed.) (1978) *Illustrated Encyclopaedia of Archeology,* Macmillan, London

D'Arcy, P. F. and Griffin, J. P. (1985) *Iatrogenic Diseases* (3rd edn) Oxford University Press, Oxford

Dauber, J. H. (1982) in *Update: Pulmonary Diseases and Disorders* (ed. A. P. Fishman) McGraw-Hill, New York

Davidson, S. and Passmore, R. (1986) *Human Nutrition and Dietetics* (8th edn) Churchill-Livingstone, Edinburgh, London and New York

'Davidson's Principles and Practice of Medicine' (14th edn) (1984) see Macleod, 1984

Davies, P. (1960) *Ann. Intern. Med.* **53,** 1250

De Caprio, A. P., Olajos, E. J. and Weber, P. (1982) *Toxicol. Appl. Pharmacol.* **65,** 440

Dench, W. (1981) *Association of the British Pharmaceutical Industry News,* **185,** 5

Dennis, V., Stead, N. and Andreoli, T. (1970) *J. Gen. Physiol.* **55,** 375

Denton, D. A. (1982) *The Hunger for Salt,* Springer Verlag, Berlin

De Santo, N. G. (1975) *J. Amer. Med. Assoc.* **234,** 841

Dixon, M. (1948) *Biochem. Soc. Sympos.* **2,** 39

Dixon, M. and Webb, E. (1979) *Enzymes* (3rd edn) Longmans, London; Academic Press, New York

Doll, R. (1977) in Hiatt, *et al.,* 1977, p. 1

Domagk, G. (1935) *Dtsch. Med. Woch.* **61,** 250

Domagk, G. (1936) *Klin. Woch.* **15,** 1585

Druckrey, H. and Küpfmüller, K. (1948) *Z. Naturforsch. Teil B,* **3,** 254

Druckrey, H. and Küpfmüller, K. (1949) *Dosis und Wirkung,* Cantor, Aulendorf-im-Württemberg

Druckrey, H., Preussmann, R., Ivankovič, S. and Schmähl, D. (1967) *Z. Krebsforsch.* **69,** 103

Dumond, D. E. (1977) *The Eskimos and Aleuts,* Thames and Hudson, London

Dunn, F. L. in Lee and DeVore (1968) pp. 221–28

Dupont, R. L. (1979) in *The International Challenge of Drug Abuse* (ed. R. C. Peterson) Government Printing Office, Washington, DC

Durnin, J. V. and Passmore, R. (1967) *Energy, Work and Leisure,* Heinemann, London

Dutkiewicz, T. and Tyras, H. (1968) *Brit. J. Indust. Med.* **25,** 243; *Int. Arch. Gewerbepathol. u. Gewerbehyg.* **24,** 253

Ebert, R. V., McNabb, McK. E., McCusker, K. T. and Snow, S. L. (1983) *J. Amer. Med. Assoc.* **250,** 2840

Ehrlich, P. (1900) *Proc. Roy. Soc. (Lond.) B,* **66,** 424

Ehrlich, P. (1909) *Ber. Dtsch. Chem. Ges.* **42,** 17

Ehrlich, P. (1911) *Theorie und Praxis von Chemotherapie,* Klinkhardt, Leipzig

Ehrlich, P. R. (1984) (pbk 1985) *The Cold and the Dark: the World after Nuclear War,* Norton, New York

Einhorn, A. (1905) *Deutsch. Med. Woch.* **31,** 1668

Einstein, N., Baker, J., Galper, J. and Wolfe, H. (1975) *Amer. J. Digest. Dis.* **20,** 282

Elion, G. B. (1967) *Fed. Proc.* **26,** 898

Elion, G. B., Furman, P., Fyfe, J., De Miranda, P., Beauchamp, E. and Schaeffer, H. (1977) *Proc. Natl Acad. Sci., USA,* **74,** 5716

Ellinwood, E. H. (1979) in *Handbook on Drug Abuse* (eds R. L. Dupont, A. Goldstein and J. O'Donnel) US Government Printing Office, National Institute on Drug Abuse, Washington, DC

Elliott, K. and Whelan, J. (eds) (1977) *Health and Disease in Tribal Societies,* Elsevier Amsterdam

Ember, L. R. (1986) *Chem. Eng. News,* **64** (April 14th), 8

Entomological Society of America (1981) *Pesticide Handbook: 'Entoma'* (29th edn) (eds R. Caswell, K. Devold and L. Gilbert) ESA, College Park, Maryland

Epstein, M. A. and Achong, B. G. (eds) (1979) *The Epstein-Barr Virus,* Springer-Verlag, Berlin

Erickson, J. D. (1978) *New Engl. J. Med.* **298,** 1112

Evans, I. A., Jones, R. S. and Mainwarning-Burton, R. (1972) *Nature (Lond.)* **237,** 107

Everett, A., Lowe, L. and Wilkinson, S. (1970) *Chem. Comm., Chem. Soc. (Lond.)* p. 1020

Everitt, A. V., Porter, B. D. and Wyndham, J. R. (1982) *Gerentology,* **28,** 168

Eyre, E. J. (1845) *Journals of Expeditions of Discovery into Central Australia and Overland from Adelaide to King George's Sound, in the years 1840–1,* Boone, London

Falco, E. A., Goodwin, L. G., Hitchings, G. H., Rollo, I. M. and Russell, P. B. (1951) *Brit. J. Pharmacol. Chemother.* **6,** 185

FAO (Food and Agricultural Organization of the United Nations) (1977) *Dietary Fats and Oils in Human Nutrition,* FAO, Rome, Italy

FAO/IAE/WHO (Food and Agricultural Organization of the United Nations/ International Atomic Energy Agency/World Health Organization) (1981) Joint Expert Committee's Report, *WHO Tech. Reports,* **557,** WHO, Geneva, Switzerland

FAO/WHO (1980) Joint FAO/WHO Expert Committee on Food Additives, *24th Tech. Rep.* **648** (reports from other years are specified on pp. 80–81)

Farber, S. (1952) *Blood,* **7,** 107

Farmer, E. H., Bloomfield, G. F., Sundralingham, A. and Stutton, D. A. (1942) *Trans. Farad. Soc.* **38,** 348

Fassett, D. W. in NAS (1973) p. 7

Fastier, F. N. (1949) *Brit. J. Pharmacol.* **4,** 315

Fazio, T. (1984) in Lawrence (1984) p. 395

FDA, see Food and Drugs Administration

Federation of American Societies for Experimental Biology (1976) *Evaluation of Sucrose as a Food Ingredient,* FASEB, Bethesda, Maryland

Federation of American Societies for Experimental Biology (1978) *Evaluation of the Health Aspects of Vitamin D_2 and D_3 as Food Ingredients,* FASEB, Bethesda, Maryland

Federation of American Societies for Experimental Biology (1978a) *Evaluation of the Health Aspects of Caffeine as a Food Ingredient,* FASEB, Bethesda, Maryland

Federation of American Societies for Experimental Biology (1978b) *Evaluation of the Health Aspects of Protein Hydrolysates as Food Ingredients,* FASEB, Bethesda, Maryland

Feingold, B. F. (1975) *Why Your Child is Hyperactive*, Random House, New York

Feingold, D. S. (1970) *New Engl. J. Med.* **283,** 1384

Feldmann, R. J. and Maibach, H. I. (1970) *J. Invest. Dermatol.* **54,** 435

Feldmann, R. J. and Maibach, H. I. (1974) *Toxicol. Appl. Pharmacol.* **28,** 126

Ferebee, S. H. (1970) *Adv. Tuberc. Res.* **17,** 28

Ferencz, B. B. (1979) *Less Than Slaves*, Harvard University Press, Cambridge, pp. xix, xxiv, 17–20, 30, 59

Ferguson, L. R., Van Zijl, P., Holloway, W. D. and Jones, W. T. (1985) *Mutation Research,* **158,** 89

Fernstrom, J. D. and Wurtman, R. J. (1972) *Science,* **178,** 414

Feron, V. C. (1972) *Cancer Res.* **32,** 28

Ferone, R., Burchall, J. and Hitchings, G. H. (1969) *Molec. Pharmacol.* **5,** 49

Festenstein, H. and Garrido, F. (1986) *Nature, (Lond.)* **322,** 502

Fieser, L. and Fieser, M. (1935) *J. Amer. Chem. Soc.* **57,** 491

Finkel, M. J. (1961) *Clin. Pharmacol. Ther.* **2,** 794

Finley, J. W. and Schwass, D. E. (eds) (1983) *Xenobiotics in Foods and Feeds*, American Chemical Society, Washington, DC

Finley, J. W. and Schwass, D. E. (eds) (1985) *Xenobiotic Metabolism: Nutritional Effects*, American Chemical Society, Washington, DC

Fischman, M. W. and Schuster, C. R. (1982) *Fed. Proc.* **41,** 241

Flath, R. K. and Forrey, R. R. (1970) *J. Agr. Food Chem.* **18,** 306

Florey, H. W., Chain, E. B., Heatley, N., Jennings, M. and Sanders, A. G. *et al.* (1949) *Antibiotics*, Oxford University Press, Oxford

Food and Agricultural Organization, see FAO

Food and Drug Administration (1978) *Federal Register, Washington* **43,** 60883

Food Standards Committee (1965) *Report on Flavouring Agents*, HMSO, London

Forman, D., Al-Dabbagh, S. and Doll, R. (1985) *Nature, (Lond.)* **313,** 620; **317,** 676

Fox, B. and Fox, M. (1984) *Antitumor Drug Resistance*, Springer-Verlag, New York

Frankel, E. N., Smith, L. M., Hamblin, C. L., Creveling, R. K. and Clifford, A. J. (1984) *J. Amer. Oil Chem. Soc.* **61,** 87

Franklin, T. J. (1971) *Biochem. J.* **123,** 267

Franks, N. and Lieb, W. (1982) *Nature, (Lond.)* **300,** 487

Franks, L. M. and Teich, N. (1986) *Introduction to the Cellular and Molecular Biology of Cancer*, Oxford University Press, Oxford

Friberg, L., Piscator, M., Nordberg, G. F. and Kjellstrom, T. (1974) *Cadmium in the Environment* (2nd edn) CRC Press, Cleveland, Ohio

Friedberg, E. (1985) *DNA Repair*, W. H. Freeman, CA.

Fulöp-Miller, R. (1927) *Rasputin, the Holy Devil* (tr. F. S. Flint and D. F. Tait) Garden City Publishing Co., New York

Furia, T. E. (1979–80) *Handbook of Food Additives* (2nd edn, 2 vols) CRC Press, Boca Raton, Florida

Furia, T. E. and Bellanca, N. (eds) (1975) *Fenaroli's Handbook of Flavor Ingredients*, CRC Press, Cleveland, Ohio

Garrow, J. S. (1978) *Energy Balance and Obesity in Man* (2nd edn), North Holland, Amsterdam; Elsevier, New York

Gessner, P. K. (1979) in *Biochemistry and Pharmacology of Ethanol* (Vol. 2) (eds E. Majchrowicz and E. P. Noble) Plenum, New York

Gibaldi, M. (1984) *Biopharmaceutics and Clinical Pharmacokinetics* (3rd edn) Lea and Febiger, Philadelphia

Gibson, G. G. and Ioannides, C. (eds) (1981) *Safety Evaluation of Nitrosable Drugs and Chemicals*, Taylor and Francis, London

Gibson, G. G. and Skett, P. (1986) *Introduction to Drug Metabolism*, Chapman and Hall, London

Gibson, G. G. and Walker, R. (eds) (1985) *Food Toxicology – Real or Imaginary Problems*, Taylor and Francis, London

Gilbert, R. M. (1976) *Research Advances in Alcohol and Drug Problems*, **3**, 49, Wiley, New York

Gillette, J. R. (1966) *Adv. Pharmacol.*, **4**, 219

Gillette, J. R. and Mitchell, J. R. (1975) *Concepts in Biochemical Pharmacology*, Part 3, Springer-Verlag, Berlin

Gilligan, D. and Plummer, N. (1943) *Proc. Soc. Exper. Biol. Med.* **53**, 142

Gilman, A. G., Goodman, L. S., Rall, T. W. and Murad, F. (1985) (eds) *'Goodman and Gilman's Pharmacological Basis of Therapeutics'* (7th edn) Macmillan, New York

Ginnings, P. and Baum, R. (1937) *J. Amer. Chem. Soc.* **59**, 1111

Glatt, H., Protić-Sabljić, M. and Oesch, F. (1983) *Science*, **220**, 961

Glave, W. and Hansch, C. (1972) *J. Pharm. Sci.* **61**, 589

Gleibermann, L. (1973) *Ecol. Food Nutrit.* **2**, 143

Glueck, C. J., McGill, H. C., Shank, R. E. and Lauer, R. M. (1978) *Circulation*, **58**, 381A

Goering, P. L. and Klaassen, C. D. (1984) *Toxicol. Appl. Pharmacol.* **74**, 308

Goldacre, R. J. and Phillips, J. N. (1949) *J. Chem. Soc.* p. 1724

Goldman, P., Ingelfinger, J. A. and Friedman, P. A. (1977) in Hiatt (1977) *A*, p. 465

Goldman, P. G. (1973) *Der Hautarzt*, **24**, 149

Goldstein, A., Aronow, L. and Kalman, S. M. (1974) *Principles of Drug Action* (2nd edn) Wiley, New York

Goldstein, J. L., Kite, T. and Brown, M. S. (1983) *New Engl. J. Med.* **309**, 288

'Goodman and Gilman's Pharmacological Basis of Therapeutics' (1985) see Gilman, *et al.* (1985)

Goodwin, D. W. (1976) *Is Alcoholism Hereditary?* Oxford University Press, New York

Gorrod, J. W. (1981) *Testing for Toxicity*, Taylor and Francis, London

Gosselin, R. (1984) *Clinical Toxicology of Commercial Products: Acute Poisoning* (5th edn) Williams and Wilkins, Baltimore.

Gough, M. (1986) *Dioxin, Agent Orange: The Facts* Plenum Press, New York

Gould, J. (1957) *Nature, (Lond.)* **180**, 282

Goutières, F. and Aicardi, J. (1977) *Brit. Med. J.* **2**, 663

Grasso, P. (1979) *Chem. Indust., (Lond.)* p. 73

Grasso, P. (1983) in Conning and Lansdown (1983) pp. 122–40

'Gray's Anatomy' 1983 see Leonard (1983)

Greden, J. F. (1981) in *Substance Abuse: Clinical Problems and Perspectives* (eds J. H. Lowinson and P. Ruiz) Williams & Wilkins Co., Baltimore

Green, A., Heale, D. and Grahame-Smith, D. (1977) *Psychopharmacology*, **52**, 195

Green, J. H. (1976) *An Introduction to Human Physiology* (4th edn) Oxford University Press, Oxford

Greenlee, W. F., Sun, J. D. and Bus, J. S. (1981) *Toxicol. Appl. Pharmacol.* **59**, 187

Gregoriadis, G. (1977) *Nature, (Lond.)* **265**, 407

Grey, Sir George (1837) *Journals of two Expeditions of Discovery in North-West and Western Australia during the Years 1837, 1838 and 1839* (2 vols) Boone, London

Griffiths, R. R., Bigelow, G. E. and Liebson, E. (1983) *Arch. Gen. Psychiatry*, **40**, 865

Gull, K. and Trinci, A. (1973) *Nature, (Lond.)* **244**, 292

Gustafssen, B. E., Quensel, C. E., Lanke, L. S., Lundquist, C., Grahnén, H. *et al.* (1954) *Acta. Odontol. Scand.* **11**, 232

Haber, L. I. (1986) *The Poisonous Cloud: Chemical Warfare in the First World War*, Clarendon Press, Oxford

Habermann, E. (1974) *Ann. Rev. Pharmacol.* **14**, 1

Haenzel, W. and Kurihara, M. (1968) *J. Natl Cancer Inst.* **40**, 43

Haest, C. W., De Gier, J., Op den Kamp, J. A., Bartels, P. and Van Deenen, L. L. (1972) *Biochim. Biophys. Acta*, **255**, 720

Haley, T. J. (1975) *J. Toxic. Envir. Health*, **1**, 47

Hammett, L. (1970) *Physical Organic Chemistry* (2nd edn) McGraw-Hill, New York

Hanawalt, P. C., Cooper, P. K., Ganesan, A. K. and Smith, C. A. (1979) *Ann. Rev. Biochem.* **48,** 783

Hancock, J. L., Applegate, H. G. and Dodd, J. D. (1970) *Atmos. Environ.* **4,** 363

Hansch, C. (1968) *J. Med. Chem.* **11,** 920

Hansch, C. (1969) *Accounts Chem. Res.* **2,** 232

Hansch, C. (1971) *Drug Design,* **1,** 271 (review)

Hansch, C. (1976) *J. Med. Chem.* **19,** 1

Hansch, C. and Fujita, T. (1964) *J. Amer. Chem. Soc.* **86,** 1616

Hansch, C. and Leo, A. (1979) *Substituent Constants for Correlation Analysis in Chemistry and Biology,* Wiley, New York

Hansch, C., Steward, A., Anderson, S. and Bentley, D. (1968) *J. Med. Chem.* **11,** 1

Hanson, D. J. (1986) *Chem. Eng. News,* **64** (June 2), 7

Hansten, P. D. (1985) *Drug Interactions,* (5th edn) Lea and Febiger, Philadelphia

Harlan, J. R. (1975) *Crops and Man,* American Society of Agronomy, ASA, Wisconsin

Harper, A. E. (1973) in NAS (1973) p. 130

Harris, R. H., Page T. and Reiches, N. A. (1977) in Hiatt, *et al.* (1977) p. 309

"Harrison's Principles of Internal Medicine' (10th edn) (1983) (see Petersdorf, *et al.* 1983)

Harvey, J. and Colin-Jones, D. G. (1981) *Brit. Med. J.* **282,** 186

Hathway, D. E. (1984) *Molecular Aspects of Toxicology,* Royal Society of Chemistry, London

Hay, A. (1982) *The Chemical Scythe,* Plenum Press, New York

Hay, A. (1983) *Nature, (Lond.)* **306,** 8

Hayden, J. W. (1976) *Clin. Toxicol.* **9,** 169

Haynes, R. C. and Murad, F. (1985) in Gilman, *et al.* (1985)

Hayes, W., Durham, W. and Cueto, C. (1956) *J. Amer. Med. Assoc.* **162,** 890

Hecht, G. (1936) *Arch. Exper. Path. Pharmakol.* **183,** 87

Heffernan, A. G. A. (1964) *Amer. J. Clin. Nutrit,* **15,** 5

'Heilbron's Dictionary of Organic Compounds' (5th edn) (1982, plus supplementary volumes) (ed. J. Buckingham) Chapman and Hall, London and New York

Heiser, C. B. (1981) *Seed to Civilization: The Story of Man's Food,* (2nd edn) Freeman, San Francisco

Helweg, P., Larsen, P., Hoffmeyer, H., Kieler, J., Thaysen, E. H. *et al.* (1952) *Acta Med. Scand. suppl.* **274**

Henderson, P. J. and Lardy, H. A. (1970) *J. Biol. Chem.* **245,** 1319

Hennekens , C. H. (1979) *Lancet,* **1,** 1390

Herbert, V. (1975) in *Proc. Western Hemisphere Nutrit. Cong.,* **4,** 84, Publishing Sciences Group, Acton, MA

Herbert, V. (1979) *Amer. J. Clin. Nutrit.* **32,** 1121

Herbert V. and Jacob, E. (1974) *J. Amer. Med. Assoc.* **230,** 241

Hetzel, B. S. and Frith, H. J. (eds) (1978) *The Nutrition of Aborigines in Relation to the Ecosystem of Central Australia,* Commonwealth Scientific and Industrial Research Organization, Melbourne

Hiatt, H. H., Watson, J. D. and Winsten, J. A. (eds) (1977) *Origins of Human Cancer, A,* Cold Spring Harbor Laboratory, Long Island, NY

Higginson, J. and Muir, C. S. (1979) *J. Natl. Cancer Inst.* **63,** 1291

Higuchi, T. and Stella, V. (eds) (1975) *Pro-Drugs as Novel Drug Delivery Systems,* American Chemical Society, Washington, DC

Hill, D. L. and Grubbs, C. J. (1982) *Anticancer Res.* **2,** 111

Hillman, R. S. (1985) in Gilman, *et al.* (1985) p. 1332

Hillman, R. S. and Finch, C. A. (1985) in Gilman, *et al.* (1985) p. 1308

Himmelweit, F. (ed.) (1956) *The Collected Papers of Paul Ehrlich, with Biography,* Pergamon Press, Oxford

Hinson, J. A., Pohl, L. R., Monks, T. J. and Gillette, J. R. (1981) *Life Sci.* **29,** 107

Hirayama, T. (1978) *Preventive Med.* **7**, 173

Hirom, P. and Millburn, P. (1981) in *Foreign Compound Metabolism* (ed. D. Hathway) The Chemical Society, London

Hirono, I. (1973) *J. Natl Cancer Inst.* **50**, 1367

HM Stationery Office (1969) *Methods for the Detection of Toxic Substances in Air: Hydrogen Sulfide*, HMSO, London

Hodge, H. C. and Smith, F. A. (1965) in *Fluorine Chemistry*, **4**, 247

Hodgkin, A. (1964) *The Conduction of the Nervous Impulse*, Liverpool University Press, Liverpool

Hodgson, E. and Guthrie, F. E. (1980) *Introduction to Biochemical Toxicology*, Blackwell Scientific Publications, Oxford

Hoekstra, W. G., Suttie, J. W., Ganther, H. E. and Merts, W. (eds) (1974) *Trace Element Metabolism in Animals*, University Park Press, Baltimore

Hoffman, R. E., Paul, A. S., Webb, K. B., Evans, R. G., Knutsen, A. P. *et al.* (1986) *J. Amer. Med. Assoc.* **255**, 2031

Holan, G. (1971) *Nature, (Lond.)* **232**, 644

Holbrook, J. H. (1983) in Petersdorf, *et al.* (1983) p. 1302

Holloway, W. D., Tasman-Jones, C, and Lee, S. P. (1978) *Amer. J. Clin. Nutrit.* **31**, 927

Holmstedt, B. (1980) *Arch. Toxicol.* **44**, 211

Hölscher, P. M. and Natzschka, J. (1964) *Dtsch. Med. Wochenschr.* **89**, 1751

Hoover, R. N., McKay, F. W. and Fraumeni, J. F. (1976) *J. Natl Cancer Inst.* **57**, 757

Hoover, R. N. and Strasser, P. (1980) *Lancet*, **i**, 837

Hough, L. (1985) *Chem. Soc. Rev.* **14**, 357

Hueper, W. C. (1948) *US Publ. Health Rpts, suppl.* 209

Hueper, W. C. (1961) *Cancer Research*, **21**, 842

Hueper, W. C. (1961a) *Path. Microbiol., (Basel)* **24**, 77

Hueper, W. C. and Conway, W. D. (1964) *Chemical Carcinogenesis and Cancers*, Thomas, Springfield, Illinois

Hughes, P., Barker, N., Crawford, G. and Jaffe, J. H. (1972) *Amer. J. Public Health*, **62**, 995

Hurwitz, J., Furth, J., Malamy, M. and Alexander, M. (1962) *Proc. Natl Acad. Sci., USA*, **48**, 1222

Hutson, D. H. and Roberts, T. R. (eds) (1986) *Progress in Pesticide Biochemistry and Toxicology*, Wiley, Chichester, England (this is the fifth volume of a multivolume work that began in 1981)

IARC (International Agency for Research on Cancer) (1976) *Monographs on the Carcinogenic Risk of Chemicals to Man*, **10**, IARC Lyon, France; also vols **17** (1978), **22** (1980), **29** (1982) and **37** (1985)

Iida, M., Yamamoto, H. and Sobue, I. (1973) *Igaku No Ayumi*, **84**, 199

Ing, H. R. (1936) *Physiol. Rev.* **16**, 527

International Labour Office (1983) *Encyclopedia of Occupational Health and Safety* (3rd edn, 2 vols) Geneva, Switzerland

International Military Tribunal (1947) *Major War Criminals before the International Military Tribunal*, Nuremburg, pp. 415–6

Ioannides, C., Lum, P.and Parke, D. V. (1984) *Xenobiotica*, **14**, 119

Irvine, F. R. (1957) *Oceania*, **28**, 113

Itakura, M. and Holmes, E. W. (1979) *J. Biol. Chem.* **254**, 333

Iversen, L. (1985) *Nature, (Lond.)* **316**, 108

Jackson, W. A., Steel, J. S. and Boswell, V. R. (1967) *Amer. Soc. Hortic. Sci.* **90**, 349

Jaffe, J. H. (1985) in Gilman *et al.* (1985) p. 532

Jaffe, J. H. and Jarvik, M. E. (1978) in *Psychopharmacology: a Generation of Progress* (eds M. A. Lipton, A. DiMascio and K. F. Killam) Raven Press, New York

Jaffe, J. and McCormack, J. (1967) *Molec. Pharmacol.* **3**, 359

Jaffé, W. G. in NAS (1973, p. 106)

Jaffé, W. G. in Liener (1980) p. 73

Jayaraman, K. S. (1986) *Nature*, (*Lond.*) **319,** 7

Jenkins, D. J. A., Goff, D. J., Alberti, K., Gassull, M., Leeds, A. R. *et al.* (1976) *Lancet*, **ii,** 172

Jenkins, D. J. A., Hockaday, T. D. R., Howarth, R., Apling, E. C., Wolever, T. M. S. *et al.* (1977) *Lancet*, **ii,** 779

Jeri, F. R. (ed.) (1980) *Cocaine, 1980, Proceedings of the Inter-American Seminar on Medical and Sociological Aspects of Coca*, Pacific Press, Lima, Peru

Jick, H. and Dinan, B. J. (1981) *Lancet*, **ii,** 92

Joffe, A. Z. (1978) in *Mycotoxic Fungi, Mycotoxins, Mycotoxicoses* (eds T. D. Wyllie and L. G. Moorehouse) **3,** Marcel Dekker, New York, p. 21.

Johnson, G. (1978) *Ann. Rev. Pharmacol.* **18,** 269

Kalow, W. (1962) *Pharmacogenetics, Heredity and Response to Drugs*, Saunders, Philadelphia

Kalow, W. (1980) *Trends Pharmacol. Sci.* **1,** 403

Kaplan, S. D. and Morgan, R. W. (1981) *Rev. Environ. Health* **3,** 329

Karlin, A. (1967) *J. Theoret. Biol.* **16,** 306

Katan, I. J. (1985) in Gibson and Walker (1985)

Kay, R. M. and Truswell, A. S. (1977) *Amer. J. Clin. Nutrit.* **30,** 171; *Brit. J. Nutrit.* **37,** 227

Kelly, F. C. and Snedden, W. W. (1960) *Endemic Goitre*, WHO Monograph Series No. **44,** WHO, Geneva

Kendall, M. J. (1982) *Brit. J. Clin. Pharmacol.* **13,** 393

Keys, A., Brozek, J., Henschel, A., Mickelsen, O. and Taylor, H. L. (1950) *The Biology of Human Starvation* (2 vols) Oxford University Press, Oxford; Minnesota University Press, Minnesota

Kini, M. and Cooper, J. (1962) *Biochem. J.* **82,** 164

Kinlen, L. and Doll, R. (1981) *J. Epidemiol. Commun. Health,* **35,** 239

Kinosita, R. (1937) *Trans. Soc. Path. Japan*, **27,** 665

Kirk, R. L. (1981) *Aboriginal Man Adapting*, Oxford University Press, Oxford

Klaassen, C. D. (1985) in Gilman, *et al.* (1985)

Klaassen, C. D., Amdur, M. O. and Doull, J. (eds) (1985) *'Casarett and Doull's Toxicology: The Basic Science of Poisons'* (3rd edn) Macmillan, New York

Klayman, D. L. (1985) *Science*, **228,** 1049

Klein, E., Milgrom, H., Stoll, H., Helm, F., Walker, H. *et al.* (1972) in *Cancer Chemotherapy* (eds I. Brodsky and S. Kahn) Grune and Stratton, New York

Klimek, M. (1966) *Photochem. Photobiol.* **5,** 603

Kmet, J. (1970) *J. Chronic Dis.* **23,** 305

Knightley, P., Evans, H., Potter, E. and Wallace, M. (1979) *Suffer the Children: the story of Thalidomide*, Viking Press, New York

Knox, E. G., Armstrong, E. and Lancashire, R. (1980) *Community Medicine*, **2,** 190

Knox, J. B. and Shapiro, C. S. (1986) *Nature*, (*Lond.*) **321,** 22

Knudson, A. G. (1977) in Hiatt, *et al.* (1977) p. 45

Krier, J. E. and Ursin, E. (1972) *Pollution and Policy*, University of California Press, Berkeley

Krishna, G., Pohl, L. R. and Bhooshan, B. (1978) *Toxicol. Appl. Pharmacol.* **45,** 238

Krueger, H. and O'Brien, R. (1959) *J. Econ. Entomol.* **52,** 1063

Krüger-Thiemer, E. (1960) *Klin. Woch.* **38,** 514

Krüger-Thiemer, E. (1966) *J. Theoret. Biol.* **13,** 212

Krüger-Thiemer, E. and Bünger, P. (1961) *Arzneim. Forsch.* **11,** 867

Krüger-Thiemer, E. and Bünger, P. (1965) *Chemotherapia*, **10,** pp. 61, 129

Kubic, V. and Anders, M. (1975) *Drug Metab. Dispos.* **3,** 104

Kuhn, R., Möller, F., Wendt, G. and Beinert, H. (1942) Ber. Deutsch. Chem. Ges., **75,** 711

Kuper, L. (1981) *Genocide*, Yale University Press, New Haven, p. 134

Kyte, J. (1981) *Nature*, *(Lond.)* **292,** 201

La Du, B. N., Mandel, H. G. and Way, E. L. (eds) (1971) *Fundamentals of Drug Metabolism and Drug Disposition*, Williams and Wilkins, Baltimore

Laing, I. G. (1986) *Chem. Indust.*, *(Lond.)* p. 231

Lambley, D. and Ware, J. (1967) *Brit. J. Urol.* **39,** 147

Langley, J. N. (1878) *J. Physiol.*, *(Lond.)* **1,** 339

Lansdown, A. B. G. (1983) in Conning and Lansdown (1983) p. 98

Lansdowne, R. and Yule, W. (eds) (1986) *The Lead Debate*, Croom Helm, Beckenham, UK

Larkin, T. (1976) *Food Consumer*, **10,** 4

Laug, E. P. and Kunze, F. M. (1948) *J. Indust. Hyg.* **30,** 256

Laughlin, W. S. (1963) *Science*, **142,** 633

Laughlin, W. S. (1968) in Lee and DeVore (1968) pp. 242, 316

Lawrence, J. F. (ed.) (1984) *Food Constituents and Food Residues, Their Chromatographic Determination*, Marcel Dekker, New York

Laws, E., Curley, A. and Biros, F. (1967) *Arch. Environ. Health*, **15,** 766

Lederberg, J. (1957) *J. Bact.* **73,** 144

Lederberg, J. and Lederberg, E. (1952) *J. Bact.* **63,** 399

Lee, R. B. (1979) *The !Kung San, Men, Women, and Work in a Foraging Society*, Cambridge University Press, Cambridge

Lee, R. B. and DeVore, I. (eds) (1968) *Man the Hunter*, Aldine, Chicago

Lehninger, A. (1982) *Principles of Biochemistry*, Worth, New York

Leibkowitz, J. O. (1970) *The History of Coronary Heart Disease*, University of California Press, Berkeley

Leo, A., Hansch, C. and Elkins, D. (1971) *Chem. Rev.* **71,** 525

Leo, A., Panthananickal, A., Hansch, C., Theiss, J., Shimkin, M. *et al.* (1981) *J. Med. Chem.* **24,** 859

Leonard, C. H. (reviser) (1983) '*The Concise Gray's Anatomy*', Omega Books, Ware, UK

Leopold, A. C. and Audrey, R. (1972) *Science*, **176,** 512

Lerman, L. (1961) *J. Mol. Biol.* **3,** 18

Lerman, L. (1964) *J. Cell. Compar. Physiol.* **64** (Suppl. 1), 1

Lessof, M. H. (ed.) (1984) *Allergy*, Wiley, New York

Levitzki, A. (1973) In *A Guide to Molecular Pharmacology* (ed. R. Featherstone) Marcel Dekker, New York, p. 305

Levitzki, A. (1986) *Trends Pharmacol. Sci.* **7,** 3

Levy, D. and Boiron, M. (1969) *Bull. de Cancer, France* **56,** 365 (in French)

Lewis, B. (1976) *The Hyperlipidaemias. Clinical and Laboratory Practice*, Blackwell Scientific Publications, Oxford

Lewis, R. J. and Tatken, R. L. (1980) *Registry of Toxic Effects of Chemical Substances*, The National Health Institute for Occupational Safety and Health, US Dept. Health, Cincinnati, Ohio

Li, A. P. (ed.) (1985) *Toxicity Testing, New Approaches and Applications in Human Risk Assessment*, Raven Press, New York

Lieberman, M. W., Baney, R. N., Lee, R. E., Sell, S. and Farber, E. (1971) *Cancer Res.* **31,** 1297

Liener, I. E. (ed.) (1980) *Toxic Constituents of Plant Foodstuffs*, (2nd edn) Academic Press, New York

Lincoff, G. and Mitchel, D. H. (1977) *Toxic and Hallucinogenic Mushroom Poisoning: Diagnosis and Treatment*, Van Nostrand-Reinhold, Cincinnati

Liska, K. (1986) *Drugs and the Human Body*, Macmillan, New York

Loewi, O. and Navratil, E. (1926) *Pflugers Arch. Ges. Physiol.* **214,** 689

Loo, J. and Riegelman, S. (1968) *J. Pharm. Sci.* **57,** 918

Lovenberg, W. (1973) in NAS (1973) p. 170

Lowenstein, L. and Ballew, D. H. (1958) *Canad. Med. Assoc. J.* **78,** 195

McBrien, D. and Slater, T. (eds) (1982) *Free Radicals, Lipid Peroxidation and Cancer,* Academic Press, London

McCance, R. A. and Widdowson, E. M. (1978) see Paul and Southgate (1978)

McCarrison, R. (1922) *J. Amer. Med. Assoc.* **78,** 1

McCay, C. M., Sperling, G. and Barnes, L. L. (1943) *Arch. Biochem.* **2,** 469

McClellan, W. S. and Du Bois, E. F. (1930) *J. Biol. Chem.* **87,** 651

McClure, G. M. (1984) *Brit. J. Psychiatry,* **144,** 134

McGandy, R. B., Hegsted, D. M. and Myers, M. L. (1970) *Amer. J. Clin. Nutrit.* **23,** 1288

McGilvery, R. W. and Goldstein, G. W. (1983) *Biochemistry: A Functional Approach* (3rd edn), Saunders, Philadelphia

McKinney, L. L., Picken, J. C., Weakley, F. B., Eldridge, A. C., Campbell, R. E. *et al.* (1959) *J. Amer. Chem. Soc.* **81,** 909

Macleod, J. (ed.) (1984) '*Davidson's Principles and Practice of Medicine*' (14th edn) Churchill Livingstone, London

McMichael, A., Spirtas, R., Kupper, L. and Gamble, J. (1975) *J. Occup. Med.* **17,** 234

McNeil, N. I. (1984) *Amer. J. Clin. Nutrit.* **39,** 338

MacPhee, D. G. and Hall, W. (1985) *Search, Australia,* **16,** 146

Magee, P. N. (1971) *Food Cosmet. Toxicol.* **9,** 207

Mager, J., Chevion, M. and Glaser, G. (1980), see Liener (1980) p. 265

Maltoni, C. (1977) *Environ. Health Perspect.* **21,** 1

Mandel, H. G. and Cohn, V. H. in Gilman, *et al.* (1985) p. 1573

Mansour, T. and Bueding, E. (1954) *Brit. J. Pharmacol. Chemother.* **9,** 459

Mantle T. J., Hayes J. D. and Pickett C. B. (1987) *Glutathione S – Transferases and Carcinogenesis,* Taylor and Francis, London

Marcus, R. and Coulston, A. M. (1985) in Gilman, *et al.* (1985) p. 1567

Marquart, M. (1949) *Paul Ehrlich,* Heinemann, London

Marshall, E. K. (1937) *J. Biol. Chem.* **122,** 263

Martin, C. E. (1967) *Amer. J. Public Health,* **57,** 803

Marzulli, F. N. and Brown, D. W. C. (1972) *J. Soc. Cosmet. Chem.* **23,** 875

Mason, H. S., North, J. C. and Vanneste, M. (1965) *Fed. Proc.* **24,** 1172

Masoro, E. J. (1985) *J. Nutrition,* **115,** 842 (review on ageing)

Masoro, E. J., Yu, B. P., Bertrand, H. A. and Lynd, F. T. (1980) *Fed. Proc.* **39,** 3178

Massachusetts Institute of Technology (1978) Report on Contract No. 223–74–2181, *Study of Dietary Nitrite in the Rat,* FDA, Washington, DC

Masuda, Y., Mori, K. and Kurastune, M. (1966) *Gann,* **57,** 133

Masuda, Y., Kuroki, H., Yamaryo, T., Haraguchi, K., Kuratsune, M. *et al.* (1982) *Chemosphere,* **2,** 199

Mato, J. M. and Konijn, T. M. (1979) in *Biochemistry and Physiology of Protozoa,* Vol 2 (2nd edn) (eds M. Levandowski and S. H. Hutner) Academic Press, New York, p. 181

Matthews, D. A., Bolin, J. T., Burridge, J. M., Filman, D. J., Volz, K. W., *et al.* (1985) *J. Biol. Chem.* **260,** 381

Matthews, W. B. and Miller, H. (1979) *Diseases of the Nervous system* (3rd edn) Blackwell Scientific Publications, Oxford

Mattocks, A. R. (1986) *Chemistry and Toxicology of Pyrrolizidine Alkaloids,* Academic Press, New York

Mattson, F. H. (1973)in NAS (1973) p. 200

Meehan, B. (1982) *Shell Bed to Shell Midden,* Australian Institute of Aboriginal Studies, Canberra

Megaw, J. V.S. (ed.) (1977) *Hunters, Gatherers and First Farmers beyond Europe,* Leicester University Press, Leicester, UK

Melhorn, D. K. and Gross, S. (1969) *J. Lab. Clin. Med.* **74,** 789
Meltzer, J. B., Frankel, E. H., Bessler, T. R. and Perkins, E. G. (1981) *J. Amer. Oil Chem. Soc.* **58,** 779
Mendelson, J. and Mello, N. K. (1983) in Petersdorf, *et al.* (1983) p. 1282
'Merck's Index' see 'The Merck Index'
Metcalf, R. (1980) *Ann. Rev. Entomol.* **15,** 219
Meyer, H. (1899) *Arch. Exper. Path. Pharmacol.* **42,** 109
Miles, W. R. (1922) *J. Pharmacol. Exper. Ther.* **20,** 265
Miller, E. C. and Miller, J. A. (1981) *Cancer,* **47,** 2327
Miller, E. C., Miller, J. A. and Hartmann, H. (1961) *Cancer Res.* **21,** 815
Miller, J. A. (1973) in NAS (1973) p. 530
Miller, J. W. and Winter, P. M. (1981) *Int. Anaesthesiol. Clin.* **19,** 179
Miller, R. W. (1968) *Pediatrics,* **41,** 257
Milner, J. A. (1985) in Finley and Schwass (1985)
Ministry of Agriculture, Fisheries and Food (UK) (1978) *Report of Committee on Food Additives and Contaminants,* HMSO, London
Minney, R. J. (1972) *Rasputin,* Cassell, London
Mitchell, J. R. and Horning, M. G. (eds) (1984) *Drug Metabolism and Drug Toxicity,* Raven Press, New York
Mitchell, J. R., Thorgeirssen, U. and Black, M. (1975) *Clin. Pharmacol. Ther.* **18,** 70
Mitra, K. (1942) *Indian J. Med. Res.* **30,** 91
Mitsuhashi, S. (1982) *Drug Resistance in Bacteria,* Georg Thieme Verlag, Stuttgart
Moertel, C. G., Fleming, T. R., Creagen, E. T., Rubin, J., O'Connell, M. J. *et al.* (1985) *New Engl. J. Med.* **312,** 137
Moertel, C. G., Fleming, T. R., Rubin, J., Kvols, L. K., Sarna, G. *et al.* (1982) *New Engl. J. Med.* **306,** 201
Moffat, A. C. (ed.) (1986) *'Clarke's Isolation and Identification of Drugs'* (2 vols, 2nd edn) Pharmaceutical Press, London
Montgomery, R. D. (1980) in Liener (1980) p. 143
Moorhouse, E. C. (1969) *Brit. Med. J.* **2,** 405
Morley, A., Blenkinsopp, J., Nicholls, J. R. and Nicholls, J. L. (1986) *Pharm. J., (Lond.)* **236,** 619
Morley, J. E. and Levine, A. S. (1985) *Ann. Rev. Pharmacol. Toxicol.* **25,** 127
Morrison, A. S. and Buring, J. E. (1980) *New Engl. J. Med.* **302,** 537
Mosher, L. R. (1970) *Amer. J. Psychiat.* **126,** 1290
Muir, R. (1921) *Proc. Roy. Soc. B,* 92, 1
Müller, F. (1979) *Auschwitz Inferno,* Routledge and Kegan Paul, London
Mulvaney, D. J. (1970) *Australian Aboriginal Prehistory* (pamphlet) Nelson, Melbourne
Murad, F. and Haynes, R. C. (1985) in Gilman, *et al.* (1985)
Näf-Müller, R. and Willhalm, B. (1971) *Helv. Chim. Acta,* **54,** 1880
Nagataki, S. (1974) in *Handbook of Physiology, Vol. 3, Endocrinology,* American Physiological Society, Bethesda, Maryland
NAS (National Academy of Sciences) (1956–1959) *Handbook of Toxicology (5 vols) NAS,* Washington, DC
NAS (1973) *Toxicants Occurring Naturally in Foods* (2nd edn) (1st edn appeared in 1966), NAS, Washington, DC
NAS (1982) *Diet, Nutrition and Cancer,* NAS, Washington, DC
Nater, J. P. and De Groot, A. C. (1985) *Unwanted Effects of Cosmetics Used in Dermatology,* Elsevier, The Netherlands
National Cancer Institute (1979) *Progress Report to the Food and Drugs Administration Concerning the National Bladder Cancer Study,* NCI, Bethesda, Maryland
National Heart, Lung and Blood Institute (1984) *J. Amer. Med. Assoc.* **251,** pp.351, 365
National Research Council (US), see NRC

National Science Foundation (1966) *Chemicals and Health,* Government Printing Office, Washington, DC

Neal, J. and Rigdon, R. H. (1967) *Tex. Rep. Biol. Med.* **25,** 553

Needham, J. (1954) *Science and Civilization in China,* Cambridge University Press, Cambridge.

Nelson, E. (1961) *J. Pharm. Sci.* **50,** 181

Nelson, E. and O'Reilly, I. (1960) *J. Pharmacol.* **129,** 368

Newberne, P. M. (1985) in Finley and Schwass (1985)

Newbold, R. and Overell, R. (1983) *Nature, (Lond.)* **304,** 648

Nishio, Y. and Fukushima, S. (1986) *Science,* **231,** 843

Norway (Royal Norwegian Ministry of Agriculture) (1975) *On Norwegian Food and Nutrition Policy,* Royal Norwegian Ministry of Agriculture, Oslo

Notari, R. (1973) *J. Pharm. Sci.* **62,** 865

NRC (National Research Council) (1971) *Fluorides,* NAS Washington, DC

NRC (1980) *Recommended Dietary Allocwances* (Food and Nutrition Board (9th edn), National Academy Press, Washington, DC

NRC (1982) *Diet, Nutrition and Cancer* (Commission on Life Sciences) National Academy Press, Washington, DC

NRC (1984) *Asbestiform Fibers: Nonoccupational Health Risks,* National Academy Press, Washington, DC

Nyhan, W. L. (ed.) (1974) *Heritable Disorders of Amino Acid Metabolism,* Wiley, New York

O'Brien, J. S. (1967) *J. Theoret. Biol.* **15,** 307

O'Dell, B. L. (1976) *Med. Clin. North Amer.* **60,** 687

Offe, H., Siefken, W. and Domagk, G. (1952) *Naturwiss.* **39,** 118

Oliver, T. K. (1958) *Amer. J. Dis. Child.* **95,** 57

Orlova, A. (1981) *Music and Letters* **62,** 125

Orme, B. (1977) in Megaw (1977) p. 46

Overton, E. (1901) *Studien über die Narkosen,* Gustav Fischer, Jena pp. 195

Padmanabam, G. (1980) in Liener (1980) p. 239

Palca, J. (1986) *Nature, (Lond.)* **320,** 476

Palca, J. (1986a) *Nature, (Lond.)* **321,** 554

Paracelsus (1538) (Theophrastus von Hohenheim) (1493–1541), *The Works of Paracelsus* (1965), (5 vols) (ed. W. Peuckert) **2,** Schwabe & Co., Basel p. 510

Parfitt, A. M. (1972) *Orthop. Clin. North. Amer.* **3,** 653

Parke, D. V. and Ioannides, C. (1984) *Arch. Toxicol. Suppl.* **7,** 183

Parsons, W. and Flinn, J. (1957) *J. Amer. Med. Assoc.* **165,** 234

Passmore, R. (1951) *Lancet,* **ii,** 303

Passmore, R., Nicol, B. M., Rao, M. N., Beaton, G. H. and De Maeyer, E. M. (1974) *Handbook on Human Nutritional Requirements,* FAO Nutritional Series No. 28, FAO, Rome (also issued as WHO Monograph No. 61)

Paton, W. D. M. (1961) *Proc. Roy. Soc., B,* **154,** 21

Patwardhan, V. N. and White, J. W. (1973) in NAS (1973) p. 477

Paul, A. A. and Southgate, D. A. T. (eds) (1978) *'McCance and Widdowson's: The Composition of Foods',* HMSO, London (also Supplements)

Pauling, L. (1968) *Science,* **160,** 265

Payne, J. and Hughes, R. (1981) *Brit. J. Anaesth.* **53,** 45

Pearn, J. (1983) *Med. J. Austral.* **2,** 16

People of the State of California v. Ernst Krebs and Malvina Cassese (1977) *Documents G. 14673 and G. 14670 of the Municipal Court of the State of California,* San Francisco

Perez-Reyes, M., Di Guiseppi, S., Davis, K. H., Schindler, V. H. and Cook, C. E. (1982) *Clin. Pharmacol. Ther.* **31,** 617

Perkins, H. C. (1974) *Air Pollution,* McGraw-Hill, New York

Perlman, F. (1980) in Liener (1980) p. 295

Petersdorf, R. G., Adams, R. D., Braunwald, E., Isselbacher, K. J., Martin, J. B. and Wilson, J. D. (eds) (1983) *'Harrison's Principles of Internal Medicine'* (10th edn) McGraw-Hill, New York

Pitt, H. A. and Costrini, A. M. (1979) *J. Amer. Med. Assoc.* **241,** 908

Poland, A. and Kimbrough, R. D. (eds) (1984) *Biological Mechanisms of Dioxin Action*, Cold Spring Harbor Laboratories, Long Island, NY.

Poland, A. and Knutson, J. (1982) *Ann. Rev. Pharmacol. Toxicol.* **22,** 517

Pott, P. (1775) *Chirurgical Observations*, Hawes, Clarke and Collins, London

Prakash, N., Schechter, P., Mamont, P., Gove, J., Koch-Weser, J. *et al.* (1980) *Life Sci.* **26,** 181

Price, J. M., Biava, C. F., Oser, B. L., Vogin, E. E., Steinfeld, J. *et al.* (1970) *Science,* **167,** 1131

Propping, P. (1978) *Rev. Physiol. Biochem. Pharmacol.* **83,** 123

Puck, T. (1977) *Proc. Natl Acad. Sci., USA* **74,** 4491

Purchase, I., Longstaff, E., Ashby, J., Styles, J., Anderson, D. *et al.* (1976) *Nature, (Lond.)* **264,** 624

Ragelis, E. P. (ed.) (1984) *Seafood Toxins*, American Chemical Society, Washington, DC

Rall, T. W. (1985) in Gilman, *et al.* (1985) p. 589

Rapoport, S. (1976) *The Blood-Brain Barrier in Physiology and Medicine*, Raven Press, New York

Rawls, R. (1980) *Chem. Eng. News,* **58** (April 7), 27

Read, P. P. (1974) *Alive, the Story of the Andes Survivors*, Martin Secker and Warburg, London

Reeve, V. C. (1979) State of California Department of Justice, Division of Law Enforcement, Sacramento, USA

Reeves, A. L. (1981) *Toxicology: Principles and Practice* (2 vols) Wiley, New York

Regan, J. D. and Setlow, R. B. (1973) in *Chemical Mutagens* (ed. A. Hollaender) Plenum Press, New York, p. 151

Reinhold, D. and Rice, D. (1970) *Arctic Anthrop.* **7,** 83

Rekker, R. F. (1977) *The Hydrophobic Fragmental Constant*, Elsevier, Amsterdam

Renzoni, A. (1977) *Environ. Conserv.* **4** (1), 21

Reynolds, J. (ed.) (1982) *'Martindale, the Extra Pharmacopoeia'* (28th edn) Pharmaceutical Press, London

Richards, W. H. G. (1970) *Adv. Pharmacol. Chemother.* **8,** 121

Ringold, H. (1961) in *Mechanisms of Action of Steroid Hormones* (eds C. Villee and L. Engels) Pergamon Press, Oxford

Ritchie, J. M. (1985) in Gilman, *et al.* (1985) p. 372

Roberts, H. R. (ed.) (1981) *Food Safety*, Wiley, New York

Rodricks, J. V., Hesseltine, C. W. and Mehlman, M. A. (1977) *Mycotoxins in Human and Animal Health*, Pathotox Publishers, Park Forest South, Illinois

Roitman, J. N. (1981) *Lancet,* **i,** 944

Rosenthal, G. (1971) *J. Amer. Med. Assoc.* **215,** 1671

Roth, B. and Cheng, C. (1982) *Progr. Med. Chem.* **19,** 270

Roth, B., Falco, E. A. and Hitchings, G. H. (1962) *J. Med. Pharm. Chem.* **5,** 1103

Rounsaville, B. J., Weissman, M. M., Kleber, H. and Wilber, C. (1982) *Arch. Gen. Psychiatry,* **39,** 161

Rowland, I. R. and Walker, R. (1983) in Conning and Lansdown (1983)

Royal College of Physicians (London) and the British Cardiac Society (1976) Report of Joint Working Party on Coronary Disease, *J. Royal College of Physicians,* **10,** 213

Royal Commission on the Use and Effects of Chemical Agents on Australian Personnel in Vietnam (1985) *Final Report* by Commissioner P. Evatt, (9 vols) Australian Government Publishing Service, Canberra

Royal Society (1972) *Report of Committee on Metrication in the Nutritional Sciences*, The Royal Society, London

Rubbo, S. D., Albert, A. and Gibson, M. I. (1950) *Brit. J. Exper. Path.* **31,** 425

Ruckpaul, K. and Rein, H. (eds.) (1985) *Cytochrome P-450,* Taylor and Francis, London

Ruge, F. (1974) *Rommel in Normandy,* Macdonald and Janes, London

Rumack, B. H. and Burrington, J. P. (1977) *Clin. Toxicol.* **11,** 27

Rumack, B. H. and Lovejoy, F. H. (1985) in Klaassen, Amdur and Doull (1985)

Russell, R. M. (1980) *Amer. J. Clin. Nutrit.* **33,** 2741

Ryan, C. (1966) *The Last Battle,* Collins, London p. 37

Sachs, L. (1965) *J. Natl Cancer Inst.* **35,** 641

Safe, S. H. (1986) *Ann. Rev. Pharmacol. Toxicol.* **26,** 371

Sagan, C. (1985) *Nature, (Lond.)* **317,** 485

Sandberg, A. A. (ed.) (1982) *Sister Chromatid Exchange,* Alan Liss, New York

Sander, J., Schweinsberg, F. and Menz, H. (1968) *Z. Physiol. Chem.* **349,** 1691

Saunders, B. C. (1957) *Some Aspects of the Chemistry and Toxic Action of Organic Compounds containing Phosphorus and Fluorine,* Cambridge University Press, Cambridge

Saunders, P. A. H. (1986) *Nature, (Lond.)* **319,** 532

Sax, N. I. (1984) *Dangerous Properties of Industrial Materials* (6th edn) Van Nostrand-Reinhold, New York

Schaefer, H., Zesch, A. and Stüttgen, P. (1982) *Skin Permeability,* Springer-Verlag, Berlin

Schanker, L. S. (1961) *Ann. Rev. Pharmacol.* **1,** 29

Schanker, L. S. (1978) *Biochem. Pharmacol.* **27,** 381

Schantz, E. J. (1973) in NAS (1973)

Schaumburg, H., Kaplan, J., Windebank, A., Vick, N., Rasmus, S., Pleasure, D. *et al.* (1983) *New Engl. J. Med.* **309,** 445

Scheline, R. R. (1973) *Pharmacol. Rev.* **25,** 451

Schilling, R. F. (1953) *J. Lab. Clin. Med.* **42,** 860

Schmiedeberg, O. (1912) *Arch. Path. Pharmakol.* **67,** 1

Schneider, E. L. and Reed, J. D. (1985) *New Engl. J. Med.* **312,** 1159

Schopf, J. W. (ed.) (1983) *Earth's Earliest Biosphere: its Origin and Evolution,* Princeton University Press, Princeton, NJ

Schrader, G. (1963) *Die Entwicklung neuer Insectizider Phosphorsäure Ester* (3rd edn) Verlag Chemie, Weinheim

Schrauzer, G. N. and White, D. A. (1978) *Bioinorgan. Chem.* **8,** 303

Schul, W. J., Otake, M. and Neel, J. V. (1981) *Science,* **213,** 1220

Schultz, F. (1940) *Z. Physiol. Chem.* **265,** 113

Searle, C. E. (ed.) (1984) *Chemical Carcinogenesis* (2 vols) (2nd edn) American Chemical Society, Washington, DC

Seevers, M. H. and Deneau, G. A. (1963) *Physiol. Pharmacol.* **1,** 565 (review)

Seinfeld, J. H. (1986) *Atmospheric Chemistry, and Physics of Air Pollution,* Wiley, New York

Seydel, J. (1981) *J. Quant. Chem.* **20,** 131

Shamberger, R. J. and Frost, D. V. (1969) *Canad. Med. Assoc. J.* **100,** 682

Sharp, C. W. and Carroll, L. T. (eds) (1978) *Voluntary Inhalation of Industrial Solvents* (compiled for the National Institute on Drug Abuse) Pubn ADM 79–779, US Government Printer, Washington, DC

Shellard, E. J. (1986) *Pharm. J. (Lond.),* **237,** 495

Shilotri, P. G. and Bhat, K. S. (1977) *Amer. J. Clin. Nutr.* **30,** 1077

Shirota, F., DeMaster, E. and Nagasawa, H. (1979) *J. Med. Chem.* **22,** 463

Shorofsky, M. A. and Lamm, N. (1977) *N. Y. State J. Med.* .**77,** 217

Shtenberg, A. I. and Gavrilenko, E. V. (1970) *Vopr. Pitan.* **29,** 66

Sijpesteijn, A. K. and Janssen, M. (1959) *Antonie van Leeuwenhoek,* **25,** 422

Simonen, O. and Laitinen, O. (1985) *Lancet,* **ii,** 432

Simpson, G. R. and Shandar, A. (1972) *Med. J. Austral.* **2,** 1060

Singer, S. and Nicolson, G. (1972) *Science*, **175**, 720

Singleton, V. L. and Kratzer, F. H. (1973) in NAS (1973)

Sittig, M. (1985) *Handbook of Toxic and Hazardous Chemicals and Carcinogens* (2nd edn) Noyes, Park Ridge, NJ

Slater, T. (1966) *Nature, (Lond.)* **209**, 36

Smith, A. H., Fisher, D. O., Pearce, N. and Chapman, C. J. (1982) *Arch. Environ. Health*, **37**, 197

Smith, D. A. and Woodruff, M. F. A. (1951) *Special Rep. Ser., Med. Research Council* (UK) No. **274**

Smith, H. W. (1969) *Lancet*, **i**, 1174

Smith, R. P. and Gosselin, R. E. (1976) *Ann. Rep. Pharmacol. Toxicol.* **16**, 189

Smith, R. T. and Landy, M. (eds) (1970) *Immune Surveillance*, Academic Press, New York

Smith, T. C., Gross, J. B. and Wollman, H. (1985) in Gilman, *et al.* (1985) p. 322

Snyder, S., Katims, J., Annau, Z., Bruns, R. and Daly, J. (1981) *Proc. Natl Acad. Sci., USA*, **78**, 3260

Sontag, J. M. (ed.) (1981) *Carcinogens in Industry and the Environment*, Marcel Dekker, New York

Spencer, P. S., Schaumburg, H. H., Sabu, M. I. and Veronese, B. (1980) *CCC Crit. Rev. Toxicol.* **4**, 279

Spring, B., Maller, O., Wurtman, J., Digman, L. and Cozolino, L. (1983) *J. Psychiat. Res.* **17**, 155

Stadel, B. V. (1985) *Lancet*, **ii**, pp. 970, 985 (cf. *New Engl. J. Med.* (1986) **315**, 405)

Starr, T. B. and Gibson, J. E. (1985) *Ann. Rev. Pharmacol. Toxicol.* **25**, 745

Stedman, E. (1929) *Amer. J. Physiol.* **90**, 528

Stefansson, V. (1960) *Cancer: Disease of Civilization?* Hill and Wang, New York

Stein, W. D. (1986) *Transport and Diffusion across cell Membranes*, Academic Press, New York

Stelmaszyńska, T. and Zgliczynski, J. M. (1981) in Vennesland, *et al.* (1981)

Sterling-Smith, R. S. (1976) *US Department of Traffic Management Report*, Contract No. DOT–HS–310–3–595, US Government Printer, Washington, DC

Stern, A. C. (1976) *Air Pollution* (5 vols) (3rd edn) Academic Press, New York

Stewart, C. P. and Stolman, A. (eds) (1960) *Toxicology Mechanisms and Analytical Methods* (2 vols) Academic Press, New York

Stimson, G. V. and Oppenheimer, E. (1982) *Heroin Addiction: Treatment and Control in Britain*, Tavistock Publications, London

Strøm, A. and Jensen, R. A. (1951) *Lancet*, **i**, 126

Strugger, S. (1940) *Jena. Z. Med. Naturwiss.* **73**, 97

Stryer, L. (1981) *Biochemistry* (2nd edn) Freeman, San Francisco

Sugerman, A. A. and Clark, C. G. (1974) *J. Amer. Med. Assoc.* **228**, 202

Surgeon General of the USA (1979) *Smoking and Health*, Department of Health, Education and Welfare Publication No. PHS 79-50066, US Government Printing Office, Washington, DC

Surgeon General of the USA (1981) *The Health Consequences of Smoking*, Department of Health and Human Services Publication, No. PHS 81–50156, US Government Printing Office, Washington, DC

Susin, M. and Herson, P. B. (1967) *Arch. Pathol.* **83**, 86

Sutherland, E. W. (1970) *J. Amer. Med. Assoc.* **214**, 1281

Swann, P. F. (1975) *J. Sci. Food Agric.* **26**, 1761

Swedish National Food Administration (1981) *Swedish Nutritional Recommendations*, Swedish National Food Administration, Stockholm

Swedish Nutrition Foundation (1971) *Famine*, Almqvist and Wiksell, Uppsala

Swintowsky, J. (1956) *J. Amer. Pharm. Assoc., Sci. Edn.* **45**, 395

Szent-Györgyi, A. (1975) *Chem. Eng. News*, **53**, (July 28) 16

Tabin, C., Bradley, S., Bargmann, C., Weinberg, R., Papageorge, A. *et al.* (1982) *Nature, (Lond.)* **300,** 143

Taeuber, C. M. (1983) *Current Population Reports,* series P-23, No. 128 Government Printing Office, Washington, DC

Takeuchi, T. and Matsumoto, H. (1969) in *Methods for Teratological Studies in Animals and Man* (ed. H. Nishimura and J. R. Miller) Igaku Shoin, Tokyo

Tannenbaum, S. R. and Correa, P. (1985) *Nature, (Lond.)* **317,** 675

Tatum, A. and Cooper, G. (1934) *J. Pharmacol.* **50,** 198

Taylor, J. R. and Calabrese, V. P. (1979) *Handbook Clin. Neurol.* **36,** 391

'The Merck Index' (10th edn) (1983) (ed. M. Windholz) Merck and Co., Rahway, NJ'

Theeuwes, F. (1975) *J. Pharm. Sci.* **64,** 1987

Timbrell, J. A. (1985) *Principles of Biochemical Toxicology,* Taylor and Francis, London

Tipper, D. and Strominger, J. (1965) *Proc. Natl. Acad. Sci., USA,* **54,** 1133

Tocchini-Valenti, G., Marino, P. and Colvill, A. (1968) *Nature, (Lond.)* **220,** 275

Todaro, G. J. and Huebner, R. J. (1972) *Proc. Natl. Acad. Sci., USA,* **69,** 1009

Tookey, H. L., Van Etten, C. H. and Daxenbichler, M. E. (1980) in Liener (1980) p. 103

Townsend, J. C., Bodner, K. M., Van Peenen, P. F. D., Olsen, R. D. and Cook, R. R (1982) *Amer. J. Epidem.* **115,** 695

Tréfouël, J., Tréfouël, Mme. J., Nitti, F. and Bovet, D. (1935) *Compt. Rend. Soc. Biol., (Paris)* **120,** 756

Trevan, J. (1927) *Proc. Roy. Soc., B,* **101,** 483

Treves, N. and Pack, G. T. (1930) *Surg. Gynec. Obstet.* **51,** 749

Truswell, A. S. (1977) in Elliott and Whelan (1977)

Tsubaki, T. and Irukayama, K. (eds) (1977) *Minamata Disease: Methylmercury Poisoning in Minamata and Niigata,* Kodansha, Tokyo; Elsevier, Amsterdam

Tunek, A., Platt, K. L., Bentley, P. and Oesch, F. (1978) *Mol. Pharmacol.* **14,** 920

Turnbull, G. J. (1985) *Occupational Hazards of Pesticide Use,* Taylor and Francis, London

Turoski, V. (ed.) (1985) *Formaldehyde: Analytical Chemistry and Toxicology,* American Chemical Society, Washington, DC

Ucko, P. J. and Dimbleby, G. W. (eds) (1969) *The Domestication and Exploitation of Plants and Animals,* Duckworth, London

UK Steering Group on Food Surveillance (1986) *Report of the Working Party on Pesticide Residues,* 1982–1985, HMSO, London

UNICEF (1987) *The State of the World's Children,* WHO, Geneva.

United Kingdom (1984) *Report of the Chief Medical Officer's Committee on Medical Aspects of Food Policy (COMA),* 'Diet and Cardiovascular Disease', Department of Health and Social Security, London

US Code of Federal Regulations (1979) Title **21,** *Foods and Drugs,* Government Printing Office, Washington, DC

US Code of Federal Regulations (1985) Title **29,** Labour (1910.1000) Government Printing Office, Washington, DC

US Department of Agriculture and Department of Health, Education and Welfare (1980) *Nutrition and Your Health,* Government Printing Office, Washington, DC

US Senate (1977) Subcommittee on Health and Scientific Resources: *Hearing on Banning of the Drug Laetrile,* Government Printing Office, Washington, DC

US Surgeon General (1979) *Report on Health Promotion and Disease Prevention,* Dept. of Health, Education and Welfare, Washington, DC

Vale, J. A. and Meredith, T. J. (1985) *A Concise Guide to the Management of Poisoning,* Churchill Livingstone, London

Van Etten, C. H. and Wolff, I. A. (1973) in NAS (1973) p. 210

Van Itallie, T. B. (1978) *J. Amer. Med. Assoc.* **240,** 144

Veldstra, H. (1956) *Pharmacol. Rev.* **8,** 339

Vennesland, B., Conn, E. E., Knowles, C. J., Westley, J. and Wissing, F. (1981) *Cyanide in Biology*, Academic Press, London

Victor, M. and Adams, R. D. (1953) *Res. Publ. Assoc. Res. Nerv. Ment. Dis.* **32**, 526

Victor, M. and Adams, R. D. (1983) in Petersdorf, *et al.* (1983) p. 1285, 1295

Visek, W. J. and Clinton, S. K. (1985) in Finley and Schwass (1985) p. 293

Vitzthum, O. G. and Wetkhoff, P. (1974) *J. Food Sci.* **39**, 1210

Vitzthum, O. G. and Werkhoff, P. (1975) *J. Agric. Food Chem.* **23**, 510

Voegtlin, C. (1925) *Physiol. Rev.* **5**, 63

Vogel, D. (1986) *National Styles of Regulation: Environmental Policy in Great Britain and the United States*, Cornell University Press, Ithaca, NY

Waddell, W. J. and Butler, T. C. (1957) *J. Clin. Invest.* **36**, 1217

Wagner, J. (1961) *J. Pharm. Sci.* **50**, 359

Wagner, J. (1967) *J. Pharm. Sci.* **56**, 489

Walker, A. R. P., Mortimer, K. L., Kloppers, P. J., Botha, D., Grusin, H. *et al.* (1961) *Amer. J. Clin. Nutrit.* **9**, 643

Walsh, B. and Grant, M. (1984) *Public Health Implications of Alcohol Production and Trade*, World Health Organization, Geneva

Walsh, D. (1984) *Internat. J. Epidemiol.* **13**, 472

Walter, W. and Weidemann, H. L. (1969), *Ernährungswiss.* **9**, 123

Walters, C. L., Carr, F. P. A., Dyke, C. S., Saxby, M. J., Smith, P. L. R. *et al.* (1979) *Food Cosmet. Toxicol.* **17**, 473

Wang, J., Kakizoe, T., Dion, P., Furrer, R., Varghese, A. J. *et al.* (1978) *Nature, (Lond.)* **276**, 280

Warburg, O. (1927), *Naturwiss.* **15**, 1 (cf. *Science*, (1956) **124**, 269)

Warnick, S. and Carter, J. (1972) *Arch. Environ. Health*, **25**, 265

Washburn, S. L. (1968) in Lee and DeVore (1968) p. 84

Washburn, S. L. and McCown, E. R. (eds) (1978) *Human Evolution, Biosocial Perspectives*, Benjamin Cummings, California

Way, A. B. (1970) *Arctic Anthrop.* **7**, 107

Way, J. L. (1981) in Vennesland, *et al.* (1981)

Weger, N. P. (1983) *Fundam. Appl. Toxicol.* **3**, 387

Weisburger, J. H. and Williams, G. M. (1984) in Searle (1984)

Wells, N. (1985) *Pharmaceutical J.* **234**, 646

White, J. W. (1976) *J. Agr. Food. Chem.* **24**, 202

White, P. (1970) *Ann. N.Y. Acad. Sci.* **174**, 23

Whitten, C. F. and Brough, A. J. (1971) *Clin. Toxicol.* **4**, 585

Williams, G. M. (1980) in *Chemical Mutagens* Vol. 6 (eds A. Hollaender and F. J. De Serres) Plenum Press, New York p. 61

Williams, R. T. (1959) *Detoxication Mechanisms* (2nd edn) Chapman and Hall, London; Wiley, New York

Willimot, S. G. (1933) *Analyst, (Lond.)* **58**, 431

Wilson, D. C. (1982) *Chem. Brit.* **18**, 499

Winter, S. L. and Boyer, J. L. (1973) *New Engl. J. Med.* **289**, 1180

Winteringham, F. P. W. (1955) *J. Sci. Food Agric.* **6**, 269

Wislocki, P. G., Miller, E. C., Miller, J. A., McCoy, E. C. and Rosenkranz, H. S. (1977) *Cancer Res.* **37**, 1883

Wittes, R. E. (1985) *New Engl. J. Med.* **312**, 178

Wogan, G. N. and Busby, W. F. (1980) in Liener (1980) p. 350

Wolff, M (ed.) (1981) *'Burger's Medicinal Chemistry'* (4th edn) Wiley, New York

Wood, R. C., Ferone, R. and Hitchings, G. H. (1961) *Biochem. Pharmacol.* **6**, 113

Woods, D. D. (1940) *Brit. J. Exper. Path.* **21**, 74

Woodwell, G. M. (1967) *Sci. Amer.* **216**, 24

World Health Organization (WHO) (1973) *Pharmacogenetics Technical Report* No. **524,** WHO, Geneva

World Health Organization (1974) *Food Additives Series* No. **5,** WHO, Geneva (see also Table 5.1)

World Helath Organization (1974a) *The Work of WHO, 1973, Annual Report of the Director-General,* Official Records No. **213,** WHO, Geneva

World Health Organization (1982) *International Nonproprietary Names (INN) for Pharmaceutical Substances* (Cumulative List, No. **6**) WHO, Geneva

World Health Organization (1985) *World Health Statistics,* WHO Geneva

Worthing, C. and Walker, S. (1987) *The Pesticide Manual: A World Compendium* (8th edn) British Crop Protection Council, Croydon, England; State Mutual Books, USA

Wray, B. B. and O'Steen, P. (1975) *Arch. Environ. Hlth* **30,** 571

Wurtman, J., Wurtman, R., Sharon, M., Tsay, R., Gilbert, W. *et al.* (1985) *Internat. J. of Eating Disorders,* **4,** 89

Wynder, E. L. and Gori, G. B. (1977) *J. Natl Cancer. Inst.* **58,** 825

Wynder, E. L. and Stellman, S. D. (1980) *Science,* **207,** 1214

Yamamoto, I. (1970) *Ann. Rev. Entomol.* **15,** 257

Yannai, S. (1980) in Liener (1980) p. 371

Young, J. Z., Jope, E. M. and Oakley, K. P. (1981) *The Emergence of Man,* The Royal Society, London

Yu, S.-Y., Chu, Y.-J., Gong, X.-L., Chong, H., Li, W.-G., *et al.* (1985) *Biolog. Trace Element Res.* **7,** 21

Zaffaroni, A. (1974) *Acta Endocrinol. Suppl.* **185,** 423

Zuelzer, W. W. (1964) *Blood,* **24,** 477

Zurer, P. S. (1985) *Chem. Eng. News,* **63** (March 4), 28

Subject index

Formula index